2008
Birthday.
from
Bonnie

THE SEVEN PILLARS of HEALTH

DON COLBERT, MD
with MARY COLBERT

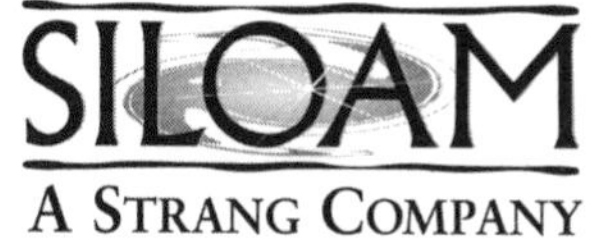

A STRANG COMPANY

The Seven Pillars of Health by Don Colbert, MD
Published by Siloam
A Strang Company
600 Rinehart Road
Lake Mary, Florida 32746
www.siloam.com

Interior design by Terry Clifton

International Standard Book Number: 978-1-59979-094-7

07 08 09 10 11 — 98765432

Printed in the United States of America

DEDICATION

I have had the opportunity to work with some well-known ministries in the United States and have had the privilege of speaking in many churches in the States. However, I attended a meeting a few years ago for the Global Pastors Network in which the late Dr. Bill Bright was speaking. He informed us that more pastors were leaving the ministry than were entering the ministry. Also, there was a high rate of depression among pastors, their wives, and their children.

I have treated many pastors in my medical practice who are literally burned out. Our pastors and ministers of the gospel are becoming an endangered species, and we need them strong mentally, physically, emotionally, and spiritually in order to help usher in the End-Time revival.

Therefore, I dedicate this book to all the ministers of the gospel of Jesus Christ—pastors, teachers, evangelists, prophets, and apostles. I pray that this book and the knowledge and wisdom it contains will educate, inspire, motivate, and enable our ministers to carry out their calling, which, in my opinion, is the highest of all.

ACKNOWLEDGMENTS

I would like to thank the people at Strang Communications Company for helping to make this book a success: Stephen Strang, Tessie DeVore, Bert Ghezzi, Lillian McAnally, Debbie Marrie, Deborah Moss, and many others at Strang Communications. I would also like to thank Joel Kilpatrick for lending his writing skills to the project and Bob Zaloba for his input.

A special thanks to Beverly Kurts for her long hours, dedication, and research that she provided. She was a tremendous help to me. Also, I would like to give a special thanks to the entire staff of Divine Health Wellness Center for their support. Thanks to Cathy Leet for her insight.

A special thanks to my mom, Kitty Colbert, and my dad, Don Colbert Sr., for being such wonderful parents and a tremendous influence in my life.

Last but not least, thanks to my wonderful wife, Mary, who has helped me present this material to churches for over a decade. She has been patient and a support to me while writing this book.

CONTENTS

INTRODUCTION

Welcome to *The Seven Pillars of Health*! This book will introduce you to the seven basic pillars of a healthy lifestyle. It is designed to become your road map for health for the rest of your life.

This book is different from other health books for several key reasons. First, most other popular health writers are not medical doctors. I am. I have been a medical doctor since 1984 and have been board certified in family practice since 1987. I treat patients and operate a thriving medical practice in Orlando, Florida. If you come to my medical office during the week you will see me in blue surgical scrubs with a stethoscope draped around my neck. I will be reviewing patients' files and meeting with patients. I dedicate my life to helping people become healthy. Living a healthy life is not just theory and research for me; it's fact.

Because I have made my career as a medical doctor, the advice I give in this book is not just something I picked up from the Internet or from other medical professionals. These are not the seven "fads" of health or the seven "theories" of health, but the seven *pillars* of health. Backed up by medical research and my actual experiences with real problems and real people that span over two decades of practice, these seven pillars have contributed health and freedom to thousands of people.

The Future of Medicine

Thomas Edison once said, "The doctor of the future will give no medicine, but will interest his patients in the care of the human frame, in diet, and in the cause and prevention of disease."

For the past ten years *The Seven Pillars of Health* has been the basis of my medical practice and my ministry. You see, Proverbs 9:1 tells us, "Wisdom hath builded her house, she hath hewn out her seven pillars." When I read this verse over ten years ago, it became the inspiration for the message you now hold in your hands. Since that time, I have taught these seven pillars to some of the largest ministries in the United States as well as in dozens of churches. Many hundreds of people have told me of major improvements in their health just from attending the one- or two-day seminars. This book includes information from those seminars, plus much more, and presents a user-friendly, easy-to-read, positive handbook on health.

Laying the Foundation

In laying the groundwork to help you obtain a higher level of health, I have implemented a couple of teaching tools. At the end of each day is a section I call "Building Blocks to a Healthy Life." In these sections are the following features:

- *Points to Ponder.* This summary highlights the principles for that particular day's material. It is something for you to reflect on throughout your day.
- *Action Step.* What we read stays with us longer when we apply what we've learned. Each day you will be able to implement some small change to help you live in divine health. Making small changes every day will make applying the principles easier.

Far from being a "don't, can't, shouldn't" book, *The Seven Pillars of Health* is designed to liberate you and help you make choices that bring you freedom in every area of your life. To withstand the storms of life—diseases, attacks, and injuries—you must build on some fundamental precepts. Those precepts are found in *The Seven Pillars of Health* and are timeless biblical truths.

Some authors write books that may leave you feeling hopeless and as if everything is gloom and doom for you. I will not cajole you, make you feel guilty, or tell you to bear heavy burdens. My purpose is simply to show you how you can become strong, healthy, energetic, disease-resistant, younger-looking, wiser, smarter, and better looking. Studies now show that we can reduce our risk of deadly diseases such as heart disease by 80 percent or more and cancer by 60 percent or more—simply by leading a healthy life.[1] I will give you knowledge about your body and how it operates so you won't be "destroyed for lack of knowledge," as an ancient prophet said. It won't take more work on your part. You will simply exchange old habits for new ones.

As just one example, many health books tell readers to avoid coffee as if it were some kind of plague. I don't say that. Instead I will show you how to have healthy, caffeinated coffee every day, if you choose. I will also show you how to sleep through the night, how to better cope with stress, how to get rid of mental fogginess, and much more. God has given us life to enjoy it. I have written *The Seven Pillars of Health* to be a handbook for enjoyable living.

Why Fifty Days?

This book is designed as a fifty-day journey, one entry per day.

On the Jewish calendar, every fiftieth year was the Year of Jubilee, when slaves were set free from their masters and debtors were released from their debts. In a similar way, this book will help to set you free from poor health, bad habits, and disease.

Over the next fifty days, read each daily entry and incorporate these valuable pillars in your life. Please do not try to rush through this program in one sitting, or you may be overwhelmed by the information. *Take it one day at a time*: digest the material you read, make notes, and pray and ask God to enlighten you. My main concern is that these seven pillars of health become your foundation for a lifetime.

Again, welcome to *The Seven Pillars of Health*! May this book change your life forever.

—Don Colbert, MD

PILLAR 1

Water

DAY 1: Water and You

My wife, Mary, and I flew into a city where I was speaking at a conference, and a local family met us at the airport. To my surprise, the husband and children hugged me, and some of the children began to cry. Never before had I received such a warm reception.

"You helped us get our mother and wife back," they said. The mother had heard a teaching I had given from my book *The Bible Cure for Headaches* and followed the recommendations, one of which is to drink two to three quarts of filtered water each day.[1] Within weeks, the headaches were gone. It was now six months later, and she was pain free. She was now able to care for her beautiful family.

Since her childhood, this woman had suffered from migraine headaches that left her unable to function and care for her family. The headaches were also interfering with her ability to practice as a professional psychologist. She had been to neurologists and doctors and tried dozens of medications, but they all failed to help her. Over time her headaches had grown worse, and even the strongest pain medicines available did not help to alleviate them.

This woman had been mildly dehydrated most of her life and never realized the cure for her headaches was as close as her glass of water.

Did You Know...?

- Your body is about 70 percent water.
- Your muscles are about 75 percent water.
- Your brain cells are about 85 percent water.
- Your blood is approximately 82 percent water.
- Even your bones are approximately 25 percent water.[2]

Why Water?

I start our study of *The Seven Pillars of Health* with water because it is the most foundational aspect of health.

Water is the single most important nutrient for our bodies. It is involved in every function of our bodies. You can live five to seven weeks without food, but the average adult can last no more than five days without water.[3]

As a Florida resident, I have lived through several periods of drought, and when we don't receive adequate amounts of rainfall, the local government rations water consumption. We can water our lawns only on certain days and during certain times on those days. Your body does a similar thing when it becomes dehydrated: it begins to ration the water.

And yet some people water their houseplants more than they do their own bodies! You are valuable; take care of yourself and properly hydrate your body.

A Miracle Cure

Many people never drink water. Some don't like the taste of water, or they were never taught the importance of drinking it. Maybe their parents gave them juice, soft drinks, milk—anything but water. As a result, many people spend their day going from one caffeinated or sugar-based drink to another. They jump-start their mornings with coffee. By mid-morning they have a soda for another boost, then drink sweetened caffeinated iced tea for lunch. Late afternoon it's another coffee-based or "10 percent juice" drink. Little do they know that all that caffeine and sugar are actually stealing water from their bodies, doing them more harm than good.

H_2O 101

Your body loses about two quarts of water a day through perspiration, urination, and exhalation.[4]

In my practice I see people all the time whose bodies are starved for clean, natural water. They are neglecting the most basic pillar of health, and their bodies and minds pay a terrible price. By the time I see them they often suffer from headaches, back pain, arthritis, skin problems, digestion problems, and other ailments. Often they have gone to another doctor, who might have given them medications that didn't address the problem but only turned off the symptoms. This is similar to a red warning light blinking on your car's dashboard, informing you to check your engine. If you simply decide to remove the fuse to turn off the warning light instead of taking your car in for service, you will eventually ruin your car's engine. That is a simple illustration of what many individuals do by taking medications instead of addressing their body's "warning light" that they are dehydrated and need an adequate intake of clean water.

Many Americans live in a mildly dehydrated state with various irritating symptoms and never realize it. I often tell patients that when they have a headache, they don't have a Tylenol deficiency. When they have joint pain, they don't have an Advil deficiency. When they have heartburn, they don't have a Pepcid deficiency, and if they are depressed, they don't have a Prozac deficiency. In each of these cases, their body is often crying out for water.[5]

Mary and I have lost count of the people who come up to us at seminars and say, "I had this or that problem, but I took your advice and started drinking water, and it went away." People tend to lose excess weight, their arthritis problems disappear, and their high blood pressure begins to return to normal levels.

If it sounds like a miracle cure, that's because it is! God created us to rely on water for our very lives. If you have ever read the Bible, you may have seen how water is a major theme in the Old Testament. People were always digging into the ground looking for water, and when they found it they gave their wells names and defended them with their lives. That's how critical water was for survival back then.

Water is just as important for you and me today.

I treat every patient I see in my practice first with water. Most of my patients get better when they simply drink as much water as their body is asking for. Drinking sufficient amounts of the right kind of water will also do more to improve your health than anything else you can do!

Take a Guess

What percentage of water does the average adult male body contain?

- a. 40–50 percent
- b. 50–60 percent
- c. 62–65 percent

Answer: c. The average adult male's body is 62–65 percent water, compared to women, who have 51–55 percent water. Men have more water in their bodies because they generally have more muscle mass, whereas women have a higher percentage of body fat.[6]

BUILDING BLOCKS TO A HEALTHY LIFE

POINTS TO PONDER: *Water is the single most important nutrient for our bodies and is considered a "miracle cure" for many health conditions. It is involved in every function of our bodies. Your body loses about two quarts of water a day through perspiration, urination, and exhalation. If you wait until you are thirsty to drink water, then you are most likely already dehydrated.*

ACTION STEP: *Instead of reaching for a soft drink or tea, drink clean, natural water.*

DAY 2: What Happens When You Don't Drink Water

A patient of mine had terrible back pain every time he got up in the morning. He had been seeing another doctor and taking anti-inflammatory medicine, but it didn't help. The pain and stiffness were worse in the morning, so he started waking up earlier and staying up since the pain would not be as intense. As he told me about his condition I could almost sense his desperation. He thought I would put him on some novel treatment or pharmaceutical regimen. But I didn't. I prescribed for him a glass of alkaline water and told him to set it on his nightstand and drink it when he woke up in the middle of the night. He wasn't convinced this would solve his problem. It seemed too simple, almost childish, but he tried it anyway—and it worked. The back pain went away.

His body was mildly dehydrated and acidic and was, in effect, "stealing" water from his facet joints, disks, muscles, and connective tissues of the back in order to "water" his important organs. This may be a very simple explanation for the complex pathophysiology that is beyond the scope of this book. However, I have decided to keep it simple so that I do not bog you down, dear reader, with medical terminology.

> **H_2O 101**
>
> Water plays a vital role in regulating body temperature, transporting nutrients and oxygen to cells, removing waste, cushioning joints, and protecting organs and tissues.[1]

A recognized physician, F. Batmanghelidj, MD, in his book titled *Water for Health, for Healing, for Life,* points out some of the benefits of maintaining your body properly hydrated:[2]

- Water is the main lubricant in the joint spaces and helps prevent arthritis and back pain.
- Water increases the efficiency of the immune system.
- Water prevents clogging of arteries in the heart and brain, and thus helps reduce the risk of heart attack and stroke.
- Water is directly connected to brain function—it is needed for the efficient manufacture of neurotransmitters, includ-

ing serotonin; it is needed for the production of hormones made by the brain, such as melatonin; it can prevent attention deficit disorder (ADD); and it improves our attention span.

- Water helps prevent memory loss as we age, reducing the risk of degenerative diseases such as Alzheimer's disease, multiple sclerosis, Parkinson's disease, and Lou Gehrig's disease.
- Water affects our appearance, making our skin smoother and giving it sparkling luster; it also reduces the effects of aging.

When your body lacks the water it needs, it goes into a sort of rationing mode, as I described in Day 1. Think of a sprinkler system whose pressure is turned too low to reach all the grass on your lawn. Some parts stay green, but other parts begin to turn brown and die. When you live in a drought condition, your body smartly manages the water you give it, keeping the vital organs well watered with nutrients.[3] I call these vital organs "the starting five," like the starting five of a basketball team. They are the:

- Brain
- Heart
- Lungs
- Liver
- Kidneys

The body keeps these organs well hydrated with water, lest you suffer serious consequences. But as a result, nonvital organs may suffer. In the body's ranking system, body parts like the skin, gastrointestinal (GI) tract, and joints are less important, and so symptoms of dehydration usually show up there first.

Health Conditions Complicated by Dehydration

Your body can't send you an e-mail message or access your voice mail, so when it gets dehydrated, it lets you know in the only way it knows how: through unpleasant symptoms. Here are some major signs you are suffering from dehydration.

Joint pains and arthritis

Joint cartilage provides the smooth surface so that joints can glide easily during movement. Cartilage is about five times slicker than ice, and that cartilage is made up of 80 percent water. If the cartilage is robbed of fluid, the joints will eventually creak, crack, and pop, like a door on a rusty hinge. The increased friction causes them to degenerate quicker, eventually leading to arthritis.

As people approach the age of fifty, back pain often becomes a real problem. And no wonder: three-quarters of the weight of the body is supported by the fluid inside the disks. When the disks in your spine lack water, they begin to degenerate and herniate more quickly. It's similar to driving a car on underinflated tires. The tires will either wear out faster or eventually blow out.

High blood pressure

When the body is mildly dehydrated, it may restrict the flow of blood to nonvital areas and concentrate it instead on the vital organs. The immediate result: your blood pressure may rise. Picture a garden hose. Constrict the water flow with your thumb, and it increases the water pressure inside.

But drink enough water, and constricted blood vessels usually begin to open up, lowering blood pressure. Sure, you could take a blood pressure medication, but why, when the safer, cheaper solution is usually to drink enough water? I've had many patients lower their blood pressure to normal with an adequate intake of water. Of course, weight loss, stress reduction, and a sensible diet are also important for lowering blood pressure.

????????

Take a Guess

Which food is highest in water content?

- a. Watermelon
- b. Lettuce
- c. Grapefruit

Answer: b. Lettuce. Although all of the foods listed have a high percentage of water content, a half cup of lettuce has the highest at 95 percent.[4]

Digestion problems

Are you a Pepcid-popper? Do you always have a roll of Tums at your desk or in your purse? Water is the hero of the gastrointestinal tract. It is the basis of every fluid your body needs for digestion, including saliva, bile, stomach acid, pancreatic juices, and even the mucus that lines our GI tract. Without adequate water, the whole digestive system goes into emergency mode, and you may get heartburn, indigestion, constipation, hemorrhoids, and even ulcers.

The mucous layer in your stomach is 98 percent water. It protects against stomach acid, and it contains bicarbonate, which neutralizes stomach acid. When your body has adequate water, the mucous layer is thick, preventing the acid from burning the stomach lining. Without a thick mucous layer, you may experience chronic burning whenever you eat.

Ulcer medications may do more harm than good; they treat the symptoms, so you feel better. But over time they reduce your stomach acid, leaving plenty of room for *Helicobacter pylori*, or *H. pylori*, the primary ulcer-causing bacteria, to run rampant.

But water keeps the digestive juices supplied and helps your body create all the acid it needs. That acid is your friend in this case, because it kills the bacteria *H. pylori* that cause ulcers, and it also improves digestion.

Asthma

Asthmatics usually have high histamine levels. Histamine is a neurotransmitter that causes the muscles in the bronchial tubes to constrict, restricting the flow of air. Your bronchial tubes need adequate hydration to prevent constriction. Animal studies have shown that histamine production goes down as water intake goes up.[5] The same goes for allergies, which are also usually associated with elevated histamine levels.

People with asthma should *slightly* increase their salt intake, provided they don't have high blood pressure or heart disease. Dr. Batmanghelidj explains the reason why salt is important to asthmatics:

> In the first stages of asthma, mucus is secreted to protect the tissues [but] there comes a time [when] that mucus...stays put, preventing normal passage of air through the airways. Sodium is a natural "mucus breaker," and it is normally secreted to make mucus "disposable." That is why phlegm is salty when it comes in contact with the tongue. Salt is needed to break up the mucus in the lungs and render it watery for its expulsion from the airways.[6]

If you are an asthmatic or tend to have allergies, water may improve your symptoms more than the latest round of inhalers or pills from pharmaceutical companies. Besides, water is cheaper, too. As I say, "Health is cheap; disease is expensive."

Today we covered the adverse conditions that dehydration can have on your body. Tomorrow I will share with you a simple antiaging secret.

BUILDING BLOCKS TO A HEALTHY LIFE

POINTS TO PONDER: *Dehydration robs from certain areas of the body to keep the brain, heart, lungs, liver, and kidneys well hydrated. Many symptoms of disease are the first sign of the body needing adequate amounts of water. Some of the symptoms of inadequate water intake may include headaches, back pain, joint aches, dry skin, allergies, heartburn, constipation, and memory loss.*

ACTION STEP: *If you are suffering from any of the health conditions listed above, identify which ones, gradually increase the amount of water you drink each day, and eventually these symptoms may start to subside.*

DAY 3: The Fountain of Youth

Located in St. Augustine, Florida, is a historical landmark known as "the Fountain of Youth," a legendary spring that reputedly restores the youth of anyone who drinks of its waters. One of the most persistent myths is that Spanish explorer Juan Ponce de León was searching for the Fountain of Youth when he traveled to present-day Florida in 1513. Each year many people visit the historical site and superstitiously drink from its water in hopes of reversing the aging process and looking forever young. The irony is that the myth is partially true: water does rejuvenate your skin, which can make you look years younger.

A few years ago I saw singer Tina Turner in a television interview, and even though she was well into her sixties, her skin looked fabulous. She said it was because she drank at least two quarts of water every day.

The Skinny on Skin

Skin…

- Is the largest organ of the body and weighs about six pounds.
- Grows faster than any other organ.
- Is tough, flexible, and waterproof.
- Stores water, fat, and vitamin D.
- Protects the body from germs, heat, cold, and sunlight.
- Is replaced approximately every thirty days.

When you don't drink enough clean water you may lose your good looks. I believe that water is the single best beauty treatment on the planet. It keeps your skin supple, your eyes bright, and your body spry. Consider this: Remove water from plums, and you get prunes. Remove water from your skin, and you get wrinkles. In a dehydrated state your skin becomes dry, flaky, and wrinkled. The skin is designed to hold in moisture, to be elastic. When you deprive it of water, the skin sags and loses its elasticity. Not even a jar of wrinkle prevention cream can cure that!

Lose Weight, Feel Great

Proper hydration has other benefits for reversing the aging process. Water will also help you to manage your weight. When you are dehydrated, your body secretes aldosterone, a hormone that causes water retention. As you drink more water, your body releases the water it was storing for "survival mode." During the first few days of drinking more water than your body is accustomed to, you are running to the bathroom constantly. This can be very discouraging, and it can certainly interfere with an otherwise normal daily routine. Take heart; it's really your body's way of getting rid of excess water and toxins. You are "flushing" out your system.

New research also shows that being dehydrated may cause your body's fat deposits to increase. Dehydration can contribute to an inefficient metabolism by affecting body temperature. When you are dehydrated, your body temperature drops slightly and causes your body to store fat as a way to help raise or maintain the temperature.[1] Also, as some savvy dieters know, drinking water reduces your appetite by giving you a full feeling.

Improve Your Memory

Have you ever felt as if you were experiencing a "senior moment"? You don't have to be resigned to the idea of losing your memory anymore. For some time, it was common knowledge that nothing could be done about memory loss. It was accepted as a part of growing old. That is, until experts discovered that humans can grow new brain cells. PET (positron emission tomography) and SPECT (single photon emission computed tomography) scans can map brain activity and measure both the destruction and growth of new brain cells. This completely changed the way we viewed memory loss. Thanks to these marvelous advances, today we know that even damaged brains can grow new cells.[3] If we know what areas of the brain can grow new cells, then we may be able to improve memory.

> **H_2O 101**
>
> As we age, our body's signal for thirst tends to decrease, which may be the reason why some elderly people don't drink as much water as they should. Their water reserves are typically lower, and their vulnerability to become more dehydrated tends to increase.[2]

One way to improve your memory is to drink a lot of water. Your brain loves water. The human brain is roughly one-fiftieth of the total body weight, and brain cells are said to be approximately 85 percent water. The brain is the only part of the body that is constantly active.[4] So to remain active, it must have water. Without adequate hydration, these processes can slow down. I believe that long-term dehydration may even contribute to Alzheimer's disease, and I believe further studies will bear this out. For further information on the use of water to prevent and treat all kinds of diseases, I strongly recommend the book *Your Body's Many Cries for Water* by Dr. F. Batmanghelidj.

Water Revives Cells

Cellular dehydration affects how our cells function. The first sign of failing health is a shift of fluid from the inside of the cell to the outside of the cell. About two-thirds of the body's fluid is inside the cells, and the rest is outside the cells. But cells die when they don't have enough energy to maintain the membrane pumps, which maintain the balance of water inside and out.

When there is more water outside the cells than there should be, it compresses blood vessels and reduces the amount of oxygen and nutrients delivered to the cells. Cells suffer. Something as simple as water can bring health back to our cells by maintaining water balance in our bodies. This is increasingly important as we age, because cells lose water as we age. Believe it or not, newborn infants are about 80 percent water, whereas older people are usually less than 50 percent water.[5]

So the next time you are tempted to try the latest expensive skin cream or pop a pill, try drinking enough water. It will keep your skin hydrated, elastic, attractive, and healthy. It will help you manage your appetite, and it will improve your memory. By giving your body the water it needs, you will maintain your youth and smarts longer.

BUILDING BLOCKS TO A HEALTHY LIFE

POINTS TO PONDER: *Water is a powerful nutrient to slow the aging process and to maintain your brain and memory. Your brain cells are mainly water—about 85 percent—and your brain is constantly active, even during sleep. Therefore, your brain needs to be well hydrated.*

ACTION STEP: *Increase your intake of salads, vegetables, and fruits since they all contain a high percentage of water.*

DAY 4: The Rap on Tap Water

As a kid you probably drank water out of the garden hose on hot days, or from the school drinking fountain, a farm pump, or maybe right out of the bathroom faucet. If so, you got it half right: we have to drink healthy amounts of water, but we need to drink the right kind of water, and tap water is not it.

I wish I could tell you that all water is the same, wherever it comes from, and that our body naturally filters out any "bad stuff." But that's not true. When there are harmful substances in our water, those substances get into our bodies and may harm us. Tap water is not as healthy anymore. Here's why.

Smokestacks and Plastics

Just a few decades ago you could find pure water right in the ground. A fifty-foot-deep well yielded plenty of pure water—that is, water free of contaminants, chemicals, and other substances our bodies consider toxic. But today, even wells two hundred feet deep may not yield pure water. They have been contaminated by the amazing increase of man-made chemicals used in industry, agriculture, and consumer products.

Industrialization and technology have introduced new, complex, and sometimes lethal pollutants into our nation's water systems. Over half a million chemicals have been developed since 1965; most are water soluble, and many are toxic.[1] In 1968 the United States manufactured its one millionth chemical, and as of February 2006, there were 8,369,447 commercially available chemicals.[2] And this number is updated daily! One government report identified more than 2,000 chemicals in our drinking water.[3] But most water-testing facilities can only perform tests for approximately thirty or forty chemicals. Municipal treatment plants neither detect nor remove most chemicals from the water supply. Our ability to filter out toxins is lagging woefully behind our ability to create chemicals.

The past few decades have taught us that it is impossible to separate our water supplies from the environment we live in. The underground aquifers that feed city water supplies may catch runoff from dump sites, landfills, and even underground storage tanks. The chemicals we pump into the air from automobiles or factories eventually settle onto the land.

Sooner or later, anything we bury, spray, emit, or flush finds its way into our drinking water. According to the Environmental Defense Group, more than four billion pounds of toxic chemicals are released into the environment each year, seventy-two million pounds of which are known carcinogens.[4] That's why about half of America's ground water is contaminated, meaning about a quarter of the population is exposed to what I consider contaminated drinking water.

Agri-Pollution

The other big offender is agriculture. Pesticides, herbicides, and fertilizers, used in massive quantities, run off from farmland and may end up in underground aquifers, which feed city water supplies. Two billion pounds of pesticides are used every year—eight pounds for every American![5] The Environmental Working Group found that a single glass of Midwestern tap water has three or more pesticides in it.[6] According to that group, farmers across the Corn Belt apply 150 million pounds of five herbicides (atrazine, cyanazine, simazine, alachlor, and metolachlor) to their corn and soybean fields every spring. Rain washes these chemicals into drinking water supplies. These chemicals are not removed by the conventional municipal drinking water treatment technologies. In many Midwestern towns and cities, children receive their lifetime dose of the herbicide atrazine, a carcinogen, in their first four months of life.[7]

Agricultural pollution is not limited to rural areas. Some of the worst contamination by insecticides has been found in urban streams.[8] Though banned in 1972, low levels of DDT have turned up recently in stream sediment and fish in major American cities.[9]

Drugs and Shampoo

Believe it or not, pharmaceutical products may end up in drinking water. How? After consuming a drug, humans or animals expel it in their waste (or sometimes people flush their medications). Wastewater treatment plants then recycle the water for use. Antibiotics, hormones, and painkillers have been found in public drinking water.[10] German scientists report that dozens of drugs can be measured in a typical water sample.[11] Fish who live downstream from water treatment plants have been shown to contain man-made chemicals from today's most popular drugs, like Zoloft, an antidepressant, and birth control pills.[12]

Personal care products like cosmetics, toiletries, and fragrances are putting chemicals into water supplies, too. For example, toluene, a chemical used in nail polish, nail treatment products (such as acrylic nails), and fragrances such as perfume and cologne, is suspected of presenting risks to human reproduction and development and has been linked to potential for reduced fertility or reduced chance for a healthy, full-term pregnancy. It is unsafe for use in cosmetics, according to the fragrance industry's International Fragrance Association.[13]

Researchers say the amount of pharmaceutical and personal care products entering the environment is about equal to the amount of pesticides.[14]

Little Critters

Finally, though cities treat water to kill most bacteria, they usually cannot kill all viruses and parasites, such as amoeba, *giardia*, and *cryptosporidium. Giardia* is a major cause of diarrhea in day-care centers and contaminates many of the lakes and streams in America. It may be showing up in water supplies more often than we think. An outbreak of the microorganism *cryptosporidium* in Milwaukee's water supply in 1993 killed more than one hundred people and sickened another four hundred thousand.[15] Some observers believe some outbreaks of intestinal flu may actually be caused by such microorganisms in tap water.

It's bad enough having chemicals and microbes in the water, but the very things that are added to tap water to "purify" it may be hurting you as well. Let's look at what most cities add to their water to make it "healthy."

Chlorine in Drinking Water

Cities add chlorine to public drinking water as a public health measure to kill microorganisms. But chlorine is not entirely safe. It can combine with organic materials to form *trihalomethanes*—a cancer-promoting substance. Bladder cancer has been linked to chlorinated drinking water in ten out of the eleven most reliable studies. One study found that 14 to 16 percent of bladder cancers in Ontario, Canada, can be attributed to drinking water that contains chlorination by-products.[16]

A study of drinking water and pregnancy outcomes in North Carolina reported a 2.8-fold increased likelihood of miscarriage among women exposed to trihalomethanes in drinking water. Chlorinated water has also been linked to birth defects and spina bifida. Many European

Chlorine, the Anti-Vitamin

Chlorinated water can destroy nutrients your body needs: vitamins A, B, C, and E, and fatty acids. Chronic skin conditions like acne, psoriasis, and eczema may clear up or improve by simply switching to unchlorinated drinking water.

cities have already abandoned chlorination in favor of oxidation to disinfect their public water supplies.[17]

Chlorinated tap water can hurt you even if you don't drink it. Those same trihalomethanes can get into your body when you shower. They evaporate out of the water, and you inhale them. A ten-minute hot shower can increase the contaminants absorbed into our bodies more than drinking half a gallon of chlorinated tap water.[18]

When you take a shower with chlorinated water, it can also make your hair brittle and dry out your skin. To avoid this, purchase a shower filter, which will remove 95 percent of chlorine from the water. (See Appendix A.)

Fluoride—Not So Healthy After All

Most cities in the United States also add fluoride to the water, even though fluoride is a proven toxin. The subject of fluoride in public drinking water has become a hot topic, as it should be. Have you ever wondered why your tube of toothpaste tells you to call a poison control center if your child swallows more than a pea-sized amount? Because fluoride is a toxin![19] The sodium fluoride that is added to toothpaste is created by aluminum smelting.[20] There are two types of fluoride: the sodium fluoride found in toothpaste and the more toxic *hydrofluosilicic acid* or *sodium silicofluoride*, most commonly used in the water systems in the United States and considered one of the most corrosive chemical agents known to man.[21]

Fluoride helps to prevent tooth decay, primarily in children, but it also partially inhibits a hundred different enzymes in the body. However, new information shows fluorinated water does not.[22] Fluoride may be linked to osteosarcoma, a rare but deadly form of bone cancer. Chester Douglass, chair of the Oral Healthy Policy and Epidemiology Department at the Harvard School of Dental Medicine (HSDM), recently came under scrutiny for allegedly submitting written testimony claiming that there was no significant link between fluoride and cancer. However, one of Douglass's doctoral students, Elise B. Bassin, using Douglass's data, came up with a different set of conclusions—she found that fluoride makes the risk of osteosarcoma five to seven times higher.[23] The outcome of the investigation is still pending at this time.

Fluoride can interfere with vitamin and mineral functions; it is also linked to calcium deposits and arthritis. The U.S. Department of Health and Human Services has said that people with cardiovascular and kidney problems, the elderly, and people with deficiencies of calcium, magnesium, and vitamin C "are susceptible to the toxic effects of fluoride."

Dr. Charles Gordon Heyd, past president of the American Medical Association, stated, "Fluoride is a corrosive poison that will produce serious effects on a long range basis."[24]

My point is to make you aware of the dangers more than to alarm you. I am not advocating poor oral hygiene or a boycott of toothpaste. Please *do not* go and throw out your fluoride toothpaste. Just make sure that you rinse out your mouth thoroughly and do not swallow your toothpaste! If you have small children, *please* take time to show them how to brush and rinse properly, and *teach them not to swallow the toothpaste.* Children are more prone to swallowing it, especially if it's "flavored."

Aluminum Problems

Cities and towns also treat ground water with aluminum to remove organic material. The aluminum coagulates organic material into clumps. It's impossible to then remove all the aluminum that has been added, so traces of aluminum remain in the drinking water. Aluminum may be worse for you than fluoride or chlorine. It has even been associated with Alzheimer's disease.[25]

Some people ask me if boiling water gets rid of the chemicals. The answer is no. Harmful bacteria may be killed, but the chemicals remain. They don't "boil out."

Your body needs water, but tap water may not be the best source. I am strongly convinced that over time it will diminish your quality of life. Even if you can't afford a two-hundred-dollar filtration system, you can begin by purchasing a pitcher filtration system or a faucet-mounted filtration system, like the ones manufactured by Brita, for as little as twenty dollars. You can find a solution within your financial means. Day 6 takes a closer look at the differences. Tap water is good for watering lawns, washing clothes, and flushing toilets, but not for drinking. You may be asking, "So what kind of water can I drink?" Tomorrow's entry compares tap water to bottled water.

Did You Know . . . ?

If you have lead pipes, *do not* drink hot water from the faucet. Hot water increases lead concentration. Flush the pipes first by running cool water before using it.[26]

DAY 4 DAY 4 DAY 4

BUILDING BLOCKS TO A HEALTHY LIFE

POINTS TO PONDER: *It's best not to drink water straight from the faucet, because tap water may contain toxins, heavy metals, pesticides, residual personal care products, bacteria, and other microbes. One of the chemicals added to our tap water is fluoride. Generally, there are two types of fluoride: the type added to toothpaste (sodium fluoride) and the type added to drinking water (sodium silicofluoride). The latter is the most toxic of the two.*

ACTION STEP: *To check your city's water supply, go the Web site www.ewg.org and click on the bar labeled "Tap Water Database: What's in your water?" Search under the tab "local findings" and select your city's name; it will generate a local water system report including any contaminants found in the water supply.*

DAY 5: Is Bottled Water Better?

Many people already drink bottled water instead of tap water, making bottled water the second most popular beverage in the United States, behind soft drinks.[1] People today consume twice as much bottled water as they did a decade ago, and the growth in the bottled water industry is "unparalleled," according to the Beverage Marketing Corporation.[2]

But is bottled water healthier for you? Does that attractive bottle with the pictures of snowy mountains and crystalline streams really mean the water inside is pure?

Bottled water is actually *less regulated than tap water* and can be just as toxic. Bottled water is considered a "food," and so it is regulated by the Food and Drug Administration (FDA). Tap water is regulated by the Environmental Protection Agency (EPA).[3] The only requirement placed on bottled water in the United States is that it be as safe as tap water. But while the EPA makes cities test public drinking water daily, the FDA requires only yearly testing for bottled water.[4]

Furthermore, cities must have their water tested by government-certified labs, but water bottlers do not. The EPA forbids the presence of bacteria, which indicate the presence of fecal material, but the FDA has no such rule, meaning bottled water can contain fecal bacteria and still be legal. Big cities using surface water have to test for *cryptosporidium* and *giardia*. Bottled water companies do not.[5]

A 1999 study of one hundred of the most popular brands of bottled water showed that a third contained arsenic, trihalomethanes, bacteria, or other contaminants. A fifth contained man-made chemicals, and one contained phthalate at twice the level acceptable in tap water. Two had high levels of fluoride, and two others had coliform bacteria.[6]

And if you think bottled water is lead free, think again. The FDA allows bottled water to contain up to five parts per billion of lead, or a third of what is permitted in tap water.[7]

Where Bottled Water Really Comes From

Brace yourself for this one. Dasani and Aquafina waters, two of the biggest brands in America, are reprocessed tap water from cities around the country. One of Aquafina's sources is the Detroit River![8] In fact, about one-fourth of bottled water is tap water, according to government and industry estimates.[9]

Clearly the words "bottled at the source" have no meaning. They are a marketing ploy. The "source" of the bottled water in your pantry could very well be the tap. As long as producers meet the FDA's standards for distilled or purified water, they don't even have to disclose the source.[10]

Did You Know...?

In 2005, the total number of bottled water brands—worldwide—is close to three thousand, conservatively, with Italy alone having more than six hundred brands.[11]

But many varieties of bottled water are very good. Penta Water, one of the top-selling bottled waters in health food stores, is considered the purest bottled water on the market. It undergoes a rigorous purification process to remove every possible impurity. It takes about eleven hours to make a bottle of Penta Water. I find it especially beneficial for my patients with fibromyalgia, chronic fatigue, headaches, arthritis, and most degenerative diseases. I usually recommend two sixteen-ounce bottles of Penta Water a day, along with one to two quarts of pure spring water.

The Problem With Plastic

The other major problem with much bottled water is that it comes in plastic bottles. Studies continue to show that some forms of plastic are not as safe as people believe. The very worst plastic used in some water bottles and food wraps, polyvinyl chloride (PVC), is a known carcinogen that emits pollutants from the moment it is created until long after it is discarded.[12] Studies clearly show that PVC leaches vinyl chloride and other pollutants, thus disrupting the hormonal balance, causing fertility problems, and damaging cells, organs, and tissues.[13]

Another common ingredient in some plastics, bisphenol A, is used in reusable water bottles. It can change the course of fetal development and cause abnormal chromosome loss or gain, which leads to miscarriage or disorders like Down syndrome. It has also been linked to obesity. Popular Nalgene water bottles—those hard, brightly colored, reusable bottles—and five-gallon bottles also contain bisphenol A.[14] Studies showed the chemical leaches into the water at room temperature.[15]

Most water bottles are made from a plastic called PET or PETE (which stands for *polyethylene terephthalate*). This kind of plastic is considered safer than PVC, but it has been shown to leach plasticizer chemicals called phthalates into the water when used repeatedly or when water is bottled for too long.[16] Phthalates disrupt the production of fatty acids and interfere with the production of sex hormones. However, these bottles appear to be safe if the water is drunk within a few months of the date the water was bottled (if the manufacturer has assigned an expiration date), and then used only once and not refilled. Otherwise, PET or PETE plastics may cause the same kinds of problems other plastics do.[17] According to a 2002 report from the FDA, the government does not require manufacturers to put expiration dates on bottled water, but the report did say that "long-term storage may result in off-odor or taste."[18]

I prefer drinking water from glass bottles or from bio-based plastics, which are made of natural products like starch, cellulose, and raw rubber. In 2005, one bottled water company, Biota, introduced the use of the first compostable bioplastic bottle. I suspect that many other companies will be following suit because as the price of oil increases, so does the price of plastic. Even Wal-Mart is planning on switching to bioplastic packaging in their stores.[19] It is fairly easy to avoid bad plastics because producers must label the bottle with the type of plastic it is made of. This labeling system is easy to follow:

1. PET or PETE: used to bottle soda, most bottled water, cooking oils, juice, salad dressing, peanut butter, and other foods
2. HDPE: milk jugs, one-gallon water bottles, some bottled foods
3. PVC: cling wraps, Reynolds Wrap, Stretch-tite, Freeze-tite (used by many grocery stores for meats), four-ounce Wesson Cooking Oil, Appalachian Mountain spring water, some plastic squeeze bottles
4. LDPE: food storage bags (like Glad and Ziploc)
5. PP: deli soup containers, most Rubbermaid containers, cloudy plastic baby bottles, ketchup bottles, other cloudy plastic bottles
6. PS: Styrofoam, some disposable plastic cups and bowls, and most opaque plastic cutlery
7. "Other" resins, usually polycarbonate, which contains bisphenol A: most plastic baby bottles, five-gallon water bottles, clear plastic "sippy" cups, some types of clear plastic cutlery, inner lining of food cans
8. PLA—bioplastic called polylactic acid[20]

The topic and debate over which plastics are safest will continue, and so will the recommendations. As for now, the safest plastics to use are PET (or PETE) and bioplastics.

Proper Usage and Storage of Bottled Water

Reusing your water bottle may seem kind to the environment, but it's terrible for your body. Studies show dangerous levels of bacteria accumulate on and in the bottle as you reuse it. The water in the bottle may become so contaminated that, if it were tap water, cities wouldn't use it![21] My recommendation: use that eight- to sixteen-ounce bottle once, then toss it.

Did You Know...?

Plastics—including baby bottles—should not go in the microwave.

Store your bottled water properly. Always keep it away from cleaning compounds, paints, gasoline, or other household or industrial chemicals. Don't store it in the garage or shed, or in direct sunlight. Store it in the refrigerator, if possible, to retard bacteria growth, or in a dark, cool place in the house.

If you are going to drink bottled water, check if the bottler is a member of the International Bottled Water Association (IBWA), which guarantees that the level of contaminants, if any, is below FDA standards. Go to the IBWA Web site at www.bottledwater.org to see which bottled water makers are members.

Also check the mineral content of your bottled water. Spring or mineral water is also important. The ideal water is water that is high in magnesium (at least 90 mg per liter) and low in sodium (less than 10 mg per liter). For example, a few waters that meet these criteria are from the same area in Northern California—Noah's California Spring Water with an incredible 120 mg of magnesium per liter, Adobe Springs water with 110 mg per liter, and BlueStar Springs, also with 110 mg magnesium per liter. For more information, go to www.mgwater.com/list5.shtml, where you will find links to these waters. Another helpful Web site that compares many different bottled waters is www.tldp.com/issue/190/Bottled%20Water.htm.

There are approximately three thousand brands of bottled waters worldwide. It is not possible to list each brand of bottled water. Two Web sites that help in finding information about different bottled waters are www.AquaMaestro.com and www.mineralwaters.org. Appendix C provides a chart that lists the pH comparisons of the various brands of bottled water.

You may be feeling overwhelmed and as if there is no hope. Be reassured hope is on the way, and there is light at the end of this tunnel!

BUILDING BLOCKS TO A HEALTHY LIFE

POINTS TO PONDER: *Some bottled waters contain more toxins than tap water and are not as closely regulated as tap. If you drink bottled water, check if the manufacturer of the bottled water is a member of the IBWA (International Bottled Water Association). Always properly store your bottled water. Keep it away from chemicals, and store it in a refrigerator if possible. If the container is plastic, check the expiration date or bottling date.*

ACTION STEP: *Purchase clean bottled water, preferably alkaline and in glass containers rather than plastic. Penta Water, however, is extremely pure water even though it comes in a plastic bottle.*

DAY 6: Filtered Water

One of the best kinds of water to drink is filtered water. Using a water filter in your home can be a big step toward restoring health to your drinking water. Some people use filtration pitchers or faucet-mounted carbon filters, some use full-home filtration systems, and others use reverse-osmosis under-the-counter systems and distillation. These may sound mysterious and expensive, but a good water filter probably costs less than you currently spend on soft drinks every month.

But not all filtration systems do the same things, cost the same, or create better water. Let's examine the pros and cons of each, and then I'll recommend what I think is the healthiest kind of water.

Carbon Filters

Carbon filters are the "entry-level" filters: inexpensive, reliable, and common. They come in many forms, from a base model water-filtering pitcher that costs around twenty dollars, to a faucet-mounted filter, which costs a bit more, all the way to the kind that attaches near your water main and filters water for the entire house.

There are two types of carbon filters. One uses granulated carbon; the other uses a solid carbon block. The solid block filter costs more, lasts longer, and does a much better job at filtering out microorganisms. The only disadvantage is that the flow rate is slower than with loose charcoal filters.

A pitcher filter, which uses granulated charcoal, removes most chlorine and 90 percent of the lead. However, many toxins are not filtered out. Because it is so convenient and inexpensive, for some people this is the best filter to use—if the alternative is to use no filter at all.

But there are drawbacks to all carbon filters. Carbon filters are not totally effective for heavy metals, and they don't remove fluoride, viruses, pharmaceuticals, or personal care products.[1] Also, if you don't change the filters as the instructions direct, they can become more of a hazard than a help. Old filters collect the "garbage" in the water and may actually begin to breed bacteria.[2]

If you choose a carbon filter, you will remove some, but not all, of the impurities from your tap water. It's an inexpensive but incomplete option, in my opinion.

A Water Distiller

Water distillers are extremely effective at removing everything, unfortunately even good minerals, from water. Distillers use electricity to heat tap water to the boiling point, separating impurities from the "steam," which becomes your clean drinking water.[3]

The drawback with distilled water is that there are no beneficial minerals left in it! The water is mineral free. A growing body of evidence suggests that completely mineral-free water is worse for your body than water with dissolved minerals in it. Distilled water is absorbent water, meaning it absorbs carbon dioxide, which may make your body acidic. A distiller will get you halfway to your goal. You won't have anything bad in your water, but it can adversely affect your health in other ways. A good water distiller can remove heavy metals, pesticides, herbicides, organic compounds, bacteria, and some viruses.

Reverse Osmosis

In terms of price, reverse-osmosis systems are the "optimum level" of water filters. They filter water through an extremely fine membrane. It's a slow process, and the cost ranges anywhere from a couple of hundred dollars to many hundreds of dollars, but, like distillers, they remove virtually everything from water: chlorine, fluoride, bacteria, parasites, chemicals, and heavy metals like lead and mercury.[4] Reverse-osmosis systems are commonly used by water bottlers to create their waters. They often add back minerals at the end of the process.

Like distilled water, most reverse osmosis creates acidic water. The water it produces is similar to distilled water. It is 95 percent mineral-free acidic and therefore aggressive—meaning it pulls minerals from anything with which it comes into contact. Because the water is acidic, it may keep your tissues acidic.[5]

Nevertheless, both distilled and reverse-osmosis water are the purest water. If you use these filters, make sure that you take adequate minerals. It's also a good idea to add an alkaline booster to the water. A couple of drops in an eight-ounce glass of water will raise the alkalinity to a healthy level. (See Appendix A for more information.) You may purchase the drops that alkalinize the water from most health food stores.

What to drink, then? Let's get to my recommendations.

Alkaline Water Filters

Your body thrives in an alkaline environment since it is able to detoxify more efficiently than in an acidic environment. In an alkaline environment your tissues get rid of impurities more efficiently. When cancer patients come into my office to begin nutritional treatment, their bodies are almost always very acidic and toxic. My first task is to get their tissues alkalinized with alkaline water and alkaline foods.

Alkalinity and acidity are measured in terms of pH. On the pH scale of 1 to 14, a pH of 7.0 is considered neutral. Anything under 7.0 is acidic; anything over 7.0 is alkaline. Blood has a constant pH of 7.4—it's alkaline. But most Americans' tissues are very acidic (as indicated by an acidic urine pH), meaning their bodies are less efficient at removing toxins. Many health problems are associated with being too acidic, including chronic fatigue, fibromyalgia, arthritis, arteriosclerosis, most cancers, diabetes, autoimmune disease, osteoporosis, and practically all degenerative diseases.[7]

Did You Know...?

Snow water from the Alps or the Caucasus Mountains is some of the very best water to drink. That's because the melted snow water usually travels down mountains, gaining energy and oxygen.[6] But I advise not to drink snow water from anywhere else, especially in cities where pollution is a problem.

I have had countless numbers of patients with painful osteoarthritis on many different medications for arthritis. Many have been pain free within a couple of months after adjusting their urine pH to 7.0 to 7.5 simply by consuming adequate amounts of alkaline water and alkaline foods. As a result, many are able to go off their anti-inflammatory medications.

By drinking alkaline water, you start to bring your tissues back to an alkaline state. Some spring waters are alkaline, but you can create alkaline water from tap water or spring water by using an alkalizing filter. These filters sit on your kitchen counter and use activated charcoal and an electrolysis process to produce two types of water: one is alkaline, which you drink, and the other acidic, which you can discard or use for washing clothes, watering the lawn, or showering.

I use an alkalizing filter in my home and office. Because water alkalizers use an electromagnetic process to separate acidic water from alkaline water, the water you put into it must be rich in minerals and not distilled or reverse-osmosis water.

Some alkalizer filters also make the water clustered or "hexagonal," meaning that at a molecular level, it is denser, richer, and more energetic. All of these attributes benefit health in many ways. Clustered water moves easily within the body and aids nutrition absorption and waste removal. It is more readily taken up by the cells and is therefore more hydrating to the cells and helps them to detoxify. I also use clustered water in my practice.

Dr. Mu Shik Jhon, who has conducted extensive research on hexagonal water and its many benefits, says, "Hexagonal water moves easily within the cellular matrix of the body, helping with nutrient absorption and waste removal."[8] Some of the benefits of hexagonal water are:

- Greater energy
- Rapid hydration
- Heightened immune function
- Better nutrient absorption
- Longevity
- Weight loss
- Greater metabolic efficiency

I have recommended alkaline, hexagonal water to even my youngest patients. In 2005, a ten-year-old girl and her parents came to my office from South Carolina. The girl had crippling juvenile rheumatoid arthritis and weighed only fifty-two pounds. Her hands were swollen like mitts, and her knees were swollen as large as softballs. I put her on hexagonal, alkaline water, one to two quarts a day. A week and a half later she was pain free, and her swelling was significantly diminished. We were giving her nutritional products as well, but not until two weeks later. When she arrived she was wheelchair-bound, but she was actually able to walk without pain after only a week and a half of drinking the hexagonal, alkaline water. Her parents were ecstatic. We raised the pH of her tissues. After a month, her hands were almost normal size. Hexagonal, alkaline water is especially effective in treating those with chronic disease. (See Appendix A.)

Certain bottled waters are also alkaline. Evamor and Abita waters are just a few of the alkaline bottled waters.

I use a variety of filters and spring waters because each has its unique benefits. I always start with spring water that is alkaline because it supplies minerals in their natural form. For normal, everyday drinking I use Mountain Valley Spring brand bottled water, from a glass bottle, and I treat it with my Vitalizer Plus machine, which converts it into hexagonal water. When I go to the gym, I take a bottle of Penta Water with me. Now, I realize that very few people are able to do what I do, but I'm frequently asked what type of water I drink. This is my regular practice.

When I make coffee I use an alkalizing filter, because coffee is more acidic. At home I use reverse-osmosis water in my ice machine. I also have a large filter outside of the house that filters all water entering the house. I encourage you to examine the benefits of each filter, do your research, decide what you're going to do—and then do it! In my opinion, there is nothing more important to your health than water.

Acid Test

If you would like to know how acidic your body is, buy pH strips at the drugstore. Collect your first morning urine and dip pH paper into it. It will indicate your urine's pH level with a change of color. The change of color can then be matched to a numerical reading. A card is included in the pH paper that correlates a color to a pH number. It is similar to checking the pH of a swimming pool.

Most people will have a pH test reading of about 5.0, which means their bodies are very acidic. It should be between 7.0 to 7.5. Close enough doesn't count. Even though five is only two points less than seven, a pH of 5.0 is actually a hundred times more acidic than a pH of 7.0. It may take you a while to achieve this pH, but keep at it. Continue drinking alkaline water and eating alkaline foods (such as fruits and vegetables), and take supplements discussed later in the book. Be patient, and know that by implementing each of these pillars you can achieve it.

So how much should you drink, and when? We will cover that tomorrow.

BUILDING BLOCKS TO A HEALTHY LIFE

POINTS TO PONDER: *Filtered water is one of the best waters for your body. When choosing a filter, remember that carbon filters are the "entry-level" type of filter and the least expensive. Distilled water and reverse-osmosis water are the purest water. However, they are also the most acidic. In my opinion, alkaline water filters are one of the best types of filters because our bodies thrive best in an alkaline environment, which helps our systems function at an optimum level.*

ACTION STEP: *Start to look for a home water filter system. If you are on a limited budget, start with a pitcher filter or a faucet-mounted filter.*

DAY 7: How Much, and When, to Drink

Once when my niece, Kennedy, who was three years old at the time, was visiting, I noticed how much she liked to drink sodas. So I went to the store and bought some small bottles of pure spring water. I gave her some, and, surprisingly, she drank it to the last drop.

Not long after, she said, "Mommy, Mommy, more water!" My sister was amazed. "How on earth did you get her to drink that water? She's never liked water at home." I knew my sister only gave her tap water at home.

The answer is that our bodies yearn for pure, clean water. But one of the most common questions I hear is, "How much water should I drink?" I'm going to give you the answer to that question. To determine how much water your body needs, take your body weight (in pounds) and divide it by two. That's how many ounces of water you need every day.

How Much Should I Drink?

Take your weight in pounds and divide it by two. The result is how many ounces of water you should drink daily.

____ Weight ÷ 2 = ______ ounces per day

Usually that amounts to two to three quarts a day. Picture a one-gallon container of milk, and imagine it three-quarters full. If you are an average-sized person, that's about how much water your body needs *daily*. If you weigh 120 pounds, you will need 60 ounces of water; if 220 pounds, you'll need 110 ounces. Most people have no idea they require that much.

But you won't consume it all in liquid form. Simply by eating lots of fruits and vegetables—as you should—you will get a quart a day. Foods such as bananas are 70 percent water; apples, 80 percent water; tomatoes and watermelons are more than 90 percent water; and lettuce is 95 percent water. If you eat an inordinate amount of starches, like breads or pastries, you will need more water, because these foods add little water to your body.

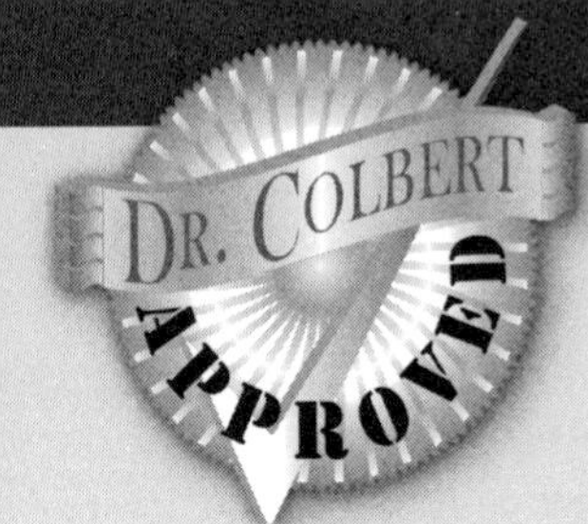

Dr. Colbert Approved Coffee

Here's a recipe for healthy coffee. Use unbleached (brown) filters, organic coffee, alkaline water, and stevia instead of sugar. If you must have a creamer, use organic skim milk or rice milk, and never use a Styrofoam cup, as styrene, considered a possible human carcinogen, tends to migrate into food and beverages more quickly if they are hot.[1]

Is Caffeine Bad?

Too much coffee, cola, and tea are not substitutes for water, but recent studies also show that caffeine isn't all bad for you. It helps prevent Parkinson's disease and cirrhosis of the liver, and it helps with male fertility. It has also been shown to protect the brain, possibly from diseases like Alzheimer's.[2] A Harvard study showed that the risk for developing type 2 diabetes is lower among regular coffee drinkers.[3] Coffee also is linked to lower rates of suicide, colon cancer, high blood pressure in women, and heart disease.[4] Coffee has more than one thousand antioxidants, which is more antioxidants than green tea. It is the top source of antioxidants in the American diet.[5]

People who drink decaffeinated coffee also show reduced diabetes risk, though at half the benefit of those drinking caffeinated coffee.[6]

The key, as with anything, is moderation. One or two cups a day won't hurt you, and research shows that it will probably help you. But three to four cups may be too much. You can drink iced tea all day and still be mildly dehydrated, because the caffeine is a diuretic, meaning it takes (or removes) water from the body. Some individuals with arrhythmias of the heart, fibrocystic breast disease, and migraine headaches should probably avoid caffeinated beverages altogether.[7]

If you don't like coffee—and even if you do—you should drink organic green tea. It has been a favorite in Japan for over a thousand years. Its antioxidant activity is two hundred times more potent than that of vitamin E and five hundred times more potent than vitamin C. This decreases the risk of cancer. Have two or three cups of organic green tea a day. And if you don't like green tea, try regular tea. The fact is, tea can be good for your mental health. One study on depression by a group of Finnish researchers found that individuals who drank five or more cups a day were not depressed, while those who drank no tea at all had the highest rate of depression.[8]

Climate Matters

If you live in a warmer or drier climate, you will need more water. I recently had a patient who worked outside in lawn maintenance in Florida. He would sweat so much he could wring a cup or two of sweat from his shirt. He was drinking four to five quarts of water a day, a little over a gallon, to keep up with his body's water requirement. Most of us lose about a pint of water a day through perspiration. Our bodies also lose water through exhalation (about a pint a day), and through urination and stool (about one to two pints a day).[9] Two pints equal one quart, so our bodies lose about one and a half to two quarts a day. However, this doesn't account for excessive perspiration.

When to Drink Water

Most people wait to drink until they are thirsty or until they have a dry mouth. By that time you are most likely already mildly dehydrated. A dry mouth is one of the last signs of dehydration.

Other people only drink during meals—another mistake. When you drink too much with a meal, it washes out the hydrochloric acid, digestive juices, and enzymes in your stomach and intestines, which delays digestion. Fluids, and iced drinks in particular, quench the digestive process similarly to pouring water on a fire.

You can drink some water with a meal. I usually drink room-temperature bottled water with a slice of lemon or lime squeezed into it or unsweetened tea. But don't go overboard. Meals are not the time to get most of your fluids. Stick to four to eight ounces with a meal.

Here's a typical timetable for healthy water consumption:

Start with an eight- to sixteen-ounce glass half an hour before breakfast. If you usually have juice, coffee, or tea with breakfast, don't eliminate them. The point of this pillar of health is not to take the fun out of life. You don't want to feel like a slave to water, but do limit coffee to one or two cups a day if you can. Organic green tea and organic black tea only have a small amount of caffeine, 30 and 50 mg per

When's a Good Time to Drink Water?

Here are some rules of thumb about when to drink water:

- Drink fifteen to thirty minutes before meals or two hours after.
- Only drink four to eight ounces of room-temperature water at meals.
- Do not drink much water past 7:00 p.m., because it may interfere with your sleep.

eight-ounce serving, respectively. So you can have a few glasses of tea a day, though not late in the evening, as it may interfere with your sleep.

A couple of hours after breakfast drink another eight- to sixteen-ounce glass of water. As you near lunch time, repeat your breakfast schedule. If your goal is to lose weight, drink more water before meals to give yourself a "full" feeling, which lessens your appetite.

Two hours after lunch have another eight- to sixteen-ounce glass of water. Then thirty minutes before your evening meal drink your next glass. If dinner is your largest meal of the day, try drinking sixteen to twenty-four ounces (or if lunch is your big meal, drink sixteen to twenty-four ounces before then). I predict that you won't eat as much.

Finally, two hours after dinner have another eight-ounce glass and another before bedtime, unless you have a hiatal hernia, reflux disease, or an enlarged prostate. In those cases, do not drink anything else after dinner.

Is it possible to drink too much water? Yes. There is a psychiatric condition called *psychogenic polydipsia,* which is drinking excessive amounts of water. It can cause potassium and electrolyte levels to become dangerously low.

Water is the first and most important pillar upon which to build a healthy life. The next most important pillar is a good night's sleep and a little "R&R," which we will begin tomorrow.

Let me end this section with a recommended blessing you can use to bless your water. Jesus blessed His food and thanked God the Father for it when He was on earth. We too should thank God for everything we take into our bodies and bless it beforehand.

> *Thank You for my clean, healing water. Mark 16:18 says that if I drink any deadly thing it shall not harm me. By faith, I thank You for cleansing this water from any toxic chemicals, bacteria, viruses, parasites, etc., and for protecting me supernaturally from any harm. I bless the water according to Exodus 23:25, which says that God shall bless my water and take sickness away from the midst of me.*
>
> *I drink this water with thanksgiving. Because God loves me and desires me to be healthy, I receive this water with gratitude and rejoice as it goes to every cell in my body. As I drink this water, my cells, tissues, and organs are cleansed, strengthened, and renewed like the eagle. I see myself healed, and I keep this vision before my eyes. In the name of Jesus, amen.*

BUILDING BLOCKS TO A HEALTHY LIFE

POINTS TO PONDER: *Don't wait until you are thirsty to drink water. If you wait until you're thirsty, you've waited too long. You're probably already dehydrated. Drink at least two quarts of clean water per day. Drink thirty minutes before meals or two hours after meals. Try not to drink excessive amounts of water past 7:00 p.m. Doing so may interfere with your sleep.*

ACTION STEP: *Use the formula on page 31 to figure out how much you should drink based on your body weight (in pounds).*

PILLAR 2

Sleep and Rest

DAY 8: Restoring Your Body With Sleep

Every night when the Walt Disney World theme parks close their gates and the crowds go home, the most important hours of the Disney day begin. Big lights go up, and massive crews of workers repair and clean every ride, every walkway, and every concession stand. When the gates open the next morning, the parks are completely renewed. The trash from the previous day is gone, and the roller coasters are in top condition again.

A similar thing happens every night in your body. During those precious hours your body shuts down and repairs itself. Your immune system recharges. Your major organs are restored. Old cells are being replaced with new ones. Your mind relaxes and orders its thoughts, creating a healthy mental state.

That's why this second pillar of health is wonderful, nourishing, restorative sleep and rest.

Edge of Collapse

What if Walt Disney World stayed open all night or let people in at 3:00 a.m., cutting short the repair time? The park would eventually be unsafe, unsanitary, and unappealing. It would end up a run-down shadow of itself, careening toward financial disaster and, worse, causing injuries or deaths on rides that were not maintained properly.

Lack of sleep is just as disastrous for you as an individual. A good night's sleep is free. A bad night's sleep is costly, because it takes a toll on your health.

But just as many Americans live in a state of unrecognized dehydration, an estimated fifty to seventy million also live on the brink of mental and physical collapse because of lack of sleep.[2] Researchers found that in one year alone about forty-two million sleeping pill prescriptions were filled for American adults and children.[3] An estimated sixty million Americans suffer from insomnia and other sleep disorders. More than half of all American adults suffer from insomnia at least a few times each week. As

> **Did You Know...?**
>
> Getting enough sleep will help you to learn new physical skills. Studies have shown that sleep builds procedural memory. What you practice during the day, you continue to learn while you sleep.[1]

a result, over 50 percent of the American population will experience daytime drowsiness.[4]

It's the same in my practice. The number one complaint I hear from patients who come into my office is, "I'm tired." They slump forward in their chairs, peering at me from under the weight of fatigue. I fear to send some of them out of my office because they don't seem awake enough to drive home!

We live in a world where day and night no longer matter. Thanks to modern technology, we can work and play around the clock. This is not the way our bodies or minds were made to operate. God gave us a promise of deep, restorative sleep. Psalm 127:2 (NIV) says, "He grants sleep to those he loves." To those who are tired, He says, "Come to me, all you who are weary and burdened, and I will give you rest" (Matt. 11:28, NIV).

Sleep and rest are so important because of what they do for your health.

Transportation Safety and Sleep Deprivation

When the Exxon Valdez ran aground in 1989, causing $1.85 billion in damage to the environment, the third mate was at the helm and had slept only six hours in the previous twenty-four.[5]

The crash of Korean Air Flight 801 in 1997 killed 228 people. The cockpit voice recorder picked up the pilot uttering the words "…really…sleepy…" as he made his final approach. The pilot's fatigue was ruled as a major contributor to this tragedy.[6]

1. *Sleep regulates release of important hormones.* When you sleep, growth hormone is secreted. This causes children to grow, and it regulates muscle mass and helps control fat in adults. When you don't sleep enough, this hormone's function is disrupted. Perhaps lack of sleep is partially to blame for the fact that two-thirds of Americans are overweight or obese. Leptin, another hormone, is secreted during sleep and directly influences appetite and weight control. It tells the body when it is "full." A person who doesn't have enough of this regulating hormone often has a runaway appetite.
2. *Sleep slows the aging process.* The term "beauty rest" is literally true. Sleep slows the aging process, and some say it is one of the most important "secrets" for averting wrinkles. How well a person sleeps is one of the most important predictors of how long a person will live.
3. *Sleep boosts the immune system.* People who sleep nine hours a night instead of seven hours have greater than nor-

mal "natural killer cell" activity. Natural killer cells destroy viruses, bacteria, and cancer cells.

4. *Sleep improves brain function.* One study shows that short-term sleep deprivation may decrease brain activity related to alertness and cognitive performance.[7]

5. *Sleep reduces cortisol levels.* Excessive stress raises cortisol levels, which disrupt neurotransmitter balance in the brain, causing you to be more irritable and prone to depression, anxiety, and insomnia. High cortisol levels are associated with many diseases, but the cure is as close as your pillow. Sufficient sleep helps to reduce cortisol levels.

Good sleep is one of the best "health principles" available to you, and yet relatively few people get adequate sleep. As a society, Americans are chronically sleep deprived. One in six claim that insomnia is a major problem for them. By not sleeping, they degrade and even ruin their health.[8]

What Happens When You Don't Sleep

The medical research is clear about what happens when you don't get sufficient sleep.

1. *You increase your risk of developing type 2 diabetes.* One study published by the medical journal *Lancet* revealed that even in young, healthy individuals, a sleep deficit of three to four hours a night over the course of a week affected the body's ability to process carbohydrates, leading some people into a prediabetic state.[9]

2. *You become clumsy and "sleep drunk."* Lack of sleep slows your reaction time, shortens your attention span, and impairs your memory, your decision-making process, and your coordination. People who go for up to nineteen hours without sleep score significantly worse on performance and alertness tests than people with a blood alcohol level of .08, which is legally drunk.[10]

3. *You jeopardize your job.* According to the National Commission on Sleep Disorders at the National Institutes of Health in Bethesda, Maryland, sleep deprivation costs an estimated $150 billion a year in higher stress and reduced workplace productivity.[11]

A third of America's adult workers either missed work or made mistakes at work in the past three months because of a lack of sleep.[12] Nobody drinks on the job, but plenty of people come to work after pulling all-nighters or getting too little sleep, thus functioning as if they were drunk.

4. *You endanger your life and the lives of others.* Sleep deprivation is responsible for at least 100,000 crashes and 1,500 fatalities a year, according to a 2002 report from the National Highway Traffic Safety Administration. Half of Americans admit to driving while drowsy. Studies show huge peaks in the number of accidents caused by people falling asleep at the wheel in the middle of the night and smaller peaks in the middle of the afternoon.[13]

Sleep Myth
FACT or FICTION?

You can "cheat" on the amount of sleep you get.

☐ Fact

☐ Fiction

Answer: Fiction. *Sleep experts say most adults need between seven and nine hours of sleep each night for optimum performance, health, and safety. When we don't get adequate sleep, we accumulate a sleep debt that can be difficult to "pay back" if it becomes too big. The resulting sleep deprivation has been linked to health problems such as obesity, high blood pressure, negative mood and behavior, decreased productivity, and safety issues in the home, on the job, and on the road.*[15]

5. *You reduce your sex drive.* Sleep deprivation raises cortisol levels, which blocks the normal response of the testicles to testosterone and decreases the production of hormonal precursors to testosterone. This is one reason young men in military boot camp generally have a lower sex drive, believe it or not.[14]

6. *You invite diseases.* A host of physical conditions are associated with insomnia, including chronic fatigue, fibromyalgia, chronic pain syndrome, autoimmune diseases, hypertension, obesity, depression, and other forms of mental illness. Adults with commonly diagnosed health conditions such as high blood pressure, arthritis, heartburn, and depression say they rarely get a good night's sleep, showing an association between sleeplessness and disease. People with these

conditions are nearly twice as likely to experience frequent daytime sleepiness as those who don't have the conditions.[16]

7. *You jeopardize your marriage.* Studies show higher rates of divorce among people who don't get adequate sleep.[17]

Getting the adequate amount of sleep is beneficial to you, and it benefits those around you. The next daily entry will show you the causes of insomnia, and later we will learn about what steps you can take toward getting successful sleep every night.

BUILDING BLOCKS TO A HEALTHY LIFE

POINTS TO PONDER: *A good night's sleep restores, repairs, and rejuvenates your body. Sleep is important because it is vital for your immune system and your overall health. Sleep also slows down the aging process. Lack of adequate sleep increases your risk of developing type 2 diabetes as well as a host of other diseases.*

ACTION STEP: *Make sure you get at least seven to nine hours of sleep tonight.*

DAY 9: What Causes Insomnia

One time I developed a shoulder injury while lifting weights. During the day the pain was annoying, but I could ignore it. At night the pain became major because every time I tried to sleep, I eventually rolled over on that shoulder and woke up. That went on for months, and I became an unwilling insomniac until the shoulder healed. I felt like a walking zombie!

Many of you know exactly how I felt. Everybody wants to sleep well, but many of us can't, for reasons that range from troubling life situations to physical problems to poor eating habits. If you have difficulty sleeping, you are not alone, but this pillar of health will help you to get the sleep you need regularly.

First, see if any of these common sleep thieves apply to you.

What's Robbing You of a Good Night's Sleep?

Stress and anxiety. By far the biggest cause of insomnia is stress. People lie awake trying to work out their life's problems, mourning the past, and worrying about the future.

Painful physical conditions. Arthritis, chronic back pain, tension headaches, degenerative disk disease, bursitis, tendonitis, and virtually any other painful condition can rob an otherwise healthy person of sleep.

Caffeine. Many people doom their sleep by consuming caffeine in coffee, soft drinks, chocolate, and over-the-counter headache medicines like Excedrin. Caffeine increases the stress hormones adrenaline and cortisol. Caffeine can remain in the body for up to twenty hours. More than 80 percent of all Americans consume caffeine regularly, and the average American drinks about three cups of coffee a day. For some people, that's a recipe for sleepless nights.

Did You Know . . . ?

The top three factors that rob women of sleep:

- Stress related to work or family
- Ailments such as an allergy or cold
- Uncomfortable mattress or pillows[1]

CAFFEINE-CONTAINING BEVERAGES[2]	
Quantity and Substance	**Amount of Caffeine**
8 ounces brewed coffee	135 mg
8 ounces instant coffee	95 mg
Starbucks coffee, grande (16 ounces)	550 mg
12 ounces Coca Cola	34.5 mg
12 ounces Mountain Dew	55.5 mg
8 ounces black tea	50 mg
8 ounces green tea	30 mg
2 Excedrin capsules	130 mg

Cigarettes and alcohol. Nicotine and alcohol can interfere with sleep. Some people think alcohol helps you to fall asleep, but in fact, alcohol can disrupt the stages of sleep, causing you to sleep lighter and to awaken feeling less refreshed. Nicotine from cigarette smoking is a stimulant that causes adrenaline to be released, which often causes insomnia.

Medications. Decongestants, appetite suppressants, asthma medications (such as theophylline), prednisone, thyroid medications, hormone replacement, some pain relievers, some blood pressure medications, and certain antidepressants may all cause insomnia.

Food insomnia. Many people eat too much sugar and highly processed foods before bed, keeping their nightly date with a bowl of ice cream, piece of cake, or bag of popcorn. These carbohydrates stimulate excessive insulin release from the pancreas. The result is a "sugar high" of energy. But later, usually in the middle of the night, your blood sugar hits a "low," which triggers the adrenal glands to produce more adrenaline and cortisol. Suddenly, you are awake and feel hungry again.

Low-carb diets. These diets can also create a low-blood-sugar reaction, causing you to awaken in the middle of the night. Even if you fill up your stomach with healthy foods at bedtime, it may affect the quality of your sleep. When you eat too much protein or eat too late, you generally will need more sleep. This is especially true when you eat too much meat. That's the reason why animals, like lions and tigers, usually require up to twenty hours a day of sleep—their bodies are having to digest and assimilate all the protein in their bellies.

Exercise. People who exercise within three hours of going to sleep raise their levels of stress hormones, which may interfere with sleep.

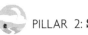

A bad mattress or pillow. Is there anything more frustrating than a mattress that is too saggy or too hard, or an overstuffed pillow?

A snoring spouse. My neighbor came to me one day and said, "Please give my husband something to stop his snoring! I can't even sleep in the same bed anymore. He snores so loud that our kids in the other bedrooms wake up scared in the middle of the night." Many people feel that desperate. A snoring spouse wrecks many people's sleep. I'll share my remedies for snoring in a later section.

Hot flashes or menstrual cramps. Women over fifty often know the aggravation of being kept awake by hot flashes or night sweats. Other women have such severe cramping that they become insomniacs every month when their period arrives.

It's a Fact

Snorers cause their sleeping partners to lose an average of forty-nine minutes of sleep a night.[3]

Enlarged prostate. Some men over fifty find themselves on a there-and-back-again loop to the bathroom when they should be fast asleep.

Newborn babies. As welcome as they are, babies can ruin sleep patterns. Breast-feeding mothers know how an active nighttime routine can make their brains and bodies feel like jelly.

Environment. Noisy neighbors and their dogs, the room too hot or too cold, bright lights shining through your bedroom window, or trucks, planes, trains, or motorcycles passing by can all disrupt sleep patterns.

Each of these sleep thieves is responsible for countless hours of lost sleep, lost productivity, lost creativity, and lost mental health. Today we identified the main things that rob you of sleep. Tomorrow we will talk about how much sleep you need as we begin building sleep patterns on this pillar of health.

BUILDING BLOCKS TO A HEALTHY LIFE

POINTS TO PONDER: *Insomnia affects many people, robbing them of sleep—and, in the long run, good health. Some causes of insomnia are stress, anxiety, depression, chronic pain, caffeine, and medications. Be careful not to eat sugary or high-processed foods before bedtime because they may cause low blood sugar, which makes it difficult for you to sleep.*

ACTION STEP: *Discover which factors are affecting your sleep (stress, pain, caffeine, a snoring spouse, a bad mattress or pillow, a noisy environment, a warm bedroom, etc.).*

DAY 10: How Much Sleep You Really Need

When President Clinton first ran for the presidency, he declared that he went the last forty-eight hours of his campaign without sleep because of his passion to become president.[1] But later, after a series of scandals, Clinton changed his mind about sleep. He said that every important mistake he had made in his life, he made because he was too tired. In fact, former White House counsel Beth Nolan blamed one Clinton-era scandal on sleep deprivation. She told Congress that she had been going on a couple of hours of sleep most nights that week, as had the president. "Had I been operating on more sleep, had the president been operating on more sleep...there would have been more calls made," she said.[2]

Red Bull Generation

Many people in everyday life brag that they only need four or five hours of sleep a night. It's usually the same people who chug energy drinks, like Red Bull, and pop energy pills for breakfast. Anyone who thinks they are getting the most out of life with just a few hours of sleep is kidding himself. It means, rather, that he has learned to function at a much lower level of mental and physical capacity, sustained artificially and temporarily by the adrenal glands and his caffeinated drink of choice.

> **Dr. Colbert Says...**
>
> Get seven to nine hours of sleep every night!

Evidence suggests that inadequate rest and sleep may shorten life span by eight to ten years, which means you can beat the clock now, but the clock will beat you later.[3]

A well-known minister who is a good friend of mine told me, "Before I heard your teaching on sleep, I thought I could live on six hours of sleep a day. Now I wake up early, look at my watch, and think, *Hmm. I've got to lie here for two more hours.* But I feel more refreshed. My mind is clearer."

Many patients come into my office complaining of fatigue and tell me they get six or seven hours of sleep a night. I give them the cell phone analogy. Your phone (or your iPod or Blackberry) won't last as long if you don't totally recharge it. These people, like their gadgets, run out of energy in the middle of the day.

Most adults need seven to nine hours of sleep a night without interruption. Infants need more—about fourteen hours a day.[4] A five-year-old needs twelve hours a day. Most people find that eight hours is perfect. Any less and you feel drowsy at some point during the day. Any more and you may feel unnaturally sluggish.

Are You Getting Enough Sleep?

How do you know you are getting enough sleep? Here's a quick quiz:

1. Do you need an alarm clock to wake up in the morning?
2. Do you get drowsy while driving short distances or while waiting at traffic lights?
3. Do you run out of steam in the middle of the day?
4. Are you irritable and agitated? (Ask your spouse to answer!)
5. Are you a light sleeper and wake up easily at every noise?
6. Are you unable to get persistent worries out of your mind?

If you answered "yes" to even some of these, you are probably lacking sleep. If you're still not sure, try sitting in a comfortable chair in a darkened room for five minutes. If you can't do this without falling asleep, it's a sign that you need more sleep.

Sleep Stages

It's not just the length of sleep that matters, but the depth of sleep and the number of cycles you go through are also important. Normal sleep occurs in cycles, with most people experiencing five to six sleep cycles during a normal night. Each cycle lasts sixty to ninety minutes and has two parts. The first part is broken down into four stages, with stages three and four being the most restful part of sleep.[5]

Did You Know...?

By sleeping less, you increase your chances of suffering from heart attack, stroke, diabetes, weight gain, and premature aging.[6]

The second part of the cycle is rapid eye movement (REM) sleep, which is when dreaming occurs. Usually during the first ninety-minute cycle, only a few minutes are spent in REM sleep. But with each successive ninety-minute cycle, less time is spent in the first part of the cycle and more in the second, so that before awakening in the morning, REM sleep takes up a major part of the cycle.[7]

Even though 25 percent of your dreams occur in non-REM sleep, you're most likely to have a vivid memory of your dreams if you awaken during the REM stage.

Sleep and dreams play a huge part in your mental health. REM sleep is responsible for memory consolidation. During sleep, our brains take different memories and examine how well they fit or don't fit together. Dreams serve to bring mysterious images from the unconscious soul to the wakeful consciousness where we can lay them out in front of us, examine them, dissect them, and glean meaning from them. These images often reflect issues we need to address in order to become whole. There are many biblical examples of how God used dreams to make people aware of important matters in their world and to help them prepare solutions to forthcoming challenges. Today, dreams can serve the same purpose for us. They connect us with our internal intelligence, our true selves, our souls. They are images that have the ability to bring wellness and wholeness.

Broken Sleep

Middle-aged and elderly people tend to spend less time in deeper sleep than younger people. The elderly generally secrete lesser amounts of certain chemicals that regulate the sleep/wake cycle. Both melatonin and growth hormone production decrease with age. For older people, sleep becomes more shallow, fragmented, and variable in duration. The elderly wake up more frequently than younger adults.[8]

How do you get the right amount of sleep? Tomorrow we will plan your perfect night of sleep, but for now, pleasant dreams.

BUILDING BLOCKS TO A HEALTHY LIFE

POINTS TO PONDER: *As a nation we have become too dependent upon energy drinks and medications to keep us awake longer. We need to realize that when we cheat the body from getting the sleep it needs, we may eventually suffer the consequences healthwise. There are stages to our sleep cycle, with stages three and four being the most restful part of sleep. Dreams are important to restore the mind.*

ACTION STEP: *For the next seven days, keep track of your sleeping pattern using the sleep journal on the next page.*

MY SLEEP JOURNAL

Write down the time you went to bed, the time you arose, how many hours you slept, and how you felt when you woke up. In the notes column, write down anything that might help you discover a pattern for good or poor sleep, such as what you ate, any physical pain, and so on.

Day	Bedtime	Wake-up Time	No. of hours slept	I felt...	Notes
SUN.					
MON.					
TUE.					
WED.					
THUR.					
FRI.					
SAT.					

DAY 11: Planning Your Perfect Night of Sleep

We've looked at what can rob you of a good night's sleep. We have also learned that getting the right amount of sleep is vital to optimal performance on a daily basis. Now let's go through your ideal night of sleep and sleep preparation together, starting in the afternoon.

Getting Ready for Nighttime

Preparing for sleep at night begins during the daytime. Engage in some sort of aerobic exercise such as brisk walking in the afternoon or early evening. Daily exercise is one of the best ways to improve the quality of your sleep because it helps you fall asleep faster and sleep longer. People who exercise spend a greater amount of time in stage three and four sleep, the most restorative and repairing stages of sleep.

But don't go overboard and rev up your body with exercise within three hours of bedtime. It heats up your body and raises the stress hormones. Not long ago I took a sauna too close to bedtime and got so hot that I couldn't sleep well. What a mistake!

Eat a modest, healthy dinner four hours before bedtime. You may eat a light evening snack before bed—even better is a snack that is correctly balanced with proteins, carbohydrates, and fats. This snack will help stabilize blood sugar through the nighttime hours. Some people can handle caffeine; others can't. If you fall in the latter category, then quit drinking or eating caffeinated products by noon.

As the sun goes down, your body will relax naturally. You are designed hormonally to stay in sync with the cycles of nature. When the light fades, the hormone melatonin is released into your bloodstream, making you sleepy. The amount of melatonin your body produces is affected by the amount of light going into your eyes. That's why you are more alert and energetic on sunny days and more lethargic on cloudy days. It's also why some people can work all night staring at a computer or television screen, because they are feeding light into their eyes.

Follow your body's signal. Turn down the lights. Light messes up our hormonal response at night. I tell patients to buy dimmer switches so they can bring the lights down. If you have the money and time, get a massage in the late afternoon. If you don't have the money, but you do have a spouse, exchange massages with him or her. If you don't have

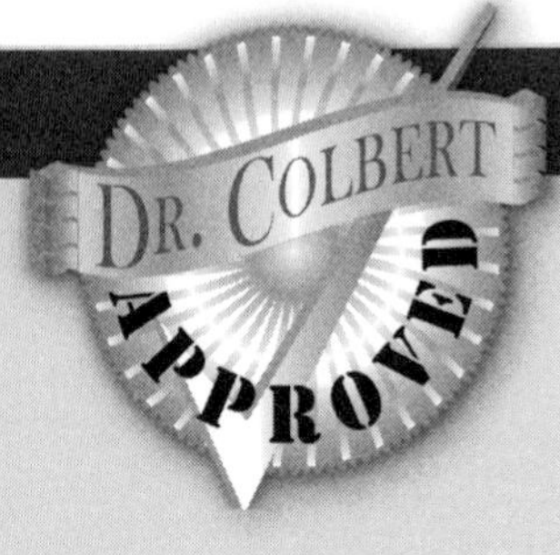

Dr. Colbert Approved Bedtime Snacks

- A piece of fruit, like a small apple, grapefruit, 4 ounces of berries or kiwi with a small handful of nuts (walnuts, almonds, or pecans)
- One serving of low-fat, whole-grain crackers or one piece of whole-grain bread with about a teaspoon of organic peanut butter or two ounces of turkey
- One-half cup organic skim milk or low-fat cottage cheese or low-fat, no-sugar yogurt (if not sensitive to dairy) with fruit added
- A small bowl of whole-grain cereal (about ½ cup) with organic skim milk

a spouse, buy a handheld massager at a store like Brookstone or The Sharper Image.

Corral Your Thoughts

Don't watch an action-packed movie or even the late local news program, which tends to play up violent news stories. Watch something calming, play your favorite soothing music, or perhaps watch a funny TV show or movie since laughter helps to relax you. Take a warm shower or bath, adding soothing salts or lavender oil. (Epsom salt has magnesium, which relaxes the body.) Get all your senses involved. Dim the lights, listen to music, and relax.

In the fall season, I break all these rules once a week because of a sports tradition I can't let go of: Monday Night Football. I unrepentantly watch the game and get all worked up, and my sleep takes a hit that night, especially when the game goes into overtime. To me it's worth it, and I usually recover fine because I sleep properly the other six nights of the week. But as a doctor, I don't recommend getting hooked on habits that interfere with sleep.

As the evening goes on and your mind wanders over the events of the day, don't let anxiety derail you from your goal. Switch from the "worry" channel to the "appreciation and praise" channel. Make a list of things for which you are thankful, and then dwell on those instead.

One woman I treated had gone through a divorce and developed a serious sleep problem. She would wake up at 2:00 or 3:00 a.m., and she would lie in bed and rehash the whole failed relationship—every detail, what she did, what he did, what she should and shouldn't have done. She could not figure out why he left her. She wanted a sense of peace, but her mind would not let her sleep.

Mary and I had to teach this divorced woman how to change her thoughts. I gave her a prescription—to read the Bible. I had her write out promises from the Bible and keep them by her bedside. Before she turned in, she read them and laid her problems in God's hands. I had her memorize verses from the Bible, so when she woke up she wouldn't have to turn on the light—which would stimulate her mind—but could quote the Bible from memory. Instead of focusing on her problems, I had her corral her thoughts and focus on God's Word, which is the answer. I had her meditate on 1 Corinthians 13:4–8, which is the love walk. I'll have more tips on handling stress and anxiety in pillar seven, which is "Coping With Stress."

Did You Know . . . ?

Before Thomas Edison invented the light bulb in 1879, Americans slept an average of ten hours a night.[1]

When to Head to Bed

In my opinion, sleep before midnight is better than sleep after midnight. If you can't bear the idea of going to sleep that "early," remember that your very health is at stake. Ninety to 95 percent of your 60 to 100 trillion cells are replaced each year, and much of that occurs during sleep that comes early in the night. Not only that, but while you sleep your body rejuvenates itself.[2] Sleep and water are the two best antiaging secrets I have found. If you value your looks and your life span, getting to bed at 10:00 p.m. won't be difficult. For many patients with chronic disease, the most important recommendation I can give them is to be in bed by 9:00 p.m. and to sleep at least eight hours. God designed us to fall asleep when it is dark and to wake up when the sun rises.

BUILDING BLOCKS TO A HEALTHY LIFE

POINTS TO PONDER: *Maintaining a bedtime ritual is essential to a good night's sleep for children* and *adults. Exercise is one way to improve the quality of your sleep. However, exercising within three hours of sleep may interfere with sleep because exercise raises the levels of stress hormones. Eat a light, bedtime snack. (See the suggested list on page 50.) Corral your thoughts, and take time to relax.*

ACTION STEP: *Make an appreciation list, and recite it when you have trouble falling asleep. (See the appreciation list on the next page.)*

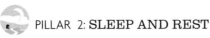

Appreciation List

1. Before you get out of bed in the morning, begin each day by saying, "Today is the best day of the rest of my life. I choose to be happy and to enjoy this day."
2. Make a list of things for which you are thankful. Include:
    a. Your physical being—eyesight, hearing, taste, smell, ability to touch, ability to walk. Be grateful that you have the use of your fingers, hands, arms, legs, and so on.
    b. Modern-day conveniences—a car, running hot water, air conditioning/heater, a working computer, telephone, and so on
    c. Everyday needs—food, a job, water, shelter, and so on
    d. People—spouse, children, relatives, friends, co-workers, and so on (even your pets!)
    e. Nature—flowers, weather, fresh air, or anything in nature that makes you grateful to be alive
3. Review the list daily.
4. Recite it aloud frequently.
5. Update the list periodically.

I AM THANKFUL FOR:

DAY 12: Your Bedroom—Storage Unit or Sleep Haven?

When you walk into your bedroom it should look like an inviting place of rest, not a storage unit. Some women use their bedrooms for all their projects, surrounding the bed with stacks of magazines, sewing supplies, half-finished blankets, books, and family photos waiting to be put in albums. Then they cover the bed with the laundry they did earlier and the outfits they considered wearing that morning. This scene causes clutter stress. If you wonder why you and your husband start arguing as soon as you walk into your bedroom, maybe it's the clutter that assaults your eyes.

Men are just as bad. Some men turn their bedroom into their home office or video game room. Nestled conspicuously in the corner is a computer desk, a whirring CPU, stacks of receipts, and important papers. Small wonder that when you walk into the room, your mind is conflicted: "Is this where I sleep, work, or play?" All that stress comes on you at precisely the wrong time.

Make your bedroom a haven for sleep and unwinding. Have some rules: No eating, no computers, no harsh clock lights, and no televisions, if you can stand it. No studying, no sewing projects, no stacks of laundry waiting to be folded and put away, no piles of junk you shoved in there when the neighbor came over to visit. Pleasure reading is acceptable, and television is tolerable, provided it helps you and your spouse get in a drowsy state of mind. Your bedroom should say one thing: sleep!

Setting the Stage for Sleep

Your bed should be more comfortable than your couch. After all, you don't spend eight hours a day on the couch, but you do on your mattress. One of the best investments you can make for your health is a mattress you thoroughly enjoy and look forward to lying on. The same goes for your pillow. Treat these like a secret source of happiness, which you anticipate every day.

A mattress that is too firm does not adequately allow for the right alignment of the spine. A mattress that is too soft will allow the spine to sag and may cause a backache. When you shop for a mattress, don't just lie on your back; also lie on your side and your stomach. Slide your hand, palm down, between the mattress and the small of your back as you try lying on your back. If you are able to get your entire hand through the small of your back, the mattress is too hard. If while lying flat on the bed the base of the spine is lower than your heels, the mattress is too soft.

If your pillow is too hard, too soft, too large, or too small, your quality of sleep may suffer. Select the right pillow for you. A pillow should be soft enough to conform to the contours of your head and neck, but also thick enough to support the head and neck in a neutral position.

Sleep Myth
FACT or FICTION?

A 1999 Mayo Clinic sleep disorders study found that when a partner snores, the non-snoring partner wakes up twenty times per hour, even if only briefly. It's a fact.[1]

The room should be as dark as you can reasonably make it. Don't have nightlights, and don't let streetlights shine through the window. Line the drapes, or pull down a dark shade if you need to. If you are routinely awakened by sirens, car alarms, horns, roaring motorcycles, coyotes, airplanes—whatever noisemakers roam freely in your area during the night—invest in double-pane windows or maybe a good set of soft earplugs. Or buy a sound generator that makes waterfall or raindrop sounds. If you tend to get unwanted calls, get the call block feature from your phone service provider or take the phone off the hook.

I noted earlier that some people wake up because their blood sugar level drops. Eat some of the snacks mentioned in the previous daily entry. That will balance out your blood sugar level for the evening.

The room should be at a comfortable temperature, usually around 70 to 75 degrees Fahrenheit. Some people like to open the windows, especially if they live in the mountains or at the beach, and let the cool air come in while they huddle under warm blankets. Others like a warmer ambient temperature. Some prefer the feeling of a ceiling fan, which improves airflow. Figure out what works best for you and your spouse, and stick with it.

The Curse of the Snoring Spouse

Many of my patients complain about their spouse's snoring problem. For them it's an annoyance, but snoring can actually be a sign of sleep apnea. If your spouse snores, make sure he or she gets it checked out by a doctor.

Dr. Colbert Recommended

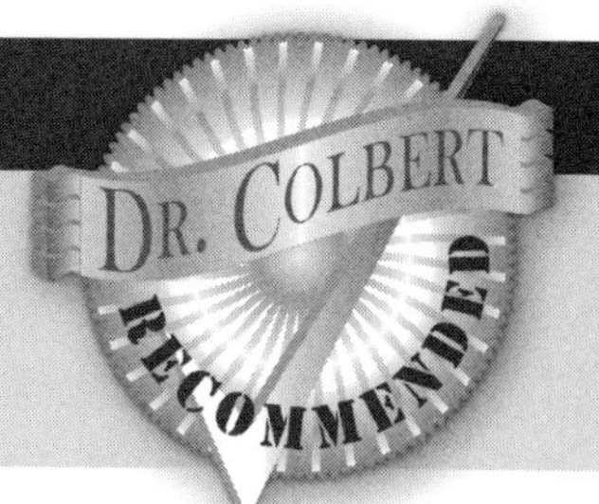

The kind of mattress that I have and that has helped many of my patients with chronic back pain is a pressure-relieving memory foam mattress.

Why do people snore? They often have anatomical differences, such as an obstructed nasal passage, an elongation of the uvula (the soft tissue that hangs down the back of the throat), or a sagging soft palate. Enlarged tonsils or adenoids can also cause snoring, as can poor muscle tone in the tongue and throat. Most snorers tend to be overweight. They typically have increased girth around their neck and poor muscle tone of their tongue and throat. Simply losing weight and exercising may be their best cure for snoring. A weight loss of only ten to fifteen pounds can make a big difference.

Snoring can also be helped if a person avoids using alcohol, muscle relaxants, tranquilizers, or sleep medications. These tend to relax the muscles of the throat and can worsen snoring. Snorers who have nasal congestion might try a product such as Breathe Right strips.

Changing positions while sleeping can also help. People who sleep on their sides or stomachs snore less. There are also dental appliances and "snore alarms" that can help. In the meantime, if you are the suffering spouse, use earplugs or a sound generator that produces white noise, or have your spouse try an anti-snore spray like Snore Eze.

You should sleep soundly and awaken at dawn.

Did You Know . . .?

There is a fairly new procedure using radio frequency waves to help shrink the uvula and soft palate. The U.S. Food and Drug Administration has approved a treatment for snoring that uses radio waves to shrink tissue in air passages and eliminate snoring. The procedure is called *radiofrequency volumetric tissue reduction of the palate.* The radiofrequency treatment involves piercing the tongue, throat, or soft palate with a special needle (electrode) connected to a radio frequency generator. The inner tissue is then heated to 158 to 176 degrees in a procedure that takes approximately half an hour. The inner tissues shrink, but the outer tissues, which may contain such things as taste buds, are left intact. Several treatments may be required.[2]

Something I like to do is meditate on 1 Corinthians 13:4–8, Psalm 1, or Psalm 23. And I recall Isaiah 26:3, which says, "Thou wilt keep him in perfect peace, whose mind is stayed on thee: because he trusteth in thee."

Each of these suggestions for your sleep routine will increase the likelihood of your sleeping soundly through the night.

DAY 12 DAY 12 DAY 12

BUILDING BLOCKS TO A HEALTHY LIFE

POINTS TO PONDER: *Your bedroom is a place to retreat, relax, revive, and rejuvenate. For a more sleep-conducive environment, try the following: keep the room dark, filter out noise, get a good mattress and pillow, and make sure the room temperature is comfortable. Pleasure reading or watching TV is acceptable, provided they help you (and your spouse) relax and do not add stress.*

ACTION STEP: *Eliminate light from shining through your bedroom window, and keep the room dark. Install room-darkening drapes or vertical blinds.*

DAY 13: Sleep Aids

I had a major sleep problem some years ago when my son was in rebellion and when we were having financial stresses. I'd lie in bed at night and ask myself, *What if this happens? What if that happens?* I did a combination of things: I took 5-HTP and L-theanine, meditated on the Word of God, and trusted Him. "He will keep him in perfect peace" became very real to me. I also ate a little bedtime snack so my blood sugar wouldn't drop too low.

Ten million people take a prescription medication to sleep,[1] but the very best sleep aid is the Word of God. I don't mean that the Word is so boring it will put you to sleep; rather, it puts all things in perspective and offers perfect peace. Nothing else comes close. Billions of dollars could be saved if people would stop taking both prescription and nonprescription sleep medications and simply meditate on God's Word.

Acceptable Sleep Aids

In general, sleep medications are to be avoided. Most are addictive and disrupt natural sleep cycles. But sometimes natural sleep aids can give a gentle nudge that we need in times of crisis or while traveling and waiting for our bodies to adjust to a new time zone. Some natural sleep aids have proven to be helpful in getting to sleep faster and achieve a more restful state of sleep.

Valerian

Valerian is an herb that has been used for centuries in Europe for sleep. Several clinical studies have demonstrated valerian's ability to relieve insomnia. One double-blind study of twenty patients with insomnia received a combination of valerian (160 mg) and *Melissa officinalis* (lemon balm, 80 mg) or benzodiazepine (triazolam, 0.125 mg) or a placebo. The group receiving the valerian and *Melissa officinalis* had a comparable response to the sleep medication but did not have the daytime drowsiness.[2] In general, clinical studies with valerian extracts suggest that the mild sleep-inducing effect of valerian decreases the time it takes to fall asleep and improves sleep quality.[3]

Valerian may be combined with other herbs, such as lemon balm and passionflower, to potentiate its effect. It can be taken as a tincture, a tea,

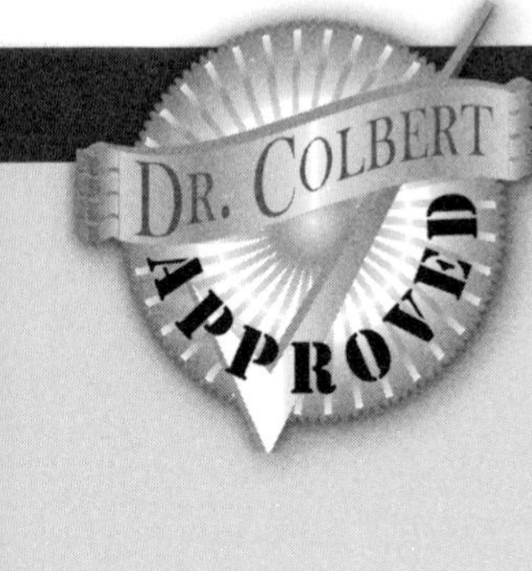

Dr. Colbert Approved

If you're having trouble falling asleep, try drinking a cup of Celestial Seasonings Sleepytime Extra Wellness Tea or Yogi Bedtime Tea one to two hours before bedtime. They are all-natural, no-caffeine herbal teas. Sleepytime Tea contains chamomile, tilia estella, and 25 mg of valerian. Yogi Bedtime Tea contains organic skullcap leaf. However, do not give these teas to children. If you are pregnant, nursing, or on medications, consult with your physician before drinking the tea.

or fluid extract; however, the taste is very unappealing. Therefore I recommend a valerian extract in capsules 150 to 300 mg taken one hour before bedtime. (See Appendix A for recommended products for aiding sleep.)

5-HTP

The body manufactures serotonin from the essential amino acid L-tryptophan. This amino acid is converted into 5-hydroxytryptophan (5-HTP). Individuals who are chronically stressed, anxious, and depressed usually are low in serotonin. These same individuals usually suffer from insomnia. Supplementation with 5-HTP is very effective in raising levels of serotonin, which helps to alleviate some of these symptoms as well as improve sleep. The usual dose of 5-HTP is 150 to 300 mg taken with dinner or at bedtime. If you are taking prescription antidepressants, *consult your physician before* starting 5-HTP supplements. Do not confuse 5-HTP with L-tryptophan. In 1989 the FDA issued a nationwide recall of all over-the-counter dietary supplements containing 100 mg or more of L-tryptophan.[4] In March 1990, the FDA banned the public sale of dietary L-tryptophan completely, but it is now back on the market as a prescription drug, not as an over-the-counter dietary supplement.[5]

There is a fairly new lab test that is able to check the neurotransmitter levels. This is particularly important for patients with insomnia in order to see which neurotransmitters are imbalanced. When applying this test, I then use targeted amino acid therapy to restore the neurotransmitters.

Calcium and magnesium

For those who suffer from insomnia, an inadequate intake of calcium and magnesium can cause you to wake up after a few hours and not be able to return to sleep.[6]

Calcium is important in many processes of the body such as the contraction of muscles, the release of neurotransmitters that can support sleep, and the regulation of the heartbeat. Low levels of magnesium can lead to symptoms of fatigue, mental confusion, irritability, weakness, heart disturbances, problems in nerve conduction and muscle contraction, muscle cramps, *insomnia*, and a predisposition to stress. Large amounts of calcium alone can decrease magnesium absorption; however, calcium and magnesium work together to provide normal muscle contraction and relaxation.[7]

There are calcium and magnesium supplements that come in powder form, which you can add to a cup of tea. These can be found in most health food stores.

Taking calcium and magnesium at bedtime may help you sleep better.[8]

L-theanine

L-theanine is another amino acid that is commonly found naturally in the green tea plant (*Camellia sinensis*) and thought to contribute to the unique taste of green tea. Research has shown that in addition to its flavor properties, L-theanine also has a relaxing effect. L-theanine does not contain caffeine and actually helps prevent the side effects of caffeine.[9]

L-theanine has been shown to decrease stress, promote relaxation, calm nervousness, and decrease restlessness, possibly through its effects on serotonin, dopamine, and other neurotransmitters.[10]

It is believed that after being absorbed in the large intestine, L-theanine stimulates the generation of alpha waves in the brain. Alpha waves are associated with a calm and relaxed state. L-theanine reduces stress, promotes relaxation without drowsiness, eases nervousness due to common everyday overwork and fatigue, and reduces nervous irritability.[11]

I have used it widely and with significant success in treating ADHD children and stressed-out adults. I have also found that it helps many people who suffer with insomnia. It is able to cross the blood-brain barrier in the brain and support the activity of certain neurotransmitters in the brain. It also works to help you relax in the evening, yet it does not cause daytime drowsiness. I usually recommend 100 to 200 mg of L-theanine at bedtime. (See Appendix A.)

Melatonin

Melatonin is a hormone manufactured from serotonin and secreted by the pineal gland, which is a pea-sized gland at the base of the brain. As people age, sometimes the pineal gland will calcify, affecting levels of melatonin.

Melatonin supplementation will only help you fall asleep if melatonin levels are low. If melatonin is given to patients with insomnia who have normal melatonin levels, it will not produce a sedative effect.

Low melatonin levels are, however, a common cause of insomnia in the elderly. (See Appendix A.)

While light (or lack of it) affects the production of melatonin, there are other factors as well that may play a role in its production. Start with 1 mg, taken two hours or less before bedtime. Use it only occasionally, and do not give it to children.[12]

Did You Know...?

Light slows the production of melatonin, which is the reason you are more alert and energetic on sunny days and more lethargic on cloudy days.

When I do a lot of traveling, especially crossing time zones, I may need help falling asleep. I take 1 or 2 mg of melatonin under the tongue. It works wonders for me. Melatonin supplements are available without a prescription. I've helped many patients regain sleep with 5-HTP, calcium, magnesium, melatonin, valerian, L-theanine, or a bedtime tea. At times a combination of these natural supplements will work even better.

But prescription sleep aids are never meant as a long-term solution. They should only be used for two weeks or less. They have never been approved for *perpetual* use over long periods of time. Unfortunately, some people become addicted to sleeping pills and find they are unable to sleep well without them. Realize the main cause of insomnia is excessive stress. However, learning to cope with stress will also improve your sleep. We will learn more about how to effectively cope with stress in a later pillar. In the meantime, these natural sleep aids will enable many to get a good night's sleep.

If you are on medications, *always* consult with your physician prior to taking these, or any, natural supplements.

DAY 13

BUILDING BLOCKS TO A HEALTHY LIFE

POINTS TO PONDER: *Some people rely on sleep medications, whether over-the-counter or prescribed, which may become addictive and disrupt their natural sleep cycle. Yet nature has provided sleep aids without adding the side effects of prescription medications. Although these sleep aids, such as valerian, 5-HTP, calcium, melatonin, magnesium, L-theanine, and bedtime teas, are natural products, always consult with your health-care provider before taking them, especially if you are pregnant, nursing, or taking prescription medications. Some supplements may interfere with certain medications.*

ACTION STEP: *If you have become dependent on over-the-counter sleep aids, replace them with one or more of the natural supplements listed above.*

DAY 14: Learn to Rest

A few years ago, Mary and I gave a seminar for a major ministry. Before this minister heard our message on sleep and rest, he worked hard seven days a week without a break. But his health was plummeting. His staff was suffering physically because many worked six days a week and rarely took a break. But as he heard about the importance of sleep and rest, conviction went through him like a bullet. He knew he was guilty of never resting. He immediately mandated a day off for everyone he employed—and for himself. His health sprung back, and his ministry is much larger than before.

Busyness comes at a high price. Many people lose their health, marriages, and relationships as they strive to achieve more. But by abandoning rest we violate one of God's most basic principles: the Sabbath rest.

The Sabbath rest was God's rule for the nation of Israel. He said to rest one day out of every week. No exceptions. In fact, there is more space in the Bible allotted to the Sabbath than any other of the Ten Commandments. (See Exodus 20.) God knew what our bodies and minds are capable of and what they need to function properly. He was being merciful and wise in giving this rule. A Sabbath rest does what sleep does: it lets the body and mind relax, unwind, and recuperate. It helps to maintain our strength, energy, and youthfulness. It even humbles us by reminding us that, after all is said and done, God is the source of our strength. And it helps us rediscover the fun-loving side of ourselves.

Did You Know...?

More than half of adult Americans nap at least once a week; one-third nap at least twice a week. The average nap lasts fifty minutes for those taking two or more naps a week.[1]

But many Americans believe a day of rest is as outdated as kosher food, which stems from the Puritan work ethic. We believe it's "honorable" to work ourselves hard and long, even if it's killing us. However, there is wisdom to taking a day or two in the week to rest.

> Work shall be done for six days, but the seventh is the Sabbath of rest, holy to the LORD.
>
> —EXODUS 31:15, NKJV

Without being legalistic about it, we must recognize the health wisdom of this principle. If we don't learn to rest from working, we will suffer for it. Begin taking off one day a week for rest.

Power Naps

When I was a young exchange student in Mexico, everybody took a "siesta" (or nap) during the workday. Commerce stopped. People closed their shops and rested (or took naps). It was completely different from the go-go-go lifestyle of the United States. I found it fascinating—and healthy.

Recently I was in California at the beach at noon, and I saw a group of Hispanic men who had worked all morning in lawn maintenance sleeping soundly, right on the sand. They were being wise. They were rejuvenating their bodies with a nap.

Researchers at Loughborough University's Sleep Research Laboratory have found that people are designed for two sleeps a day—the main one at night and a nap in the afternoon.[2] Very successful men have been known to nap regularly: Winston Churchill, John F. Kennedy, Ronald Reagan, Napoleon, Albert Einstein, Thomas Edison, and George W. Bush.[3]

Dr. Colbert's Tips for Power Nappers

- Unplug phones.
- Make the room as dark as possible.
- Get in a comfortable position on a couch or recliner.
- Try to take your nap in the early afternoon or midafternoon.

Naps restore alertness and enhance performance. A study at NASA on sleepy military pilots and astronauts found that a forty-minute nap improved performance by 34 percent and alertness by 100 percent.[4] That's improvement! Naps can also extend alertness a few hours later in the day.

Siestas are not part of the American culture, but they should be. It should be normal to close the door and take a ten- to thirty-minute nap when the afternoon low hits us. Napping is better than doing poor work because you are fending off sleep.

With adequate sleep and rest you will rediscover the pleasure of life. Your body and soul will feel revived. You will restore your health as you build upon this pillar of health. For more information on this topic, please refer to my book *The Bible Cure for Sleep Disorders*.[5]

BUILDING BLOCKS TO A HEALTHY LIFE

POINTS TO PONDER: *One of the most basic principles is a day of rest. Take time to rest.*

ACTION STEP: *Take one day out of this week to do nothing but rest. For many, rest may mean going out for lunch or dinner, watching a good movie, or spending time with family and friends. Rest, however, does not mean cooking, cleaning house, or working in the yard.*

PILLAR 3

Living Food

DAY 15: Living Food vs. Dead Food

Imagine you have two shelves in your pantry, one that says "dead food" and the other "living food."

On the "dead food" shelf is a little tag that reads: "These foods will make you disease-prone, will cause degenerative diseases such as diabetes, cardiovascular disease, and arthritis, and will make you overweight. They will also make you fatigued and prone to develop hypertension and high cholesterol."

But the "living food" shelf's tag reads: "These foods will protect your body from cancer, heart disease, all degenerative diseases, and obesity, and they will sharpen your mind, energize you, and enliven you."

There's your choice. As an average American, you may be consuming up to five pounds of food each day.[1] Over your lifetime, that's around seventy tons of food that pass through your intestinal tract and are assimilated by your body.

Which shelf are you going to select food from?

Those shelves are not imaginary. They are real. In your pantry, freezer, and fridge right now are foods that lead to life and death. They are probably all mixed together, live foods next to dead foods—processed peanut butter next to extra-virgin olive oil, oatmeal next to an XXL-size bag of potato chips.

Living Longer—but Better?

Life expectancy in the United States increased to 77.6 years in 2003, according to a report by the National Center for Health Statistics at CDC. But half of U.S. residents ages fifty-five to sixty-four have high blood pressure, and two in five are obese.[2]

As we jump into the third pillar of health, living foods, I want you to understand that everything you put in your mouth has the potential to produce life or death. Food is part of a man's reward. But eating the wrong foods will bring curses of poor health. Are you at war with your health because of the foods you eat? Or are you enjoying the beautiful dance of hunger and satisfaction that centers around the divine gift of living food?

I want to make it clear from the outset that as more research is done on food and the human body, we will find that some foods may be healthier than we thought (like coffee and dark chocolate). And other foods we once considered healthy (such as margarine) are in fact very harmful to our health. I once heard a speaker say that after ten years, about half the medical knowledge we have learned turns out to be false. The problem is, we don't know which half. There will always be confusion regarding foods and their health benefits, but in this pillar you are getting the most up-to-date research and advice on how to eat for life. One principle will always stand: living foods (such as fruits, veggies, and whole grains) will always be healthier for you than processed foods.

"Why Does It Matter What I Eat?"

All foods are *not* created equal. In fact, some food should not be labeled "food" but rather "consumable product" or "edible, but void of nourishment."

Living foods were created for our consumption. They exist in a raw or close-to-raw state. Living foods include fruits, vegetables, grains, seeds, and nuts. They are beautifully packaged in divinely created wrappers called skins and peels. Living food looks robust, healthy, and alive. No chemicals have been added. It has not been bleached or chemically altered. Living foods are plucked, harvested, and squeezed, not processed, packaged, and put on a shelf. Living foods are *recognizable* as food.

Dr. Colbert's List of Worst Fats to Consume

1. Hydrogenated and partially hydrogenated fats and trans fats
2. Excessive saturated fats
3. Excessive polyunsaturated fats

Dead foods are the opposite. They are living foods that have fallen into human hands and have been altered in every imaginable way, making them last as long as possible at room temperature and to be as addictive as possible to the consumer. That usually means the manufacturer adds considerable amounts of sugar, which is called "dextrose," "corn syrup," "fructose," "glucose," and generally any other food ending in "-ose." It also means they add man-made fats that involve taking various oils and heating them to dangerously high temperatures so that the nutrients die and become reborn as something completely different—a deadly, sludgy substance that is toxic to our bodies. That sludgy substance—which is called "hydrogenated" or "partially hydrogenated" oil—is a common ingredient in the American diet and is present in most processed foods from crackers and pastries to hamburger buns.

Life breeds life. Death breeds death. When you eat living foods, the enzymes in their pristine state interact with your digestive enzymes.

The other natural ingredients God put in them—vitamins, minerals, phytonutrients, antioxidants, fiber, and more—flow into your system in their natural state. These living foods were created for our digestive systems, bloodstream, and organs.

Dead foods hit our bodies like a foreign intruder. Chemicals, including preservatives, food additives, bleaching agents, and so on, place a strain on the liver. Toxic man-made fats begin to form in our cell membranes and become incorporated in our bodies or stored as fats. They begin to form plaque in our arteries. Fat also contains compounds called leptins. When the small intestine detects leptins, it sends a message to the brain saying, "I'm satisfied, I'm full, stop eating." However, it takes about twenty minutes from the time we start eating for the food to reach our small intestines and leptin is able to signal the brain to stop eating, and most Americans can eat a tremendous amount of food in twenty minutes. Your brain, sensing that it still doesn't have the nutrition it needs, sends out hunger signals. You eat again—more of the same dead food. Your body does its best to harvest the tiny traces of good from the food, but in the end you are undernourished, overfed the wrong foods, and overweight. You are, in other words, caught in the trap of the *standard American diet,* which is a "SAD" and toxic situation.

If you say, "Everyone around me eats 'bad' food, and they all look fine," consider that maybe everyone around you is unhealthy, in the process of becoming overweight, and disease-prone. If you want to be a healthy, vibrant, energetic person rather than someone bouncing between all-you-can-eat buffets and fast-food restaurants, take your diet seriously. Now is the time to build the rest of your life on this wonderful pillar of health—living food.

BUILDING BLOCKS TO A HEALTHY LIFE

POINTS TO PONDER: *No more living on the "SAD" diet. It's time to start choosing living foods over dead foods. Remember that from the time we start eating until the time the food reaches our small intestines, it takes twenty minutes for leptin to signal the brain to stop eating.*

ACTION STEP: *Make note of what you ate today. Compare the living foods to the dead foods. When you eat, chew your food thoroughly, put your fork down between bites, and eat slowly. Give your brain time to send the "stop" signal.*

DAY 16: Your Body Is a Temple

Years ago a friend of mine borrowed my small Ford Ranger pickup truck. When he brought it back, the whole bed was sagging. "I went to a marble show at the convention center, and they gave me lots of free samples," he said. But the weight was way too much for my little pickup. It messed up the shocks and cost me some money to replace them. My friend was totally unaware that anything was wrong with the truck.

Millions of people do to their bodies what my friend did to my poor little truck. They load up their bodies with extra weight, more than their frames were designed to carry. Then they wonder why their knees and hips are wearing out and they're developing arthritis, ankle problems, heel spurs, lower back pain, bunions, degenerated disks, and more. That's their body's way of saying, "Quit putting so much weight on me!"

A Nation of Diabetics

A new study indicates that more than one out of three Americans has either impaired fasting glucose (pre-diabetes) or diabetes. Incidence of diabetes was estimated at 9.3 percent of the population, and impaired fasting glucose at 26 percent of the population. Impaired fasting glucose increases the risk of diabetes.[1]

Why can't Americans lose weight and keep it off? There are some basic reasons.

Bad foods are a habit. Some people who were raised on regional/ethnic cooking, like southern food, habitually eat fried foods, gravy, fatback, biscuits, apple pie, cake, butter-soaked grits, and worse. My mother raised me on southern food, and after frying bacon she would pour the bacon grease into a cup and add the grease to green beans, butter beans, and many of the vegetables we ate.

Bad foods are convenient. To my knowledge, there isn't a fast-health-food chain in America.

Bad foods are a vicious cycle. People fall into a cycle of eating sugar, and the cycle perpetuates itself. When you eat a doughnut or a piece of cake or pie, or you drink a dessert coffee, for example, you get a sugar rush, but several hours later you get the whiplash effect. Your blood-sugar level drops, and you crave a pick-me-up. The quickest fix is something sweet or starchy, and so the cycle goes.

Hormones make bad foods look good. When women are pregnant, on their period, or going through menopause, they generally crave sweets, starches, and chocolate.

Bad foods give comfort. Excessive stress causes high cortisol levels, which cause cravings. When people get stressed, they reach for comfort foods: sweet, creamy, starchy, salty items. Nobody reaches for broccoli or carrots when they want comfort.

Starchy and sugary foods raise serotonin, one of the brain's feel-good chemicals. Chocolate raises dopamine levels, another feel-good chemical. Generally, when people are depressed, anxious, or just low in serotonin or dopamine, they reach for a food that pumps up these feel-good chemicals.

Food Cravings

The 2004 movie *Super Size Me* chronicled one man's switch to an all McDonald's diet. In just thirty days he went from 185 to 209 pounds, his cholesterol went up a whopping 65 points, and his body fat jumped from 11 to 18 percent. That's not even including what he suffered from mood swings, high blood pressure, and symptoms of addiction. His was an experiment, but many people treat their bodies that way by choice.

> **Did You Know...?**
>
> People who restrict their calories live longer. More than two thousand studies support the fact that a low-calorie, optimal nutrition diet can extend life by 30 to 50 percent.[2]

The main reason many Americans are obese is simply gluttony, and Christians are no exception. Think about this: How often are church functions centered around food? How many churches have doughnuts and coffee to raise attendance numbers for a Bible study or service? A study from Purdue University found that religious people are more likely to be overweight than are nonreligious people. In state-by-state comparisons, they found the percentage of obesity highest in states where religious affiliation was more prevalent.[3] Think about it! Christians often think that because they don't smoke, drink, or party, they can eat all they want! Then they reap what they sow in obesity, heart disease, cancer, hypertension, type 2 diabetes, high cholesterol, reflux disease, sleep apnea, and loss of quality of life.

Webster's dictionary defines *gluttony* as "excess in eating and drinking." The Bible equates it with drunkenness:

> Do not join those who drink too much wine or gorge themselves on meat, for drunkards and gluttons become poor, and drowsiness clothes them in rags.
>
> —Proverbs 23:20–21, NIV

The word *glutton* in this passage is defined as "ravenous eater of meat." This describes a lot of men in particular. If you want to experience the harsh reality of some people's lack of restraint, simply go to a buffet and watch how they load up their plates with meat, potatoes, and macaroni and cheese. Many will eat as if they've never seen food before. Food is not at the root of the overeating issue; it actually goes much deeper than that.

The Mind-Body-Spirit Connection

Gluttony, or overeating, is a spiritual and emotional problem first, and a dietary problem second. Gluttony is simply a lack of temperance. We may not like to think of our weight problem as gluttony, because confronting our emotional issues can be painful. Many times people who struggle with a weight problem experience self-loathing, loneliness, low self-esteem, depression, guilt, and shame, especially the latter two. In all my years of practice, I have treated numerous patients with a weight problem, and almost always the root cause is emotional. The moment they mess up by eating something they shouldn't, they feel guilty and ashamed, and they feel like quitting. In my medical office, we know that we need to treat the patient's body, mind (emotions), and spirit. We give them scriptures to confess daily aloud and meditate upon so that they begin to change their mind-set from a negative to a positive state. The Word gives them hope.

I take them through forgiveness therapy, which enables them to forgive themselves as well as others. When they forgive themselves and begin to love, respect, and accept themselves, it breaks the vicious cycle of negative feelings and emotions. Then we address the physical by making lifestyle changes—eating living foods and exercising.

Our physical bodies are precious and were created as a dwelling place for their Creator.* Yet most people pollute their temples by eating too much food and eating the wrong foods.

We must be willing to start loving ourselves and forgiving ourselves. In so doing, we can begin to exercise self-control over our physical nature. No one is going to restrain your appetite for you. You have been given *the power* to restrain yourself by having the ability to control your cravings. *You make the choice.*

Up to now you may have felt hopeless or even said, "Why try when I've tried everything?" You said it; *you tried.* The good news is that *you are not alone.* Start building on this pillar of health by practicing temperance, moderation, portion control, and self-restraint when it comes to food. Then, when you make positive changes to your diet, it will have a real and lasting effect on your health.

---

* See 1 Corinthians 3:16; 6:20.

BUILDING BLOCKS TO A HEALTHY LIFE

POINTS TO PONDER: *There are many reasons why Americans can't lose weight and keep it off; however, the main reason is that dead foods give comfort. Emotions are usually at the root of an obesity problem. However, you can exercise self-control and retrain yourself not to turn to food for comfort. You need to learn how to forgive yourself and not burden your mind with guilt and shame.*

ACTION STEP: *Read the Agreement to Lose Weight below and sign it.*

AGREEMENT TO LOSE WEIGHT

Repeat this agreement, aloud and with conviction three times a day before meals.

No longer will I only use my willpower to control my eating; instead I will use God's power infused into my willpower through the Holy Spirit. I will crucify my flesh daily and give my body what it needs and not what it craves. I covenant today that no longer will food be my comforter, but the Holy Spirit will be my Comforter.

From this day on, I refuse to pollute my body by eating junk food, sugar, fried foods, and any other food that is unhealthy.

I covenant to exercise at least every other day because I realize that I cannot lose weight and keep it off without exercise.

I CONFESS:

- I want to lose weight and keep it off.
- I deserve to lose weight and keep it off.
- Losing weight is good for me.
- Losing weight is good for others.
- It is safe for me to lose weight and keep it off.
- With the Holy Spirit's help, I will lose weight and keep it off.

____

YOUR SIGNATURE

As you begin your weight loss program, calculate your body mass index (BMI) using the chart on the next page. Which category do you fall into?

BODY MASS INDEX FOR ADULTS TABLE[4]

	Normal						Overweight					Obese									
BMI	**19**	**20**	**21**	**22**	**23**	**24**	**25**	**26**	**27**	**28**	**29**	**30**	**31**	**32**	**33**	**34**	**35**	**36**	**37**	**38**	**39**
Height (inches)	**Body Weight (pounds)**																				
58	91	96	100	105	110	115	119	124	129	134	138	143	148	153	158	162	167	172	177	181	186
59	94	99	104	109	114	119	124	128	133	138	143	148	153	158	163	168	173	178	183	188	193
60	97	102	107	112	118	123	128	133	138	143	148	153	158	163	168	174	179	184	189	194	199
61	100	106	111	116	122	127	132	137	143	148	153	158	164	169	174	180	185	190	195	201	206
62	104	109	115	120	126	131	136	142	147	153	158	164	169	175	180	186	191	196	202	207	213
63	107	113	118	124	130	135	141	146	152	158	163	169	175	180	186	191	197	203	208	214	220
64	110	116	122	128	134	140	145	151	157	163	169	174	180	186	192	197	204	209	215	221	227
65	114	120	126	132	138	144	150	156	162	168	174	180	186	192	198	204	210	216	222	228	234
66	118	124	130	136	142	148	155	161	167	173	179	186	192	198	204	210	216	223	229	235	241
67	121	127	134	140	146	153	159	166	172	178	185	191	198	204	211	217	223	230	236	242	249
68	125	131	138	144	151	158	164	171	177	184	190	197	203	210	216	223	230	236	243	249	256
69	128	135	142	149	155	162	169	176	182	189	196	203	209	216	223	230	236	243	250	257	263
70	132	139	146	153	160	167	175	181	188	195	202	209	216	222	229	236	243	250	257	264	271
71	136	143	150	157	165	172	179	186	193	200	208	215	222	229	236	243	250	257	265	272	279
72	140	147	154	162	169	177	184	191	199	206	213	221	228	235	242	250	258	265	272	279	287
73	144	151	159	166	174	182	189	197	204	212	219	227	235	242	250	257	265	272	280	288	295
74	148	155	163	171	179	186	194	202	210	218	225	233	241	249	256	264	272	280	287	295	303
75	152	160	168	176	184	192	200	280	216	224	232	240	248	256	264	272	279	287	295	303	311
76	156	164	172	180	189	197	205	213	221	230	238	246	254	262	271	279	287	295	304	312	320

	Extreme Obesity														
BMI	**40**	**41**	**42**	**43**	**44**	**45**	**46**	**47**	**48**	**49**	**50**	**51**	**52**	**53**	**54**
Height (inches)	**Body Weight (pounds)**														
58	191	196	201	205	210	215	220	224	229	234	239	244	248	253	258
59	198	203	208	212	217	222	227	232	237	242	247	252	257	262	267
60	204	209	215	220	225	230	235	240	245	250	255	261	266	271	276
61	211	217	222	227	232	238	243	248	254	259	264	269	275	280	285
62	218	224	229	235	240	246	251	256	262	267	273	278	284	289	295
63	225	231	237	242	248	254	259	265	270	278	282	287	293	299	304
64	232	238	244	250	256	262	267	273	279	285	291	296	302	308	314
65	240	246	252	258	264	270	276	282	288	294	300	306	312	318	324
66	247	253	260	266	272	278	284	291	297	303	309	315	322	328	334
67	255	261	268	274	280	287	293	299	306	312	319	325	331	338	344
68	262	269	276	282	289	295	302	308	315	322	328	335	341	348	354
69	270	277	284	291	297	304	311	318	324	331	338	345	354	358	365
70	278	285	292	299	306	313	320	327	334	341	348	355	362	369	376
71	286	293	301	308	315	322	329	338	343	351	358	365	372	379	386
72	294	302	309	316	324	331	338	346	353	361	368	375	383	390	397
73	302	310	318	325	333	340	318	355	363	371	378	386	393	401	408
74	311	319	326	334	342	350	358	365	373	381	389	396	404	412	420
75	319	327	335	343	351	359	367	375	383	391	399	407	415	423	431

BMI Categories

- Underweight = < 18.5
- Normal weight = 18.5–24.9
- Overweight = 25–29.9
- Obesity = BMI of 30 or greater

DAY 17: What the Bible Says About Food

Patients often ask me if God wanted humans to be vegetarians. The answer is yes *and* no. Originally, vegetarianism was His design for all mankind:

> And God said, Behold, I have given you every herb bearing seed, which is upon the face of all the earth, and every tree, in the which is the fruit of a tree yielding seed; to you it shall be for meat. And to every beast of the earth, and to every fowl of the air, and to every thing that creepeth upon the earth, wherein there is life, I have given every green herb for meat: and it was so.
>
> —Genesis 1:29–30

That plan changed when the Lord said to Noah, "Every moving thing that liveth shall be meat for you; even as the green herb have I given you all things" (Genesis 9:3). The only exception was this: "But flesh with the life thereof, which is the blood thereof, shall ye not eat" (verse 4). That opened up the entire world of living things as a smorgasbord for man's eating pleasure.

But in Leviticus 11 and Deuteronomy 14, the Lord gave instructions through Moses about how to eat healthy. He said which animals, birds, and fish to eat. For example, they were only allowed to eat animals that chewed the cud and had split hoofs, such as cows, sheep, and goats. These rules, we now know, have a scientific basis for health.

God's Plan for the Church

The Jews lived under those rules for centuries, and their bodies were strong and disease-resistant. The Bible says there was none feeble among all two million Jews in the wilderness (Psalm 105:37). Their phenomenal health insurance policy was based on diet alone!

Jesus also abided by those same rules, never eating pork, shellfish, catfish, or other restricted foods. He was certainly not a vegetarian, but as an observant Jew He would have followed the dietary laws. But after His death and resurrection, the dietary rules radically changed, and we are no longer under the law but under grace.

> For everything God created is good, and nothing is to be rejected if it is received with thanksgiving, because it is consecrated by the word of God and prayer.
>
> —1 Timothy 4:4–5, NIV

The apostles and elders also gave their recommendations (Acts 15:28–29) about not eating food that has been sacrificed to idols, or eating blood or the meat of animals that have been strangled. But nowhere did they say to follow the dietary laws of Leviticus 11 or Deuteronomy 14.

As a Christian, you are free to eat anything you want. Your diet will not keep you from heaven, but if you continually eat unhealthy foods, you will get there much sooner. As Paul wrote, all things are permissible, but not all things are beneficial. (See 1 Corinthians 6:12.) We must choose a diet that is good for us. Christians are supposed to be "living epistles." Non-Christians should look at us and visibly see a difference, not only in our attitude but also in our very appearance, which begins with what we eat.

Quick Quiz

Put these top three take-out foods in order of popularity among men in the United States:

- Chicken sandwiches
- Seafood
- Hamburgers

Answer (beginning with most popular): hamburgers, chicken sandwiches, seafood[1]

Back to Basics

If God is the same yesterday, today, and forever, as Hebrews 13:8 says, then what is the wisest diet for us to follow? I believe God's initial plan for vegetarianism, His first and best plan for mankind, should carry a lot of weight with us. I don't promote strict vegetarianism—and neither does God; after all, He told Peter to "get up, kill and eat" (Acts 10:13)—but I do note that vegetarians live longer and may have lower incidences of heart disease and cancer. One study showed that vegetarians under the age of sixty-five were 45 percent less likely to suffer a heart attack than meat eaters.[2] A significant study of Seventh-Day Adventists who ate little or no meat showed increased longevity of life of 7.28 years in men and 4.42 years in women.[3]

The Bible itself gives a real-life example of vegetarianism's benefits. In the Book of Daniel, Daniel and the other Hebrew children serving in the king's palace in Babylon were to be educated and nourished for three years on the king's own rich and dainty food and wine. But Daniel would not defile himself by eating the food and wine, because if he did so, he would be breaking the Hebrew health laws of Leviticus 11 and

Deuteronomy 14. He and three other Hebrews were allowed to shun the king's food and eat their choice of vegetables, grains, and water for ten days. After ten days, they looked better and healthier than all the other youths. Three years later Daniel and those three Hebrews stood before King Nebuchadnezzar and were ten times wiser than all the magicians and enchanters in the kingdom.

That's a pretty good testimony for eating vegetables, grains, and water.

Please don't misinterpret what I am saying; I am not advocating cutting meat out entirely. When people begin to command you to abstain from certain meats, realize that every creature of God is good, and you can have it as long as you bless it:

> Now the Spirit expressly says that in latter times some will depart from the faith...commanding to abstain from foods which God created to be received with thanksgiving by those who believe and know the truth. For *every* creature of God is good, and nothing is to be refused if it is received with thanksgiving.
>
> —1 TIMOTHY 4:1, 3–4, NKJV, EMPHASIS ADDED

The key here is to practice temperance, especially when eating meats. Eating the right foods makes you physically healthy and wise. Eat the wrong foods, and you fall beneath your potential.

What are those wrong foods, or "dead foods," as I call them? We will visit the dark side of the food world next and see the foods toward which we should exercise caution and temperance.

BUILDING BLOCKS TO A HEALTHY LIFE

POINTS TO PONDER: *Ask yourself this question:* What would Jesus eat? *God's initial design was for man to be a vegetarian. However, we are no longer under the law but under grace. Every creature of God is good as long as it is received with thanksgiving.*

ACTION STEP: *Beginning today, get back to the basics. Increase your intake of fruits, vegetables, and healthy nuts. Choose whole-grain breads over white breads.*

DAY 18: What to Avoid—the Dark Side of the Food World

Bear with me as you read today's segment. I realize that I am giving you a lot of information today, but it is information that is vitally important for you to understand. If you only come away with one concept from today's reading, I want you to understand that the foods we need to avoid are not the "unclean foods" listed in Leviticus and Deuteronomy; the foods we need to avoid are the man-made foods—processed foods, fast foods, excessive sugars, and toxic fats. These foods are the real killers in the American diet.

A woman walked into my office weighing nearly three hundred pounds. It was the first time I'd seen her. Her back was slightly bent with osteoporosis, and she was suffering from arthritis and shortness of breath so severe that she had to move very slowly. I examined her, performed lab work, a chest X-ray, and an EKG, and I found she had angina, heart disease, high blood pressure, arthritis, type 2 diabetes, and other obesity-related problems. Her cholesterol was even over 300.

"I eat the four basic food groups," she told me. "I don't understand why I gained fifty pounds over the past year."

I asked her what specifically she ate. "Well, I fast every morning," she began. "I miss breakfast. Then for lunch I have my four food groups—a Quarter-Pounder with cheese, lettuce, and tomato on a bun. Sometimes I have a jelly sandwich made with strawberry preserves, too. So I get my fruit.

"For dinner," she said, "I'm a meat-and-potatoes woman. I get my vegetables from potatoes, and I love T-bone steaks. So that satisfies my meat group requirement. I always include bread for my grains, and I put lots of butter on it to meet my needs for the dairy group. And I like a tall glass of orange juice or grape juice for my fruit group needs."

I was stunned almost to silence. No wonder she was obese and had a host of medical problems. Many people like this woman have visited my office. Those who chose "life-giving" foods have gone on to live long and healthy lives.

The Plague of Processed Foods

On the first day of this pillar I described dead foods as those that have been processed beyond recognition, the life sucked out of them and man-made chemicals added to extend their shelf life. I like to call them "Franken-foods." Your first rule of thumb is this: limit your intake of processed food (white bread, instant white rice, crackers, chips, and so forth). It enriches the food company's bottom line but usually constipates your body. If processing food made it healthier, I would be its biggest advocate, but it is without exception higher in depleted flours, sugar, salt, food additives, and usually toxic fats. The "creation" process that produces this "Franken-food" strips away valuable vitamins, minerals, fiber, enzymes, phytonutrients, and antioxidants. You see, they remove the fiber and wheat germ, which are rich in nutrients, and sell them to health food stores. Most processed foods have a high glycemic index and raise your blood sugar, causing weight gain and setting the stage for most degenerative diseases. Most contain little to no nutrition and actually put a drain on your digestive enzymes.

With dead, processed food you get the worst and lose the best. And yet food companies hire the brightest minds and chemists to make their foods as addictive as possible, so you can't eat just a little bit. They know how to create the eye appeal, tastes, textures, feels, and smells people find irresistible. Your five senses get so attached to these foods that the foods become your comforter and friend. Food companies also hire very bright marketers to package and promote their products in a way that appeals to you and your children—like putting toys in cereal boxes and cartoon characters on the outside of the boxes.

But it's time for you to boot dead foods out of your life. Here are the main ones you need to kick out or reduce dramatically.

MSG

A common ingredient in processed foods—as well as one of the most dangerous and best disguised—is MSG (monosodium glutamate). MSG is the sodium salt of an amino acid, glutamic acid, and looks similar to sugar or salt. MSG doesn't alter the actual taste of food the way salt and other seasonings do. Instead it "enhances" taste by increasing the sensitivity of your taste buds. In other words, it tricks your brain into thinking the food tastes good by stimulating your taste buds. Many food manufacturers add MSG to stimulate your appetite.

> **A Rule of Thumb**
>
> Generally, the more salty or processed a food is, the more MSG or "free glutamate" the food contains.

They want you to become addicted to their products for life.

Glutamate, or glutamic acid, comes in a bound form and a free form. Both are found in natural protein-rich foods, such as most meats, most dairy products, seaweed, mushrooms, tomatoes, fermented soy products, yeast extracts, hydrolyzed proteins, nuts, and legumes. Only the "free" form can enhance the food's flavor. Free glutamic acid is metabolized to MSG in the body.

Most of our MSG intake is found in the processed foods we consume, such as soups, gravies, salad dressings, bouillon products, soy sauce, Worcestershire sauce, dry milk powder, processed meats, frozen entrees, ice cream, and the list goes on. Not only is it hidden in most of the store-bought processed foods, but it is also in many of the processed foods in restaurants, such as fried chicken products, sausage, scrambled egg mix, and grilled chicken fillet.

As I said earlier, MSG is one of the most well-disguised food additives on the market. Food manufacturers are getting more creative with their labeling of MSG. Now it comes under the guise of names like hydrolyzed vegetable (or plant) protein, autolyzed yeast, yeast extract, soy protein isolate, natural flavors, artificial flavors, and autolyzed plant protein, to name a few.

So why the big fuss over MSG? We've known about some of the symptoms when consumed in large quantities, but there are new conditions associated with MSG—obesity and excitotoxicity.

Adverse Reactions Caused by MSG

Here is a sampling of some of the reactions that MSG-sensitive people may experience within an hour of ingesting 3 grams of free glutamic acid on an empty stomach:[1]

- Stomach cramps
- Nausea/vomiting
- Diarrhea
- Migraine headaches*
- Heart palpitations
- Rapid heartbeat
- Extreme rise or drop in blood pressure
- Shortness of breath
- Pain or tightness in the chest*
- Facial swelling*
- Numbness/burning in and around the mouth*
- Frequent urination
- Depression
- Anxiety/panic attacks
- Light-headedness/loss of balance/dizziness
- Joint pain/stiffness
- Flu-like achiness
- Blurry vision

Chinese restaurant syndrome is usually diagnosed when, after eating Chinese food, people experience the symptoms above that have been marked with an asterisk (*) . MSG has been implicated (but not proven) to be the cause of this condition.[2]

Research confirms that MSG consumed by lab animals causes brain lesions of the hypothalamus. Neuroscientists generally agree that glutamic acid (present in MSG) is neurotoxic and kills neurons by exciting them to death. The very young are most susceptible.

MSG may damage the hypothalamus, which controls appetite. A damaged hypothalamus can lead to a runaway appetite. MSG also causes the pancreas to produce more insulin. The blood sugar often drops due to the excessive insulin and typically makes you hungry. That's why many people are hungry an hour or so after eating food containing MSG.

The FDA now requires that the ingredient "monosodium glutamate" be listed on food labels. However, labels can be deceiving. MSG is also found in at least thirty-nine other labeled ingredients.

HIDDEN SOURCES OF MSG		
These ingredients ALWAYS contain MSG:		
Glutamate	Textured protein	Yeast extract
Glutamic acid	Hydrolyzed protein	Yeast food
Monosodium glutamate	Calcium caseinate	Autolyzed yeast
Monopotassium glutamate	Sodium caseinate	Gelatin
These ingredients OFTEN contain MSG or create MSG during processing:		
Artificial flavors and flavorings	Seasonings	Natural flavors and flavorings
Soy sauce	Soy protein isolate	Soy protein
Bouillon	Stock	Broth
Malt extract	Malt flavoring	Barley malt
Whey protein	Carrageenan	Maltodextrin
Pectin	Enzymes	Protease
Corn starch	Citric acid	Powdered milk
Protein-fortified ingredients	Enzyme-modified ingredients	Ultra-pasteurized ingredients

High-Sugar Foods and Beverages

Refined sugar is a man-made product, unlike the natural sugars found in living food. Why is sugar so harmful?

Sugar can make you fat.

A woman came to my office complaining of weight gain in spite of her restrictive, low-fat diet. I found she was chewing gum to keep her breath fresh at the office. Without realizing it, she was consuming lots of sugar, which was telling her pancreas to secrete insulin—a signal that tells the body to store fat.

When you overeat sugar, your body goes into fat-storage mode. That's why most diabetics gain weight when they begin taking insulin—often as much as twenty or thirty pounds. Sugar creates a cycle of demand for more sugar, which raises insulin levels. Insulin is a powerful hormone that signals the body to store fat.

Sugar impairs your immune system.

Sugar temporarily impairs your T-cells, which protect you against viruses, and also temporarily impairs the B-cells, which produce antibodies. It impairs white blood cells called phagocytes, which protect you from bacteria. Eating 100 grams of simple carbohydrates (like cookies, a large piece of cake, or a few doughnuts) can reduce the ability of white blood cells to engulf and destroy microorganisms by 50 percent for a few hours. As a result, you are more prone to bacterial and viral infections. In addition, sugar actually feeds cancer cells.

Did You Know . . . ?

A twelve-ounce can of carbonated soda contains eight to ten teaspoons of sugar.[3]

Sugar is linked to behavioral disorders.

There's a strong link between excessive sugar intake and attention-deficit/hyperactivity disorder (ADHD). Many children have become "sugar-holics." Some authorities have even linked sugar and hypoglycemia (low blood sugar) with violent behavior.[4] They believe that when individuals "come down" from a sugar "high," they become grumpy, irritable, and sometimes violent.

Sugar leads to osteoporosis.

Sugar creates an acidic environment in your tissues, which causes your body to cry out for alkaline foods. If you don't get enough calcium in your diet, your body may pull it from your bones and teeth to rebalance your pH, and you may develop bone loss and eventually osteoporosis.

Sugar aggravates yeast problems.

Yeast loves sugar. Everyone has yeast in their intestines, but after taking antibiotics and then consuming lots of sugar, you may develop yeast overgrowth in the intestinal tract, and your abdomen may swell up like a yeast roll.

Yeast infections in women are usually made worse when they eat lots of sugar. For more information on this topic, refer to my book *The Bible Cure for Candida and Yeast Infections.*[5]

Sugar leads to type 2 diabetes and elevates cholesterol.

Excessive sugar can lead to type 2 diabetes and elevated cholesterol and triglycerides. Most people understand how sugar excess can lead to diabetes by elevating insulin levels; eventually cells become resistant to insulin, which leads to type 2 diabetes. But elevated insulin levels also trigger the liver to produce more cholesterol and triglycerides. Sugar can lead to mineral imbalances in the body, leading to chromium deficiencies. Chromium is an important mineral for maintaining blood sugar control.

Sugar accelerates the aging process.

In the 1970s researchers discovered glucose amino-acid complexes that form on the surface of collagen and elastin in blood vessels and heart muscle. They named these complexes "advanced glycation end-products" (AGEs). These molecules interact with neighboring proteins and become destructive free radicals, leading to accelerated aging and disease. When AGEs interact with collagen and elastin, wrinkles and age spots appear as skin aging speeds up.

AGEs are formed within the body through normal metabolism and aging, and externally by cooking sugars with fats or proteins. Consuming externally formed AGEs has been proven to contribute to atherosclerosis, asthma, arthritis, heart disease, stroke, and diabetes-related diseases such as nephropathy, retinopathy, and neuropathy. AGEs molecules have also been found in brain tissue and have been implicated as causing damage to proteins that play a role in Alzheimer's disease.

Sugar is addictive.

When I put a patient on a low-carbohydrate diet, treating them for yeast overgrowth, they often go through sugar withdrawals, becoming intolerably irritable and cranky. One husband phoned me and said, "Dr. Colbert, you have to do something. I've never seen my wife like this!"

Sugar is highly addictive. Many people find it nearly impossible to stop eating it. In fact, eating lots of sugar may deplete the zinc in your body, which can dull your sense of taste.[6] Manufacturers know that when your taste perception is altered, you need more sugar to give you the same taste satisfaction. It becomes a vicious cycle.

Sugar sources

Back in the 1980s the average American ate six tablespoons of sugar a day. Ten years later, that average consumer ate sixteen tablespoons of sugar. Imagine eating sixteen tablespoonfuls (or forty-eight teaspoonfuls) of straight sugar every day. As of 2005, the average American consumes one hundred fifty pounds of sugar every year![7]

But before you point the finger of blame at soft drinks—which deserve some blame, as they contain about ten teaspoons of sugar per can—consider that manufacturers add stealth sugars to products you wouldn't consider "sugary" to make them more addictive. Check the labels of basic items in your fridge and pantry—start with ketchup, bread, relish, salad dressing, blended mustards, breakfast cereals, and crackers—and you will see that sugar is high on the ingredient list. It may be called "corn syrup," "dextrose," "glucose," or other words ending in "-ose" to keep the word *sugar* off the list, but the fact remains: you may be avoiding candy bars but getting just as much stealth sugar in unexpected places.

To Diet or Not to Diet Soda?

Many people think diet sodas help them lose weight, but one study showed otherwise. A study covering eight years of collected data showed that your risk of becoming overweight by drinking one to two cans of soda per day is 32.8 percent, but your risk increases to 54.5 percent if you drink one to two cans of diet soda instead.[8] That's right, ladies—you heard me correctly.

Is all sugar bad? No. Our bodies, and brains in particular, need it to function. But we don't need as much as most people eat, and especially not in man-made form. Sugar in its natural state is always combined with fiber, which prevents a blood sugar spike and excessive insulin release. All fruit has fructose or fruit sugar and an abundance of fiber. However, man has separated the fruit from the fiber and created addictive foods.

Aspartame exposed

Aspartame is made of three components: aspartic acid, phenylalanine, and methanol. Methanol is also known as "wood alcohol," and it is 10 percent of what is released from aspartame when this substance is broken down in the human digestive tract. When a beverage containing aspartame is exposed to heat, it releases methanol.

In the body, methanol is converted to formaldehyde—yes, embalming fluid—and formic acid. Methanol and formaldehyde in high amounts can cause blindness, eye damage, or neurological damage.

When broken down in the digestive tract, 40 percent of what is produced from aspartame is aspartic acid. This is known in scientific and medical circles as an excitatory amino acid or excitotoxin. An excitotoxin is a substance that overstimulates or excites nerve cells and may cause permanent damage to the nervous system. Aspartic acid has been linked to brain abnormalities, including brain tumors in research animals.[9] Aspartic acid eventually converts to glutamic acid, or MSG.

Side effects of aspartame include visual problems, headaches, confusion, depression, dizziness, convulsions, nausea, diarrhea, migraines, abdominal pains, fatigue, tightness of the chest, and shortness of breath.

According to a press release distributed by *Newswire Today* on January 17, 2006, a bill to ban the neurotoxic artificial sweetener aspartame was introduced in the New Mexico legislature by New Mexico state senator Jerry Ortiz y Pino. It is the first legislative ban in the United States on aspartame. According to the press release, a report posted on the National Institutes of Health Web site in November 2005 stated:

> The Ramazzini Foundation of Oncology's study proves aspartame to cause 6 kinds of cancer.

The press release went on to state:

> The FDA has refused to rescind its approval, thus far, so aspartame is found in coffee sweeteners, "diet" beverages, "low-fat" yogurt, "sugarless" gum—a total of 6,000 products consumed by 70% of Americans and 40% of our children.[10]

The recommendation is that industries should switch to natural sweeteners like stevia or xylitol, which I recommend as well. Be careful with xylitol, though, because it may cause excessive gas.

Splenda—not so splendid

Splenda brand sweetener is a substance called sucralose, which is made by turning sugar into a chlorocarbon. A few of the side effects of sucralose in animal studies include shrunken thymus glands, enlarged liver and kidneys, atrophy of the lymph follicles in the spleen and thymus, reduced growth rate, decrease in red blood cell count, hyperplasia of the pelvis, aborted pregnancy, decreased fetal body weights and placental weights, and diarrhea.[11] Some people have reported the conditions listed on page 84 after consuming Splenda. No long-term studies of sucralose in humans have been completed, but according to a laboratory in Oxford, England, sucralose may form trace amounts of a mutagenic agent, which may act as a carcinogen.[12] Remember, I always recommend natural products in place of artificial sweeteners.

As I was writing this book, I had a gentleman come to me after I spoke at one of my Seven Pillars seminars. He shared with me how he had used Splenda and began experiencing blurry vision and frequent urination at night. He was also diagnosed with type 2 diabetes.[13] He stopped using Splenda, and almost immediately the side effects stopped and his blood sugar normalized. His vision returned to normal and the nighttime runs to the bathroom stopped.

The "Not-So-Splendid" Side of Splenda

People who use Splenda (sucralose) may experience the following side effects:

- Bloating
- Abdominal pain
- Gas
- Nausea
- Blurry vision
- Diarrhea
- Headaches, especially migraines
- Heart palpitations (fluttering, irregular heartbeats)
- Shortness of breath
- Frequency to urinate at night
- Depression or overwhelming anxiety
- "Spaced-out" or drugged sensation
- Joint pain
- Dizziness[14]

White Flour

White bread is a poor choice for food. It is also very constipating. When water is added to white bread, it forms a sticky paste that constipates your body. Some people say it's so sticky they can almost hang wallpaper with it!

It delivers little nutrition (even with all those added vitamins and minerals they advertise on the package) and converts to sugar rapidly.

It's another example of how a wonderful, God-given food gets mugged on the way to the grocery shelf.

All bread starts out as whole grain, but to make white bread, the manufacturer removes the outer shell of the grain with all its healthy fiber and B vitamins. Then the nutrition-packed wheat germ is extracted. Both the fiber and the wheat germ are actually *resold to health food stores.* Meanwhile, the denuded white flour heads to the mainstream market to be made into white bread, buns, pastries, crackers, pasta, and so on.

White bread is created from one part of the grain head—the starchy endosperm that is ground into fine powder. Since the bran and germ are removed, approximately 80 percent of the wheat's nutrients are gone.

The milling process involves such high temperatures that the remaining grain is damaged by oxidation and has a grayish appearance. Could you imagine buying gray-colored bread?

But because consumers don't want to buy gray bread, the manufacturer bleaches it white. If there were any vitamins and minerals left, most are destroyed in the bleaching process. Then low-grade vitamins and minerals are added, along with man-made cyber-fats, sugars, food additives, and maybe a sprinkling of grains on the top, and the food is marketed to moms as healthy sandwich bread.

Any flour not called "whole wheat" or "whole oat" is white flour, even if it looks brown. White bread converts to sugar almost as fast as candy bars. When my diabetic patients switch from eating white bread to whole-grain bread, their cholesterol and blood sugar levels almost always go down. I have a saying for those who habitually consume white bread: "The whiter the bread, the sooner you're dead."

Fast Food

The typical American now consumes three hamburgers and four orders of fries per week. In 1970 Americans spent approximately $6 billion on fast food, and in 2000, we spent more than $110 billion.[15] We spend more money on fast food than we do on personal computers, computer software, new cars, and higher education combined.

Trans fats—which I will describe later in this section—are found in especially high amounts in fast food. In February 2006, a report showed that McDonald's french fries are one-third higher in trans fat than once believed. One large order of McDonald's french fries contains a whopping eight grams of trans fats![16]

Acrylamides are toxic chemicals formed by the combustion of oil and hydrocarbons. They are highly carcinogenic—particularly associated with colon cancer—and should be avoided. Acrylamides cause cellular DNA to mutate. French fries are among the worst offenders when it comes to foods containing acrylamides. So, the next time you're tempted to go to the drive-through, keep on driving!

Deadly Meats

I trained in a medical residency program operated by Seventh-Day Adventists. As a group they obey certain dietary laws, and many are vegetarians. They also live longer than most Americans and have some of the lowest incidences of heart disease and cancer.[17] Many of them are total vegetarians, eating no meat, fish, fowl, eggs, or dairy products.

Some are lacto-ovo vegetarians—meaning they sometimes eat eggs, drink milk, and use other dairy products.

I don't promote total vegetarianism since Jesus was not a vegetarian, but there are certainly meats that are best to rarely eat.

Livers and kidneys are filtering organs that filter toxins. Many toxins reside in these organs. Why would you want to eat them?

Cold cuts and packaged meats like bologna, salami, hot dogs, bacon, sausage, and processed ham are usually high in saturated fats, which are associated with heart disease and are always high in salt. They also contain lots of nitrites and nitrates—fancy names for ugly substances that may form cancer-causing chemicals called *nitrosamines* or *n-nitroso compounds.* These compounds are associated with cancer of the bladder, esophagus, stomach, brain, and oral cavity.

Because of the cancer-causing nitrosamines, it's especially important not to let children eat hot dogs and other processed meats. One study found that children who eat more than twelve hot dogs per month have nine times the normal risk of developing childhood leukemia. Another study found that children who eat hot dogs one or more times per week have a higher risk of developing brain cancer and that children whose mothers ate hot dogs during pregnancy are associated with an excess risk of childhood brain tumors. If hot dogs are a favorite in your household, please switch to brands that say "nitrite-free" or "nitrate-free" on the label.[18] Also, there is nitrite-free bacon, ham, sausage, and luncheon meats.

Nitrosamines are formed during digestion when food protein reacts with nitrite salts in the stomach. They can also be formed by frying or smoking. A general rule of thumb is that the more processed and preservative-rich the meat is, the greater the risk of nitrosamines. To lessen this risk, I recommend that you bake your own ham and turkey and slice it yourself instead of picking up cold cuts at the deli.

Bacon, sausage, and hot dogs are also high in saturated fats and chemicals. These meats are generally loaded with saturated fat.

In addition, processed meats such as hot dogs, sausage, and cold cuts are created using a process called "the advanced meat recovery system" (or AMRS). It is a process used to recover as much "meat" as possible from the bone and tissue of the carcass. It squeezes the meat through, leaving the bone and tissue on the other side.

Because of a feared connection to mad cow disease, consumer advocate groups are lobbying the government to toughen regulations on AMRS. The goal is to ban meat processors from allowing any spinal cord tissue from cows more than thirty months old to enter their processing machines. Although scientists have not yet established a direct link between spinal cord tissue in processed meat and disease in humans, I feel it would be in your best interest to limit your intake of these meats.[19]

Fats

Fats add delicious taste and "mouth feel" to foods, but often at a dangerous price. There are fats that kill (trans or hydrogenated fats and partially hydrogenated fats), fats that kill in excess but heal in moderation (saturated and polyunsaturated fats), and fats that heal (omega-3 fats and monounsaturated fats). (We'll look at "good fats" tomorrow.)

It's a Fact!

The more solid the hydrogenated fat, the more dangerous it is to your body.

The fats you should avoid are trans fatty acids, often called "trans fats," such as hydrogenated and partially hydrogenated fats. You need to limit your consumption of saturated and polyunsaturated fats. Saturated fat is found mostly in animal fats. It is solid at room temperature and significantly raises the LDL or bad cholesterol. Polyunsaturated fats are found in products such as mayonnaise, salad dressings, heat-processed safflower oil, sunflower oil, and corn oil.

Trans fats (hydrogenated and partially hydrogenated fats)

In 1902 the process of hydrogenation was patented by a German scientist. During hydrogenation the cheapest oils—soy, corn, cottonseed, and canola—are mixed with a metal catalyst, usually nickel. The oil is then subjected to hydrogen gas in a high-pressure, high-temperature reactor to force hydrogen through it until it is saturated. Emulsifiers are then added, and the oil is deodorized at high temperatures and steam cleaned. Margarine is an example of a product containing hydrogenated oils. Like the white flour I mentioned earlier, margarine must be bleached to hide its gray color and then dyed and flavored to resemble butter.

Adding hydrogen atoms to liquid fats and oils makes these oils stay in solid form at room temperature. This means that they are much less likely to become rancid, and their shelf life is greatly prolonged.

This process, however, alters the chemical structure of the fat to an unnatural "trans fatty acid," which becomes an enemy of the heart by raising LDL (bad) cholesterol levels and lowering HDL (good) cholesterol levels. Trans fats have been found to be more harmful to your arteries than saturated fat, and they are implicated in heart disease and cancer.

Trans fats, also called hydrogenated fats, are present in margarine, shortening, and most commercial peanut butters. Margarine in stick form usually has more than 20 percent trans fatty acids, whereas most tub margarine or soft margarine only contains about 15 percent.

Quick Quiz

Which Bob Evans' menu items contain the highest grams of trans fats?

a. No-sugar-added Apple Pie

b. Sausage and Cheddar Bake Breakfast

c. Turkey & Dressing Dinner

d. Chicken Pot Pie

Answer: a and c. The No-sugar-added Apple Pie contains ***thirteen grams*** *of trans fats. The Turkey & Dressing (stuffing) contains* ***thirteen grams*** *of trans fats (the* ***thirteen grams*** *of trans fats are in the dressing, not the turkey). The Chicken Pot Pie contains* ***twelve grams*** *of trans fats. The Sausage and Cheddar Bake Breakfast contains* ***eleven grams*** *of trans fats.*[20]

These bad fats are found in almost every item in the middle of a grocery store—where all the shelf-stable pastries, rolls, breakfast cereals, breakfast bars, crackers, and processed or packaged foods reside. Bad fats are also found in the bakery section in the doughnuts, pastries, cookies, cakes, pies, and other items that entice you as you walk around the grocery store. Try to avoid the middle aisles and bakeries of the grocery store so that you won't be tempted. Many salad dressings contain hydrogenated fats. However, there are healthier choices, such as Newman's Own salad dressings.

On January 1, 2006, all packaged foods sold in the United States began to list trans fat content on their Nutrition Facts labels. But observers point out a problem with the new label. Under FDA regulations, "if the serving contains less than 0.5 gram [of trans fat], the content, when declared, shall be expressed as zero."[21] That means you could eat several cookies, each with 0.4 grams of trans fats, and end up eating several grams of trans fats even though the label would say you had eaten none. A fourteen-year study found that just a 2 percent increase in trans fats elevated a person's risk of heart disease by 36 percent.[22] This is such a deadly fat that we need to avoid it entirely. The best way to avoid this is to look for the words "partially hydrogenated" or "shortening" on the label. If either of these words is on the label, don't eat the product. Just as we should avoid restaurants that allow smoking, we should also avoid restaurants that continue to cook their food in these deadly fats.

Saturated fats

Saturated fats rarely can be found in fruits and vegetables; they are primarily found in animal products. Foods high in saturated fats include most selections found at a fast-food restaurant (such as hamburgers, fried chicken strips, and so on) and dairy products such as whole-milk products, as well as commercial fried foods and processed foods such as cookies, cakes, doughnuts, pies, and pastries.

Did You Know...?

That meat drippings, such as beef tallow/dripping, lard (pork), chicken, duck, goose, bacon fat, and even turkey contain a whopping 44.8 grams of saturated fat per 3.5 oz serving. So the next time you cook those green beans, think twice about slathering them with bacon fat![23]

Saturated fats are also found in cured meat such as bacon, sausage, ham, hot dogs, cold cuts, bologna, salami, and pepperoni. Red meats, duck, and goose meat are also usually quite high in saturated fats. Some vegetable oils such as coconut oil, palm kernel oil, and palm oil are also high in saturated fats. Men, limit your intake of red meat. Men who consume high amounts of red meat increase their chances of prostate cancer by two to three times over men who do not.[24]

I recommend limited intake of these fats rather than completely avoiding them because they do provide benefits to the body when consumed in moderation. Saturated fats enhance our immune system and allow calcium to be incorporated into our bones when consumed in moderation. (*In moderation* means that no more than 7–10 percent of our caloric intake should come from saturated fats.)[25] Moderate amounts of saturated fats also protect the liver from toxins, help prevent breast cancer and colon cancer, and help promote weight loss.

Polyunsaturated fats (omega-6 fats)

Polyunsaturated fats oxidize much faster than monounsaturated fats. That is why these fats become rancid so quickly. Polyunsaturated fats are liquid at room temperature and remain in liquid form even when refrigerated or frozen. Polyunsaturated fats are divided into two families: the omega-3 fats and the omega-6 fats. I'll discuss omega-3 fats tomorrow.

When polyunsaturated oils such as corn oil, safflower oil, sunflower oil, sesame oil, commercial salad dressings, and others are used in cooking, and especially deep-frying, oxidation occurs even faster. Oxidation also occurs in your arteries as free radicals attack the polyunsaturated fats, which are carried in LDL cholesterol.

Oxidized cholesterol is much more likely to form plaque in an artery or on arterial walls. As fats are broken down through oxidation, they form substances that promote blood clotting and cause inflammation—all of which make blood flow more difficult.

Polyunsaturated fats are not the worst fats, but they aren't the best, either. They come from healthy sources, but they tend to be overprocessed by the time they reach the consumer. Eating too much polyunsaturated fat increases inflammation, which is associated with heart disease, arthritis, cancer, and Alzheimer's disease.

Polyunsaturated fats are essential for life and must be consumed daily in small amounts. I believe the best way is to consume small portions of pecans, almonds, brazil nuts, pine nuts, pistachios, and walnuts. If you must use vegetable oil, choose small amounts of *cold-pressed* polyunsaturated fats (corn oil, flaxseed oil, hemp oil, pumpkinseed oil, safflower oil, sesame oil, soybean oil, and sunflower oil), which you can find at most health food stores. (Remember—the apostle Paul says in 1 Corinthians 6:12, "'Everything is permissible for me'—but not everything is beneficial" [NIV]. Moderation is the key.) But it's best to avoid *heat-processed* oils and replace your salad dressings with extra-virgin olive oil, balsamic vinegar, and garlic oil, pressed with a garlic press. (See the recipe for "Dan's Famous Salad Dressing" on page 97.) I explain the process of expelling oil in detail on Day 19.

Now let's get to the good news and see which living foods should be the foundation of your diet.

DAY 18 DAY 18 DAY 18

BUILDING BLOCKS TO A HEALTHY LIFE

POINTS TO PONDER: *Stay on the lighter side of life by enjoying living foods. The more processed and the more sugar and toxic fats a food contains, the more harm it will do to your body. Limit your intake of fatty meats such as bacon, hot dogs, sausage, and cold cuts.*

ACTION STEP: *Begin reading labels, and avoid all trans fats, hydrogenated or partially hydrogenated fats, or shortening, which are all very dangerous fats.*

DAY 19: What to Eat—the Living Foods List

In the television program *What Not to Wear,* a crew of hip makeover artists helps a poorly dressed person learn how to dress well. The show ends with the friends and family seeing the transformed person. The before and after photos are often shockingly different.

You "wear" your food on your body every day. You really are what you eat. Your clothes may be made of cotton, polyester, rayon, or silk, but your body is made up of whatever you put in your mouth. Eyeliner and shapers can't hide an unhealthy body. It's time to make over your pantry and fridge with living foods so you can look and feel your best!

Food is a blessing from God. Exodus 23:25 (NKJV) says, "You shall serve the LORD your God, and He shall bless your bread and water. And I will take sickness away from the midst of you." The word for *bread* is also translated *nourishment.* God wants us to enjoy food. Let's see which foods He made to bless your body.

Beauty Is Skin Deep

Organic foods are often smaller and not as pretty as non-organic produce. Organic oranges appear less impressive than conventionally grown ones, but studies show that organic oranges are far more nutrient dense. Non-organic oranges are bigger and have a nicer orange color, but they are like big balls of water with fewer nutrients.[1]

Fresh Organic Fruits and Vegetables

At least half of what you eat should be living foods, preferably organic fruits and vegetables and whole grains. It is an established fact that the more fruits and vegetables you eat, the lower your chance of heart disease, cancer, and many other health problems. Even adding one serving a day can lower your heart disease risk. The current recommended daily servings of fruits and vegetables, according to the USDA, is five to thirteen servings per day, depending on your caloric intake.[2]

Many times a diet rich in fruits and vegetables is able to reduce your blood pressure as much as medications do. People who eat more than four servings a day also have significantly lower levels of bad cholesterol. Studies clearly show that for preventing cancer, fruits and vegetables are the best "medicine" you can take. The natural phytonutrients in produce protect against all kinds of cancer.[3]

Eat your fruits and vegetables raw or steamed, because food in its fresh state has all its enzymes. Enzymes are the chemical spark plugs in your body that start or speed up chemical processes that keep you alive. There are thousands of enzymes inside of you. They take proteins, fats, and carbohydrates and structure them to form your body. When you eat fruits and vegetables that still have their enzymes, you boost your body's ability to re-create itself.

It's OK to lightly steam or stir-fry your produce. But don't overcook it. One researcher found that when you cook food at temperatures above 118 degrees Fahrenheit for thirty minutes, almost all the enzymes are destroyed. It becomes dead food.[4]

Fruits and vegetables should be eaten unpeeled whenever possible because many vitamins and minerals are concentrated just beneath their skin. The outer layer of organic fruits and vegetables should be safe to eat. If you have not purchased organic items, it is imperative that you wash these fruits and vegetables carefully. For suggestions, read the section "Washing Off Produce Waxes" in my book *Toxic Relief*.[5] If no fresh products are available, choose frozen fruits and vegetables, though their nutritional value is mildly compromised. Rarely eat canned fruits and vegetables. Canned produce is usually blanched, or heated very quickly, before canning. This destroys vitamins and enzymes. It is also heated inside the can to kill microorganisms, thus destroying more vitamins.[6]

Why organic?

Organic food is defined as having been "grown with the addition of only animal or vegetable fertilizers to the soil, such as manure, bone meal, and compost." Organic foods are produced without the use of artificial pesticides and chemical fertilizers.

We will save our in-depth discussion of organic foods for our pillar on detoxification, but the bottom line is that organic foods deliver superior nutrition without the harmful chemicals or foreign substances that can wreak havoc on our bodies' health.

What kinds of fruits and vegetables?

All kinds! Carrots, tomatoes, parsley, garlic, strawberries, tangerines, grapes, blueberries—these and hundreds of other colorful, living fruits and vegetables contain antioxidants, protecting you from a myriad of diseases, including cancer. They supply vitamins and minerals in the pristine condition your body loves.

Eat nonstarchy vegetables like spinach, lettuce, cabbage, broccoli,

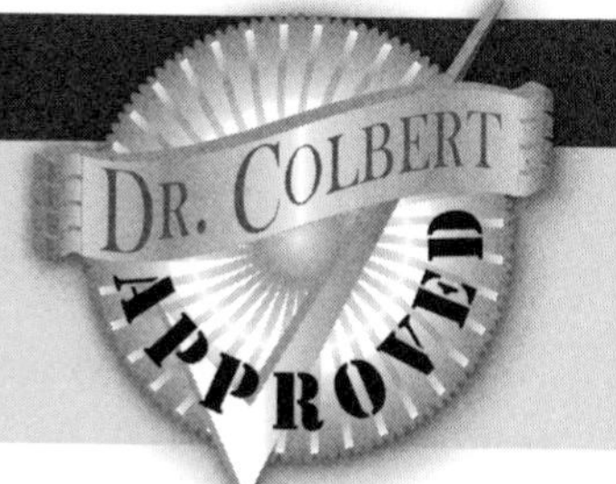

Dr. Colbert Approved—Tomatoes

According to a study by the Department of Medicine, Brigham and Women's Hospital and Harvard Medical School, frequent consumption of tomato products is associated with a lower risk of prostate cancer.[7]

asparagus, green beans, brussels sprouts, collards, mustard greens, radishes, turnips, and cauliflower. Eat colorful salads with balsamic or red wine vinegar and extra-virgin olive oil or other healthy oils from the good fats list we'll look at in a moment. Starchy vegetables like beans, peas, lentils, potatoes, and sweet potatoes are fine, though if you are overweight you will need to eat them in moderation. Coleslaw made with grape seed mayonnaise is a terrific addition to your daily diet.

Parsley is very nutritious and is a key ingredient in a Middle Eastern salad called *tabouli,* which is very tasty. Garlic has been used medicinally in Egypt for more than five thousand years and in China for more than three thousand years. It was used to treat the great plague in Europe and as a cure for dysentery during World War I. Garlic has antifungal, antiviral, antiparasitic, and antibacterial properties and can help lower blood pressure.

One of fruits' and vegetables' important ingredients is indigestible fiber, which soaks up water in the digestive system and sweeps everything out. It's nature's street sweeper for your GI tract. High-fiber diets move food, toxins, and parasites through quickly and harmlessly. When your diet is low in fiber, it gives more opportunity for parasites to attach to your intestine and for toxins to enter your bloodstream.[8]

There are two types of fiber: insoluble and soluble. Insoluble is not water soluble and includes lignin and cellulose. Bran is the most common insoluble fiber, wheat bran being the most common form. Bran also includes the bran from any grain. Most people can tolerate rice bran very well. This type of fiber increases the frequency of our bowel movements and the weight of our stool, and it helps prevent constipation, irritable bowel syndrome, hemorrhoids, diverticulosis, and other intestinal disorders. Good sources are high-fiber cereals and the skins of vegetables and fruits.

Soluble fiber is soluble in water; it helps lower cholesterol levels, stabilizes blood sugar, slows digestion, and helps bind toxins, heavy metals, and chemicals, removing them from the body. Soluble fibers are broken down by microbes in the intestines and provide the fuel for maintaining a healthy lining of the GI tract. They also bind bile salts, which prevents gallbladder disease. Good sources of soluble fiber include fruits, beans, legumes, lentils, carrots, oats, and seeds such as psyllium seed and flaxseed.

Generally speaking, the higher the fiber content the better. When taking soluble fiber, increase your fiber intake slowly, or you may experience bloating, cramping, and excessive gas.

New Recommendations

The USDA recently updated its recommendations for eating fresh foods. It used to recommend five to seven servings of fruits and vegetables every day. Now it recommends five to thirteen servings a day—almost double the previous recommendation.[9]

It's hard to go wrong with fresh, organic fruits and vegetables. They should be the major part of your diet. One note of caution, however: fruits and vegetables can be low glycemic or high glycemic. The glycemic index (GI) is a numerical system of measuring how fast a carbohydrate triggers a rise in your blood sugar. The higher the number, the greater the blood sugar response. A low-glycemic food will cause a small rise, while a high-glycemic food will trigger a dramatic spike.

I recommend eating more produce with a glycemic index of 50 or less, especially if you want to lose weight. This way you are not amping yourself up on sugar all the time.

- Low-glycemic foods are 55 or less.
- Medium-glycemic foods are 56–69.
- High-glycemic foods are 70 and above.

For people trying to lose weight, the chart below will give you glycemic values for some fruits and vegetables:[10]

GLYCEMIC INDEX VALUE	FOOD
<15	Artichoke
<15	Asparagus
<15	Avocado
<15	Broccoli
<15	Cauliflower
<15	Celery

GLYCEMIC INDEX VALUE	FOOD
<15	Cucumber
<15	Eggplant
<15	Green beans
<15	Lettuce, all varieties
<15	Peppers, all varieties
<15	Snow peas
<15	Spinach
<15	Young summer squash
<15	Zucchini
15	Tomatoes
22	Cherries
22	Peas, dried
24	Plum
25	Grapefruit
28	Peach
31	Dried apricots
32	Baby lima beans, frozen
36	Apple
36	Pear
52	Orange juice, not from concentrate
53	Banana
54	Sweet potato
55	Sweet corn
64	Beets
64	Raisins
66	Pineapple
72	Watermelon
97	Parsnips
103	Date

Whole grains

Another living foods staple is fiber-rich, living grain products like sprouted-grain breads, brown rice, whole-grain pastas, and whole-grain cereal. Whole-grain products are nutrient-dense and pass on lots of vitamins and minerals to your body. Whole grains also contain lots of fiber, which is a fabulous toxin-trapper.

When you buy grain products, look for the words *sprouted* (as in "sprouted wheat," "sprouted barley," "sprouted millet," "sprouted lentils," "sprouted soybeans," and "sprouted spelt"), *whole wheat,* or *whole oat* on the ingredient list. Don't be fooled by names like "cracked wheat," "7 grain bread," and so on. Those are meant to sound healthy, when in fact they generally use the same white flour you find in white bread. The only words that ensure you are getting a whole-grain product are *sprouted, whole wheat,* or *whole oat.* Check the ingredients label carefully. Don't be fooled by the packaging artwork.

I encourage you to go one step further than whole-wheat breads and eat sprouted breads and flat breads. Ezekiel bread and manna bread are both terrific flour-less breads made from live, sprouted grains and should be refrigerated.

Sprouted-grain products do go bad quicker, especially if you leave them on the counter, but there's nothing wrong with that. It means they aren't loaded with preservatives. The food God gave the Israelites during their sojourn in the wilderness—manna—bred worms after one day. It's characteristic of live food. You should learn to be suspicious of foods that don't go bad quickly.

Limit your consumption of whole-grain products that contain corn. We feed corn to pigs and cattle to fatten them up. Need I say more? This also includes popcorn.

Good fats

Yes, there is such a thing as good fat. Your body needs fat! The good types of fat heal the body and are necessary. You should eat fat every day for the health of your heart, brain, skin, hair, and every part of you. Good fat nourishes and strengthens cell membranes. Good fats include:

- Monounsaturated fats
- Omega-3 fats

Monounsaturated fat is found in extra-virgin or virgin olive oil that is cold-pressed (not heated). You can also get monounsaturated fats in natural organic peanut butter, avocados, olives, macadamia nuts, and especially almonds, walnuts, and hazelnuts. Raw nuts and seeds—not the roasted, salted, flavored, and candied kind—should be a mainstay of your diet. I enjoy almonds, macadamia nuts, and walnuts. Almonds are excellent because they are high in monounsaturated fats and contain about 20 percent protein. Try almond butter.

Go easy with nuts and seeds at first, or you may upset your stomach. Start out light and gradually increase them. As I said yesterday, moderation is the key. Also, if you leave nuts unsealed for thirty days, they may become rancid, doing more harm than good. Keep nuts in #1 PETE plastic or ceramic containers, and place them in the refrigerator or freezer until you are ready to use them.

Omega-3 fatty acids are found mainly in cold-water fish, some marine mammals, and algae (seaweed). Scientists believe the best way to obtain adequate omega-3 is direct consumption of DHA (docosahexaenoic acid) and EPA (eicosapentaenoic acid) from fish. DHA protects the brain, reversing signs of brain aging and protecting against development of Alzheimer's and dementia. DHA also plays a role in preventing ADHD and impaired learning. EPA protects the heart and decreases inflammation. It has anti-cancer, anti-inflammatory, and anti-hypertensive effects. EPA reduces the risk of stroke, heart arrhythmias, dementia, and heart attack.[11]

Alpha-linolenic acid (ALA) is commonly lacking in the standard American diet. The fats in flaxseed, flaxseed oil, walnuts, and different green vegetables and super foods are converted in the body into ALA. The body then uses ALA to make EPA and DHA to nourish and protect the heart and brain and to produce a powerful hormone called "PG3," which reduces pain and inflammation and prevents platelets from adhering, which reduces blood clots.

Dan's Famous Salad Dressing

My brother, Dan Colbert, has a wonderful recipe for a salad dressing. I like it so much that I wanted to share it with you.

- ¼ cup balsamic vinegar
- 2 Tbsp. Cavender's Greek seasoning
- 1 clove fresh garlic, minced
- Pinch of sea salt
- 2 Tbsp. clean, pure water
- Juice of one lemon
- ⅔ cup extra-virgin olive oil

Pour the balsamic vinegar into a glass salad dressing cruet (such as Good Seasons' mixing bottle), and add the remaining ingredients in the order listed. Refrigerate. Makes 1 cup.

TIP: Dressings prepared with olive oil may congeal when refrigerated. Let the refrigerated dressing reach room temperature before serving.

One study has found that men with the highest levels of ALA in their bloodstream are three times as likely to develop prostate cancer.[12]

Therefore, do not consume excessive amounts of flaxseeds, flaxseed oil, and walnuts.

Unfortunately, many people are unable to convert ALA to omega-3. Therefore, rather than trying to increase your intake of ALA, concentrate on getting more EPA and DHA in your diet. I recommend that you eat wild salmon as a good source of omega-3 fats or take pure fish oil supplements that contain EPA and DHA.

The canola oil controversy

Canola oil is a monounsaturated fat used primarily in cooking and food preparation. Although canola oil has been singled out by some nutritionists as having toxic properties, it is important to understand that the nutritional value of any edible oil can be destroyed and turned into poison, depending on the processing and cooking techniques used.

When canola was developed in the 1970s, oil seed from mustard rape (rapeseed), a member of the mustard family, was used. Canola today has been hybridized from rapeseed to yield a good all-purpose cooking oil with high monounsaturated fat content similar to olive oil, but with a longer shelf life.

However, there still remains controversy. Dr. Mary Enig, PhD, one of the top biochemists in the country, found that canola oil has to be partially hydrogenated or refined before it is used commercially.[13] This has led to concern over high levels of trans-fatty acids, but canola oil that has not been hydrogenated will not have significant amounts of trans fats. It is important to check the label before purchasing.

The key to choosing a healthy oil is in the extraction process. Mass-market oils are usually chemically extracted from seeds using hexane, a petroleum product that is harmful to the environment and has the potential to leave a residue on the finished product.

Expeller pressing is a much healthier alternative for processing oils. In this process, an expeller press crushes seeds with hydraulic action. This process yields less oil than chemical extraction, which is why expeller-pressed oils are usually more expensive. Still, they are the best choice for cooking and eating, and this goes for all oils.

A word about fried foods

If you enjoy fried foods, then switch to stir-frying, lightly, on low heat using organic extra-virgin coconut oil, organic butter, organic ghee (clarified butter), or organic macadamia nut oil, which has a fairly high smoke point. *Smoke point* is the point at which the oil begins to break down, releasing free radicals. This may even occur at relatively low temperatures. If you stir-fry with extra-virgin olive oil, do not stir-fry at high temperatures because it has a lower smoke point. Never cook with flaxseed oil.

Avoid frying in polyunsaturated fats such as corn oil, sunflower oil, soybean oil, or safflower oil. Frying at high temperatures converts these oils to dangerous lipid peroxides, which create tremendous amounts of free radicals. These free radicals can damage the liver and cause chromosomal damage in lab animals. Imagine the amount of damage it is doing in our bodies, and especially in the bodies of our children as we continue to feed them french fries, fried chicken strips, and onion rings.

Most vegetable oils purchased in the supermarket are heat processed. They go through various stages, and here is the process in a nutshell. The process begins by taking natural seeds, such as sunflower or sesame, and heating them to about 250 degrees. The seeds are then pressed to expel the oil. Then solvents such as hexane, a petroleum product, are added to dissolve the oil out of the seed or grain, and then heated to 300 degrees to evaporate the solvent. Next begins the degumming process, which removes most of the nutrients from the oil. The oil is left with a yellowish hue after all these processes, so it is then bleached at an even higher temperature and deodorized at temperatures of more than 500 degrees for thirty minutes to one hour. The end result is what you see on the grocery shelf—a clear, odorless oil full of dangerous lipid peroxides. See my book *What Would Jesus Eat?* for more information.[14]

Stay Alive With Living Foods

As you change your diet and build on this pillar of health, live your life and make modifications where you should. At a restaurant, choose fresh fruits and vegetables, whole grains, and lean meats that are not fried. Choose extra-virgin olive oil and vinegar on the side. There are plenty of ways to avoid bad foods, even on mostly unhealthy menus.

If you find yourself in a situation where it would be rude not to eat "dead" foods, just eat fruits, vegetables, and whole grains with it so that the fiber pushes the dead food through your system.

Tomorrow we will look at other living foods that you can eat with caution.

DAY 19 DAY 19 DAY 19

BUILDING BLOCKS TO A HEALTHY LIFE

POINTS TO PONDER: *Fruits, vegetables, whole grains, and healthy oils are all "living food." Not all fats are bad. In fact, your body needs good fat. Good alternatives are extra-virgin olive oil, almonds, macadamia nuts, and flaxseeds. Depending on the oil, you can lightly stir-fry your food. Never deep-fry.*

ACTION STEP: *Choose whole-grain breads, whole-grain pasta, and whole-grain cereals. Consume five to thirteen servings of fruits and vegetables, preferably organic, a day. Try one to two tablespoons of "Dan's famous salad dressing" on your salad today. (This salad dressing also makes a great marinade for chicken.) Add about one or two tablespoons of one of these raw nuts: almonds, walnuts, or macadamia nuts. Find out what type of oil is used in your favorite salad dressing at restaurants.*

DAY 20: What to Eat With Caution—Meat and Dairy

Yesterday's entry was about foods you can eat almost unreservedly—fresh organic fruits and vegetables, whole grains, and monounsaturated fats. Today is about foods you should eat with a little more caution—meats and dairy products.

Why Meat Is a "Caution" Food

Humans are omnivores, and meat can be an acceptable and healthy part of your diet. But many people act like carnivores. They don't understand the dangers of eating too much meat or the wrong meats. Here are the top three reasons to limit meat, red meat especially, in your diet.

Toxic fat

Red meat has a higher concentration of toxins than nearly all other foods. Any pesticide, sulfa drug, hormone, antibiotic, chemical, or other toxic residue an animal eats generally gets stored right into its fat. If you eat that fat, the same toxins go into your body and lodge in your fat. That cut of red meat on your dinner plate could be the biggest entry point of toxins into your body.

White meat is better, but not perfect. Most chickens are given antibiotics, especially tetracycline, to counter salmonella and other bacteria. In the past, it was common practice to give growth hormones and estrogens to animals to add bulk to increase their value. Fortunately, now these practices have changed.

> **Fat Caution**
>
> For a two-thousand-calorie diet, only 30 percent of your calories should come from fat.[1]

Still, the dangers of toxic meat are high. There is no such thing as fat-free meat. Everything from filet mignon to turkey breast has some fat content. When you eat any kind of animal fat, the pesticides from the meat that isn't processed and eliminated by your liver can be stored in your fatty tissue—and you may reap the damage.

Excess protein

Eating too much meat and protein (including protein from milk products, cheeses, and eggs) congests the organs and cells. It makes your tissues acidic, which, as we saw in the first pillar, makes it harder for your body to detoxify on a cellular level.

When you eat a 16-ounce steak or the equivalent in another kind of meat, you are loading your body with excessive amounts of protein. Men usually need only 20 to 30 grams of protein (3–4 ounces of meat) with each meal (or 0.8 grams per kilogram of body weight). Women usually need only 14–21 grams of protein per meal (2–3 ounces of meat). A 220-pound man would need only 80 grams of protein per day. An ounce of meat usually has 7 grams of protein. I recommend that people also get their protein by combining whole grains and beans, such as brown rice and beans, which form a complete protein.

A Good Egg

Like dairy products, eggs are a great source of protein, but they may cause allergies. When cooked, the protein changes so it's less easy to absorb or digest, and you may develop allergies or sensitivities to it. If you can "stomach" eggs, an occasional egg is good for you, especially organic eggs or the new choice eggs, which contain omega-3 fats.

Excessive protein intake may put a strain on the kidneys, and individuals with kidney failure must restrict their intake of protein, especially meats.

Irradiation

This is a problem you don't hear much about, but it is disturbing. Many foods, from meats to grains to juices, are zapped with radiation equivalent to ten to seventy million chest X-rays to kill or prevent microorganisms from growing.[2] The FDA has allowed poultry to be irradiated since 1990, and red meats since 1997.[3]

Studies of malnourished children in India showed chromosome damage after they were fed recently irradiated wheat for six weeks. When the children were taken off the diet, the condition went away.[4]

Irradiation destroys up to 95 percent of vitamin A in chicken, 86 percent of vitamin B in oats, and 70 percent of vitamin C in fruit juices.[5] It also reduces essential fatty acids, amino acids, friendly bacteria, and enzymes in food.[6]

Some public interest groups say the FDA has ignored a substantial body of evidence that suggests irradiation is unsafe, that it causes cancers, mutations, and chromosomal damage, and that it causes chemicals to be created in the food. I expect more studies to confirm or disprove this, but evidence is already in that irradiation harms foods' nutritional value.[7]

Dr. Colbert Approved Red Meats

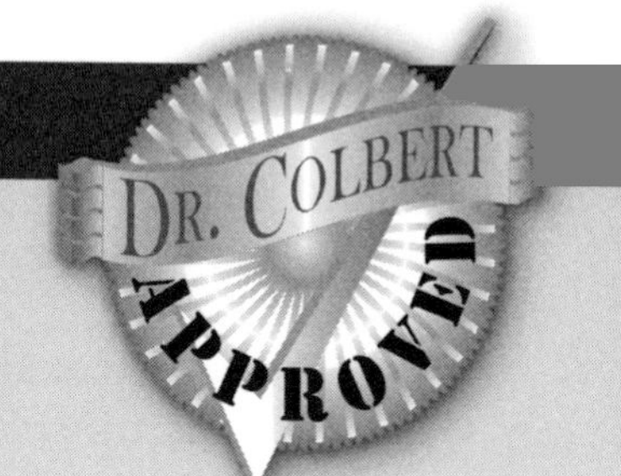

- Lean cuts
- Organically raised
- Hormone free
- Grilled without the char

You must recognize and refuse to eat irradiated meats whenever possible. Look for the Radura symbol—the international sign of irradiation—on foods you buy. Labels on packages of food that has been irradiated are legally required to carry the phrase "treated by irradiation" or "treated with irradiation." But bulk items or whole foods are only required to display the Radura symbol on the bulk container, which the consumer rarely sees. Also, the Radura label is *not* required on foods, like soups, that may include an irradiated ingredient.[8]

The Irradiation Symbol (Radura)

Starting in 2003, the USDA began allowing irradiated fruits and vegetables to be imported into the United States. All irradiated produce imported from foreign countries is supposed to be labeled, but critics say the U.S. government inspects only 2 percent of imported food and that irradiated fruits and vegetables may not be labeled as required.[9]

And since January 2004, the National School Lunch Program was allowed to include irradiated foods.[10] You might ask your school district's food services director if the schools serve irradiated foods.

Many restaurants use irradiated meats, and they don't have to declare it.[11] You might ask the manager if the restaurant where you're eating has a policy against using irradiated meats.

How to Safely Eat Meat

In spite of these dangers, you can still enjoy meat after taking some precautions.

Try to choose organic, free-range, or grass-fed meat, and always look for the leanest cuts—chicken breast, turkey breast, or very lean cuts of filet mignon or tenderloin. This will help you avoid potential toxins in the fat. Free-range meats are healthiest because the animals were not fed antibiotics. The breast of free-range chickens contains some of the lowest amounts of animal fat. Organic and free-range animals feed on grasses and have more omega-3 fats in the meat than grain-fed cattle. Grain-fed cattle are usually much fatter and contain more omega-6 fat as well as saturated fats.[12]

If you cannot afford organic or free-range meat or poultry, get the leanest cuts, trim off any visible fat, and remove any skin. Make sure the meat has not been irradiated.

Turkey is one of the best choices of meats. Turkey breast is one of the leanest meats and contains the least amount of pesticides and toxins. Other relatively safe meats include the leanest cuts of lamb, venison (U.S.), rabbit, and buffalo.

Eating Out?

Here are just a few restaurant chains that do not serve irradiated foods:

- Chili's
- Macaroni Grill
- Outback Steakhouse
- Ruby Tuesday's
- Tia's Tex-Mex
- Olive Garden

Some people worry about giving up meat because they wrongly believe they won't get enough protein in their diet. But a balanced diet that includes small amounts of lean meats and generous portions of beans and whole grains can give you the protein you need. For example, whole-grain bread and hummus make a complete protein when eaten together.

If you choose to eat red meats, limit them to only four to six ounces, once or twice a week.

When preparing poultry, peel the skin off and cut away any visible fat before it is cooked. If you leave the fat and skin on, pesticides seep into the meat. Bake, broil, grill, or lightly stir-fry your meat. (Don't deep-fry your chickens or turkeys, as some people have begun doing.) Scrape off charred portions, because char contains benzopyrene, which is a carcinogen and is associated with colorectal cancer. Cook meats thoroughly since most poultry contain dangerous bacteria such as salmonella.

Once you start buying the right kinds of meats and preparing them in a healthy way, you can fully enjoy them as part of your regular diet.

Fish

I used to recommend fish much more heartily than I do now, but new studies keep emerging about the high mercury content of fish, even fish formerly considered safe. For that reason I'm much more cautious now about fish.

Let me mention my cautions right up front. Because the oceans, lakes, and rivers have suffered from the toxic onslaught of chemicals

Dr. Colbert Recommended Fish

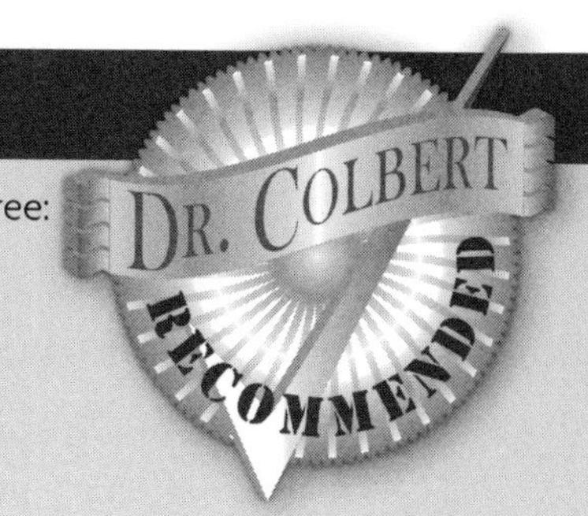

Here is a list of some fish that are usually pesticide free:

- Wild Alaskan or Pacific salmon
- Mahi-mahi (Florida)
- Sardines
- Rainbow trout (farm raised)
- Tongol tuna
- Grouper (Argentina, Chile, Mexico)

along with the rest of the environment, fish are no longer free of toxins. The American College of Obstetricians and Gynecologists recommends only two six-ounce servings of fish a week for pregnant women,[13] and the American Academy of Pediatrics recommends no more than seven ounces of fish a week.[14] This is because fish increasingly contains mercury, which is toxic for the fetus and for children's brains.

But if you are careful about which fish you eat, they can be your best source of healthy omega-3 oils, which study after study have shown is one of the best oils on the planet. Fish with the highest concentrations of omega-3 oils are Pacific herring, king salmon, wild Pacific salmon, anchovies, and lake trout. Wild Pacific salmon contains higher omega-3 fat than farm-raised Atlantic salmon.

If you have heard news reports about rising mercury levels in tuna, look into buying tongol tuna, which is much lower in mercury and comes from much smaller tuna. Most store-bought tuna comes from larger tunas, which contain much higher mercury content. Tongol tuna is generally found in health food stores.

Other good fish are tilapia, halibut, grouper, striped sea bass, and sole.

Avoid shark and swordfish. They have some of the highest levels of mercury and pesticides of any fish in the sea. Sharks will eat anything and are usually high in pesticides, PCBs, and toxic heavy metals. In many areas trout have also been subjected to contamination through industrialization. Use caution, and select fish taken from fresh, pure water areas.

If you purchase your fish from a grocery store, use wisdom. Nearly 40 percent of your grocer's fish may have already begun to spoil. Ensure the quality of your purchases by using this brief checklist:

- Look for fish that is shiny, bright, and bulging. If the scales are shiny, the fish is good.

- If your touch leaves an indentation in the flesh, don't buy it. The flesh should spring back.
- If it smells fishy, don't buy it.
- If the fish has not been kept on ice at 32 degrees, don't buy it. It is likely that it has already begun to spoil.

Certain ocean waters are known for their purity. The waters of Australia are extremely pure, as are the waters of Chile. The seas surrounding New Zealand and Greece are also extremely clean. Most types of fish you purchase from these waters should be safe to eat.

Shrimp contains higher levels of cholesterol than other seafood, but it is usually free from contamination from pesticides, though it usually contains the heavy metal cadmium, which is associated with hypertension. Most shellfish contain cadmium, so if you choose to eat shellfish, do so infrequently and eat those from less-industrialized areas where the waters remain uncontaminated. Also, be sure to cook all shellfish well, since raw or undercooked shellfish may be associated with food poisoning or hepatitis A.

Dairy products

Many people eat dairy products with great abandon because they associate milk with health, robustness, and wholesomeness. But from a physician's point of view, I'm highly aware of the problems caused by dairy products. Most children I see in my practice with chronic ear infections and sinus infections have dairy sensitivities. Other doctors I know of say that eliminating dairy products is often the only thing they need to do to stop recurrent ear problems in children. One doctor reported that, of all the children he saw who required tubes to be put into their eardrums for drainage purposes, three out of four did not need the tubes when they stopped eating dairy products.[15]

Dairy products, and cow's milk in particular, are also linked to all kinds of allergies and sensitivities, including skin rashes, eczema, fatigue, spastic colon, excessive mucus production, nasal allergies, and chronic sinus infections. Some people even have diarrhea due to lactose intolerance. If you (or especially your children) have any of these, stop all dairy products—including skim milk, butter, and even yogurt—for a week or so, and watch the improvement. Small wonder that man is the only species in the animal kingdom to drink cow's milk as an adult. Animals' instincts know better!

Another problem with milk is that it is pasteurized by heating it at 161 degrees for fifteen seconds, which denatures milk enzymes and changes its protein structure, making it difficult for our bodies to assimilate and digest.[16]

Finally, dairy products tend to have lots of saturated fat, which is associated with high cholesterol and heart disease. Butter is 81 percent saturated fat. Cheese is 75 percent fat. Regular milk is 4 percent saturated fat, which means that 48 percent of its calories come from fat—way too high for a healthy diet. And toxins are concentrated in those dairy fats. High amounts of pesticide residues are usually found in butter and cheese.

Lactose Intolerant?

Some people can't digest dairy products, so here are some other foods high in calcium:

Sardines, canned, ½ cup (3½ oz.)	314 mg
Red salmon, ½ cup (3½ oz.)	259 mg
Pink salmon, ½ cup (3½ oz.)	196 mg
Mustard greens, cooked (½ cup)	138 mg
Broccoli, cooked (1 large stalk)	88 mg
Collard greens, cooked (½ cup)	152 mg
Turnip greens, cooked (½ cup)	138 mg
Spinach, cooked (½ cup)	107 mg
Bok choy (½ cup)	126 mg

Should dairy products be banished from your diet? Not necessarily. Here are tips to eating healthy dairy products.

Consider goat milk.

Goats don't have the best image in America—we tend to think of them as obnoxious scavengers and barnyard loners—but goat milk products generally cause fewer allergies and sensitivities than cow's milk. If you don't like the idea of drinking goat milk, consider that anytime Israel was referred to as the land of milk and honey, it referred to—surprise!—goat milk, not cow's milk. Proverbs 27:27 even says, "And thou shalt have goats' milk enough for thy food, for the food of thy household, and for the maintenance for thy maidens."

Even though it is difficult to obtain organic, low-fat, or fat-free goat milk or goat cheese, it can be found in some health food stores and online. Grocery stores will often order a product for customers who request it, so don't be afraid to inquire at your local store.

If you eat or drink dairy, choose organic skim.

Skim dairy products have no saturated fat, and they are much lower in calories. Eat low-fat or nonfat organic dairy products like cheese, sour cream, yogurt, and so on. Use small amounts of organic butter or ghee, which is clarified butter.

Note: Some people choose margarine instead of butter, never realizing that it contains trans fatty acids associated with heart disease. Don't trade one problem food for another.

It's best to avoid ice cream and frozen yogurt since they are generally high in sugar, and ice cream is usually high in sugar and saturated fat.

Eat yogurt from time to time if you are not sensitive to dairy.

The best dairy product for you is low-fat organic yogurt or low-fat organic goat milk yogurt, which contains lactobacillus, acidophilus, and bifidus bacteria—good bacteria that help maintain a healthy GI tract. These good bacteria help reduce the production of cancer-causing chemicals. Eat a small container of yogurt a few times a week, but not the high-sugar, high-fat variety. Most packaged yogurt is just dessert in a yogurt cup. Instead, buy plain low-fat organic yogurt or goat milk organic yogurt and add your own fresh fruit.

The Best Diet News Ever

Good news, chocoholics! Chocolate is good for you. The *British Medical Journal* reported in 1998 that dark chocolate consumption is linked to longer life. It has been shown to reduce blood pressure and bad cholesterol. It opens blood vessels and allows blood to circulate more freely, which is good for heart health.[17]

Cacao beans are high in antioxidants. Ounce per ounce, chocolate has more antioxidants than fruits, vegetables, tea, and wine. One study showed that people who ate three ounces of dark chocolate every day for three weeks had lower blood pressure and improved insulin sensitivity.[18]

But not all chocolates are healthy. Most commercial chocolates are processed using high pressures and temperatures that destroy chocolate's benefits. And some studies show that while cacao beans are low in lead levels, the lead level skyrockets after manufacturing, perhaps because the beans easily absorb lead in the atmosphere.[19]

For All the Chocolate Lovers . . .

Provided you do not have a weight problem, eating one to three ounces per day is good for you! Eat only chocolate that has:

- 60 percent or higher cocoa content
- Low sugar levels
- All organic ingredients
- No dairy content

But if you choose your chocolate carefully and eat it in reasonable amounts, it will help you more than hurt you. Select organic dark chocolate with low sugar levels. By comparison, one commercially available bar of organic dark chocolate has four grams of sugar, while Hershey's Special Dark has twenty-one grams. That's a huge difference. Also buy organic chocolates that use unrefined sugar and no fillers (like vegetable oils). Avoid milk chocolate, which contains dairy that may interfere with chocolate's health benefits.

And don't eat too much. It's still chocolate, and it can still make you fat. One or two ounces a day are enough.

Now that you're thinking about the foods you eat and are applying the knowledge you've gained, let's see how to prepare, serve, and store food in the healthiest way.

- Bake, broil, or grill instead of deep-frying. When grilling, scrape off the charred portions, because this contains a carcinogen or cancer-causing agent.
- Limit your intake of fish, and be careful about which types of fish you choose.
- If you choose to consume dairy products, choose organic low-fat or skim dairy or goat milk products, especially yogurt.

BUILDING BLOCKS TO A HEALTHY LIFE

POINTS TO PONDER: *Foods that we used to think were good for us, in reality may be making us toxic and causing diseases, such as many of our fish and charred hamburgers and steaks. When choosing meats, choose the leanest cuts of free-range or grass-fed meats. Avoid irradiated meats; know the symbol for irradiated meats. Dark chocolate is very high in antioxidants; however, make sure it has low sugar and no vegetable oils. Avoid milk chocolate.*

ACTION STEP: *If you or another family member has frequent sinus infections, ear infections, or sore throats, eliminate all dairy products for four to twelve weeks; ; notice if you, your spouse, or your children begin to feel better. Substitute rice milk for regular milk.*

DAY 21: "Dinner's Ready!": How to Prepare and Serve Food

Dinner should be the most pleasant hour of your day, a time to slow down, relax, and gather with family and friends to enjoy food and fellowship. Here are tips for keeping food healthy all the way to the dinner table.

Preparation

Some people buy fresh fruits and vegetables and store them for days and weeks before using them. During that time much vitamin and mineral content is lost. Grapes can lose a third of their B vitamins, and tangerines can lose up to half of their vitamin C if left on the counter for a long time. Asparagus stored for one week can lose 90 percent of its vitamin C.

> **Wave Good-bye to the Microwave**
>
> A study in *Science News* in 1998 found that just six minutes of microwave cooking destroyed half the vitamin B_{12} in dairy foods and meat, a much higher rate of destruction than other cooking techniques.[1]

If you can, buy your food the day you intend to eat it, or a day or two before. Refrigerate your produce at 40 degrees to avoid vitamin loss. Keep frozen foods below zero degrees to retain maximum vitamin content. But freezing meats can destroy up to 50 percent of thiamin and riboflavin and 70 percent of pantothenic acid, so again, fresh is always best.

Cut or prepare fruits or vegetables just before you are ready to eat them. It's tempting to slice them up early for convenience's sake, but once exposed to air, they begin to lose nutrients like vitamin C, folic acid, vitamin B_{12}, biotin, and vitamins D, E, K, and A. If you must chop or cut up your vegetables, do so just before eating them when the nutritional value will still be high.

The same goes for cooking food. Though busy homemakers like to prepare meals in advance, keep in mind that reheating food and leftovers depletes them of vitamins, minerals, and nutrients. A fresh-made dish is more nutritious than one you cook and refrigerate.

Cook Healthy

Don't kill living foods by improper cooking. For example, many people don't realize that when they boil vegetables, the nutrients leach into the water. By the time the vegetables are tender enough to eat, the mineral and vitamin content of the water is greater than that of the vegetables! You have created a dead food from a living food or simply cooked it to death.

In one major test, boiling led to a 66 percent loss of flavonoids compared to fresh, raw broccoli. Pressure-cooking led to a 47 percent reduction of one of the major antioxidants—the majority was found in the cooking water.[3]

If you must boil vegetables, bring the water to a boil first, and then add your vegetables for a brief time. Do not allow them to soak in the water. Drain them immediately and serve them. If possible, just quit boiling vegetables altogether.

The Best—and Worst—Oils for Cooking

Using the most up-to-date information, here's a list of the best—and the worst—oils for cooking. They are listed in order from high to low smoke point.[2] (The lower the smoke point, the quicker the oil breaks down to create free radicals.)

Best	Smoke Point (Fahrenheit)	Worst	Smoke Point (Fahrenheit)
Rice bran oil	495 degrees	Lard	370 degrees
Grapeseed oil	420 degrees	Corn oil, unrefined	320 degrees
Macadamia nut oil	390 degrees	Soy oil, unrefined	320 degrees
Butter	350 degrees	Safflower oil, unrefined	225 degrees
Coconut oil	350 degrees	Canola, unrefined	225 degrees
Extra-virgin olive oil	320 degrees		

In the same test, microwaved broccoli lost an incredible 97 percent, 74 percent, and 87 percent, respectively, of the three major cancer-protecting antioxidant compounds (flavonoids, sinapics, and caffeoyl-quinic derivatives).[4] That's why I recommend that my patients avoid microwaved foods.

Freezing foods can also remove some nutrients. However, it is very difficult to always have fresh vegetables; eating frozen vegetables is acceptable.

Beware of fruits and vegetables grown in other countries. Many times pesticides that are banned in the United States are used in these countries. As of 2006, many countries (many of them tropical) continue to use DDT to control mosquito-borne malaria and typhus. Places such as Guyana spray it on cotton crops, and other countries such as Ecuador, Mexico, and parts of the continent of Africa continue to use it on produce crops.[5]

To fry or not to fry—that's the question

Deep-frying is a horrible way to cook because of all the free radicals it produces. For example, one study showed that canola oil releases twice the amount of one volatile pollutant, acetaldehyde, at 350 degrees Fahrenheit than extra-virgin olive oil. At 475 degrees Fahrenheit, that jumps to two and a half times as much.[6] Meat soaks up free radical fats like a sponge. The cooking oil usually contains bad fats.

Here are much better ways to cook your food:

- *Stir-fry.* This is a good method because the food is cooked so briefly that it retains most of its nutrients. Use a little bit of organic coconut oil, organic butter, ghee (clarified butter), or macadamia nut oil. Extra-virgin olive oil is also good for stir-frying but has a lower smoke point.
- *Steaming.* This is a wonderful way to cook vegetables, but do it lightly. *Lightly* steaming your vegetables causes very little loss of nutrients.
- *Grilling.* You patio chefs can still enjoy grilled meats and vegetables. Use a propane gas grill in place of charcoal or mesquite, both of which contain dangerous chemicals. Place the meat rack as high as possible, away from the flame. When meat cooks over a flame, fat drips off the meat into the fire and turns into steam. The pesticides in the fat char into the meat, and so even greater amounts of carcinogens are formed.

  Avoid charring the meat, and never eat the char. Charred meat contains a chemical called benzopyrene, which is a highly carcinogenic substance. Scrape off char. Don't even give it to the dog.

Whatever cooking method you use, don't overcook your food. Researcher Edward Howell devoted nearly his entire life to researching enzymes. He found that when food is cooked at temperatures exceeding 118 degrees for thirty minutes, almost all the enzymes are destroyed. These enzymes are the living part of the food.[7]

Dr. Colbert Approved Cookware

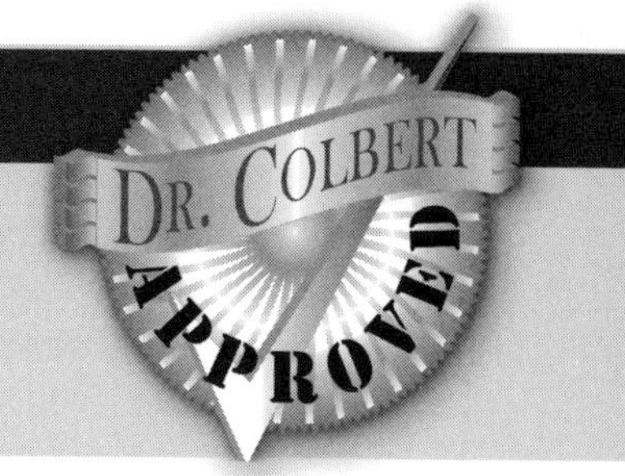

- Glass bakeware and cookware
- CorningWare and other ceramic cookware
- Pyrex or Pyrex-like glass
- Stainless steel cookware

Watch what you cook in. Teflon is possibly related to cancer. In December 2005, the DuPont Company agreed to pay $10.25 million in fines and $6.25 million for environmental projects to settle allegations by the Environmental Protection Agency that the company hid information about the dangers of a toxic chemical used to make the nonstick coating Teflon. When cooking at high temperatures using Teflon-coated cookware, PFOA (which is a chemical compound used in Teflon) is released. PFOA has been related to cancer.[8]

Among other things, the EPA said that DuPont withheld test results indicating that the chemical had been found in at least one pregnant worker from the Washington Works plant and had been passed on to her fetus.[9]

You should also avoid cooking with aluminum, which has been linked to Alzheimer's disease. This includes pots, pans, pizza pans, cookie sheets, rice cookers, and even coffee makers that have aluminum liners.

Setting the Stage for Dinner

The atmosphere at dinnertime should be completely joyful. Turn off the TV. Don't watch sporting events, the news, or suspenseful movies at dinner. Start your meal with a heartfelt blessing. Pause and consider how thankful you are. Then keep the conversation pleasant. Don't use the dinner table as a time to hold court on your children or to bring up troubling topics. Never make dinner a time to reprimand one another or argue. In Leonardo da Vinci's *The Last Supper*, you see the disciples laughing, talking, and leaning against Jesus in complete fellowship. That's a good model.

I sometimes hear people yelling and arguing in restaurants. That is the worst way to eat! When you are stressed, you can't digest well. Blood flows away from the digestive tract to the muscles for a fight-or-flight response. This shuts down the digestive juices. Food stays in the stomach longer and may cause heartburn and indigestion. Also, the food may not be digested properly, leading to bloating, gas, constipation, and even diarrhea.

If you are upset, angry, or in an irritated mood, wait to eat.

Getting back to eating meals together as a family—even if just one or two days a week—is important, especially for children. Sitting down to a meal together, especially dinner, gives parents a chance to reconnect with their children. Even if they're teenagers, you can attempt to spend time with them. The benefits will extend far beyond nutrition. Studies have found that teens who have five or more family dinners per week are three times less likely to try marijuana, two and a half times less likely to smoke cigarettes, and one and a half times less likely to drink alcohol than those who eat less often with their families. Studies also show that teens who eat with their parents are more likely to get better grades and to know that their parents are proud of them.[10]

How to Eat

Chew each bite at least twenty to thirty times, and put your fork down between bites. Your saliva contains special enzymes called ptyalin and amylase, which digest carbohydrates. Let these enzymes do their work.

Use your molars to chew. God designed humans to chew food for a long time. Don't use your canines to eat, as lions and tigers do. They have short digestive tracts and tremendous levels of hydrochloric acid to break down the meat. By contrast, you and I don't produce enough hydrochloric acid to digest half-chewed meat, so it putrefies in the intestines. Imagine setting your dinner plate on the windowsill in 98-degree weather. That's what happens in your gut when you don't chew your food thoroughly.

Some people rush through a meal as if they were orphans. They shovel in food and gulp down their beverage. Many can finish an entire meal in five minutes or less. Then they ask for an antacid!

Rushing through a meal causes hydrochloric acid to be suppressed, making digestion difficult. It also encourages you to eat more than you should. It takes about twenty minutes for your hypothalamus, located in your brain, to tell you that you are full. Many people can shovel in thousands of calories before the hypothalamus finally registers "enough."

Don't drink cold drinks with food. It dampens and dilutes hydrochloric acid, digestive juices, and enzymes. It's similar to starting a campfire and then pouring water on it.

And remember to exercise temperance. Dinner should not be the blow-out meal of the day. I tell my patients to eat breakfast like a king, lunch like a prince, and dinner like a pauper. You're giving up gluttony as part of this pillar, so eat moderate portions and feast instead on conversation and laughter.

Generally, your first deep breath toward the end of a meal is a sign that your body is satisfied and that you should stop eating. Regularly continuing to eat after this deep breath will eventually result in weight gain.

BUILDING BLOCKS TO A HEALTHY LIFE

POINTS TO PONDER: *What cookware you use to cook your food is just as important as how you cook it. Use CorningWare, glass, or stainless steel cookware when cooking. When eating, take time to chew your food instead of eating quickly. Eating too quickly sends the wrong signals to your body. Chew each bite twenty to thirty times, and set your fork down between bites. Plan your meals, cook healthy, and most of all, enjoy the company of your family or friends.*

ACTION STEP: *Eat as a family. Turn off the TV and keep the conversation pleasant. Say a blessing over your food. Below is a sample prayer.*

Blessing for Food

Thank You for my wonderful food and its healing properties. Mark 16:18 tells me that if I drink [or eat] any deadly thing it shall not harm me. Thank You for protecting me supernaturally from any harm that may be in my food. I ask that You bless the food to my body according to Exodus 23:25, which tells me that "He shall bless my food and my water and He will take sickness away from the midst of me."

I eat this food with thanksgiving. I receive His love and rejoice in the Lord as I eat my meal. As I eat this food, my cells, tissues, and organs are cleansed, strengthened, and renewed like the eagle. I see myself healed. In Jesus' name, amen.

PILLAR 4

Exercise

DAY 22: Let's Stir the Waters

Mary and I were speaking at a church in Texas, giving our presentation on the Seven Pillars of Health, and afterwards a man in his early thirties came up to me. He must have weighed 450 pounds. He said he had been on bed rest for years because of some kind of infection. Now the infection was gone, but he was having trouble regaining his health. Just by looking at him I could tell he had reached a place of lymphatic stasis—stagnation—so extreme that his legs had blown up to huge proportions. He was so full of toxins that his body was literally bulging with them.

He asked what I thought his problem might be—why he had gained so much weight and why he felt so unhealthy. I told him it was most likely because he hadn't stirred his waters with exercise.

For many people, exercise is the most difficult part of healthy living. Even people who are paid to be physically fit slack off. Public servants whose job it is to "serve and protect" the people especially need to be fit because someone's life may depend on it. In one community, a city ordinance was passed that said doughnut shops were off limits to police officers on duty because they were spending too much of their time there, and it showed in their waistlines. I once treated a police officer who weighed more than three hundred pounds. The excess weight and lack of exercise was not only putting his life in jeopardy, but it was also jeopardizing anyone whom he might have been called on to rescue.

The Case for Exercise

Stirring the waters with exercise is essential for you to prevent bodily stagnation, which is why exercise is our fourth pillar of health. We saw earlier that our bodies are approximately two-thirds water. Think of what happens when water sits for a long time in a cup, puddle, or pond. It eventually gets covered with slime and gunk, breeds disease, and becomes toxic. Think of those green algae-covered ponds you see when you drive through the country. That process is similar to what's going on in many people's bodies.

On the other hand, when water moves, life thrives. Running water is usually fresh water. Rivers and waterfalls are beautiful and inviting—alive. That's a perfect picture of what exercise does. It refreshes your body and clears it of toxins and cellular garbage, sharpening your mind and giving you strength and energy.

In ancient times, people of the Bible lived in action and motion. They didn't call it exercise, but that's what it was. People did heavy manual labor and usually walked wherever they needed to go.

Jesus did heavy manual labor as a carpenter. From the time He was five until the age of thirty, it's very likely that He walked at least 18,000 miles just on the three annual pilgrimages from Galilee to Jersualem![1] Adding up the total miles Jesus walked during His life would be at least 21,595 miles; the distance around the world at the equator is 24,901.55 miles.[2]

Bodies in Motion

Consider again that your body is mostly water. There are many references in the Bible that associate flowing water with life and healing. The Gospel of John tells about the crippled people who waited at the pool of Bethesda because they believed an angel would occasionally stir the waters, healing whomever got into the pool at that moment. To them, life was symbolized by the movement of water.*

When water moves, things grow and thrive. On the other hand, dead things are commonly associated with stagnant bodies of water. The Dead Sea in Israel is a good example. Nothing can survive and thrive in it except for microscopic bacteria, viruses, and other microbes.

Exercise is the remedy to prevent death and stir the waters of life in our bodies. If you are one of those people who use the Bible to excuse your sedentary lifestyle, that excuse is now gone. It's time to take your health into your own hands and stir the waters of life with exercise.

BUILDING BLOCKS TO A HEALTHY LIFE

POINTS TO PONDER: *Like water, when our bodies are stagnant, they become a breeding ground for disease. It's time to stir the waters of your life again and begin exercising. Exercise refreshes your body, renews your energy, and gives you strength.*

ACTION STEP: *If you haven't been exercising on a regular basis, get a walking partner and begin walking. Start by only walking for five minutes three times a week, and gradually build up to thirty minutes three times a week. Walk slow enough so you can talk but fast enough so you can't sing.*

* See John 5:2–7.

DAY 23: The Benefits of Exercise, Part I

I used to have a sports car that I loved but didn't drive much. After a while I noticed that when I took it out for a spin every few weeks, the engine wouldn't run well. I took it to the shop, and the mechanic inspected it and said, "You haven't been driving this car enough, have you? It was built to run. If you don't drive it, it will break down because you're not using it." I was ruining my car by keeping it parked.

Your body was designed to move. It needs water, rest, food, and exercise to run smoothly. When you "park" yourself in a chair and don't exercise, eventually you may ruin your engine. Many people these days are sick because they haven't stirred their waters with movement and action. They have become cesspools of disease due to stagnation. Soon they will get to the point where they can't exercise because their bodies are so broken down with heart disease, arthritis, and other degenerative diseases. "Stirring the waters" with exercise has a powerful effect on your health.

Here's how.

Exercise prevents cancer.

Studies show that approximately one-third of cancer deaths can be linked to diet and sedentary lifestyles.[1] Simple movement and exercise decrease the risk of certain cancers such as breast, colon, and possibly endometrial and prostate cancers.[2] In 2005, the National Cancer Institute reported that "physical activity at work or during leisure time is linked to a 50 percent lower risk of getting colon cancer."[3] A study published in the *Journal of the American Medical Association* found that women who engaged in the equivalent of brisk walking for about one to two hours per week decreased their risk of breast cancer by 18 percent compared with inactive women.[4]

Bottom line: exercise goes a very long way in preventing cancer.

Exercise prevents heart attacks and heart disease.

Ironically, exercise *rests* your heart. The reason is that an inactive person's heart works much harder than an active person's heart. How? Two ways.

An active person's heart usually beats about 60 to 70 times or less per minute. An inactive person's heart usually beats 80 times or more per minute because it is unconditioned and less efficient. That's like putting

33 percent more miles on your car every time you drive it. If your heart rate is 60 beats a minute, you will have approximately 86,400 beats in a twenty-four-hour period; however, if your heart rate is 80 beats a minute, it will beat 115,200 times in a twenty-four-hour period. That's quite a bit of extra mileage on your heart each day.

The only time your heart feeds itself with oxygen is between beats. The longer the pause from beat to beat, the more blood flows through the coronary arteries to nourish the heart. Regular exercise eventually enlarges the coronary arteries, improving blood flow. As the heart grows stronger, it beats fewer times, meaning the heart is at rest more often.

That's important because cardiovascular disease is the most common cause of death in the United States today.[5] Exercise protects you against it. All kinds of studies show that moderate, regular exercise is perhaps the single most important deterrent of heart-related problems. If you have coronary artery disease, regular exercise will even encourage your body to create collateral arteries, which may form a natural bypass around clogged arteries. Years ago I had a patient with an 80–90 percent blockage in his right coronary artery. After being on a regular aerobic exercise program for over one year, he actually formed a natural bypass around that plugged artery. That's what exercise can do!

Fidgeting as Exercise?

According to researchers at Mayo Clinic in Rochester, Minnesota, some people burn hundreds of calories every day...by fidgeting. Fidgeting includes crossing or uncrossing your legs, bobbing up and down, stretching or standing up often, maintaining good posture, or being generally restless.

Researchers fed subjects 1,000 extra calories per day for eight weeks. As a result, some subjects automatically began fidgeting to burn the extra calories. About 33 percent of the 1,000 extra calories consumed were burned by fidgeting and restlessness. Of the remaining calories, approximately 39 percent were deposited as fat. The participants gained from 2 to 16 pounds, but the most fidgety people gained the least amount of fat.[6]

Aerobic exercise reduces coronary risk factors. It helps lower the blood pressure, lowers blood triglyceride levels (fats), lowers the bad (LDL) cholesterol, raises the good (HDL) cholesterol, and may prevent blood clots. In a study where researchers monitored over 84,000 nurses for eight years, the nurses who exercised regularly had a 54 percent lower risk of both heart attack and stroke when compared to sedentary women.[7] Now that's reason to exercise. (And exercise costs less than Lipitor, the leading cholesterol-lowering medication, which costs more than three dollars per tablet.)

Exercise improves lymphatic flow.

The lymphatic system is a major microbe crime-fighter and cellular garbage collector in the body. It removes toxins and cellular waste, and it "keeps the peace" by rounding up bacteria, viruses, and other bad guys, bringing them to the lymph nodes where they are killed by white blood cells. Lymphatic fluid is so important that your body contains about three times more lymph than blood. The lymphatic fluid moves around via very small vessels, which usually run alongside small veins and arteries.

But the lymphatic system has a challenge: it is circulated by muscle contractions, not by your heartbeat. When you don't move, the lymphatic system becomes sluggish. But aerobic exercise can triple the rate of lymphatic flow. That means that the lymphatic system—your in-house police force and cellular garbage collector—does a much better job protecting your body from attack and removing cellular trash.

Wow! Moderate Exercise, Major Benefits

A study by Joslin Diabetes Center researchers showed that obese adults who lost just 7 percent of their weight and did moderate-intensity physical exercise for six months improved their major blood vessel function by approximately 80 percent, regardless of whether or not they had type 2 diabetes.[8]

Exercise lowers stress.

Regular exercise enhances neurotransmitter production and helps to lower cortisol levels, which helps you feel less stressed.

One researcher conducted an experiment with laboratory rats. He took some rats, shocked them with electrodes, shone bright lights, and played loud noises to them around the clock. At the end of one month, all the rats were dead from the stress. He then took another group of rats and made them exercise on a treadmill. After they were well exercised, he subjected them to a month of the same shocks, noises, and lights. These rats didn't die—they ran around well and healthy.[9]

If life is stressing you out, it's time to add exercise to your day. Exercise literally burns off those stress chemicals.

Exercise promotes weight loss and decreases appetite.

Weight training and calisthenics are exercises that increase your muscle mass, which raises your metabolic rate and enables you to burn more fat. It is perhaps the safest method of raising your metabolic rate, which is the rate at which your body converts food into energy. Realize that the basal metabolic rate decreases by approximately 5 percent for every decade of life after the age of twenty. People who are sedentary have a significant loss of muscle mass as they age. In these sedentary individuals there is about a seven-pound loss of muscle mass every ten years past the age of twenty. So by age sixty, most have lost about twenty-eight pounds of muscle and replaced it with much more *fat.*

Aerobic exercise such as brisk walking and cycling is also a very effective way to lose weight and keep it off.

Moderate aerobic exercise is also quite effective at decreasing your appetite, but you must be in your target heart rate, which you will learn about in Day 25. Individuals who exercise outside of their target heart rate by exercising too intensely may develop a ravenous appetite an hour or so after exercising due to hypoglycemia, or low blood sugar.

Exercise may help prevent diabetes and help control blood sugar in diabetics.

Exercise holds special benefits for diabetics. By helping muscles to take up glucose from the bloodstream and use it for energy, exercise prevents sugar from accumulating in the blood. By burning calories, exercise helps control weight, which is also an important factor in the management of type 2 diabetes. Exercise is also very important for individuals with type 1 diabetes; it helps to lower insulin requirements. Exercise improves the body's ability to use insulin.

Exercise increases perspiration.

Sweating is one of the body's ways of getting rid of waste products. The skin has been called "the third kidney" because it releases so many toxins from the body.

Tomorrow we will learn about eight additional benefits of exercise.

BUILDING BLOCKS TO A HEALTHY LIFE

POINTS TO PONDER: *Exercise helps to prevent many diseases and keep excess weight off. It improves the immune system, helps to maintain normal blood pressure, conditions the heart, and prevents heart disease. Exercise also helps control blood sugar in diabetics and improves lymphatic flow, which helps remove cellular waste.*

ACTION STEP: *If you don't already own a pair of good walking shoes, consider buying a pair. Look for shoes that meet the "three Fs" guideline—flexible, fit, and no flare. Make sure it's flexible, it fits comfortably with a good arch support, and it has a lower heel (no flare). Most sporting goods stores have tennis shoes that meet these requirements.*

DAY 24: The Benefits of Exercise, Part II

I once had a thirty-year-old patient, Carol, who came to see me for severe headaches, fatigue, acne breakouts, and severe constipation. She would only have a bowel movement once a week; this had gone on since her teens. I started her on two quarts of filtered water, two scoops of soluble fiber, and magnesium capsules at bedtime. However, no change occurred in her symptoms.

Since she was only thirty years old and appeared to be in good physical shape, I had failed to ask her about exercise on the first visit. However, seeing that her condition was unchanged, I questioned her and learned that she did *not* exercise. I had her start jumping on a rebounder first thing in the morning for only five minutes, gradually increasing her time as she became conditioned, and told her to continue with my previous recommendations.

Well, she has had daily bowel movements ever since. Also, her headaches went away, her skin cleared up, and she had tremendous energy. She was very happy and surprised at the healing effect of exercise.

H_2O 101

At normal activity levels, people lose two to three cups of water a day in perspiration. But during an hour of vigorous exercise, people sweat out approximately a quart of water.[1]

Exercise slows down the aging process.

In a study published in the *American Journal of Physiology*, Christiaan Leeuwenburgh, a professor at the University of Florida College of Health and Human Performance, found that antioxidant intervention, which can come from taking antioxidant supplements or from a steady routine of exercise, slows parts of the aging process. "We were surprised to see that regular exercise training was about as effective in reducing levels of oxidation as a diet of antioxidants," Leeuwenburgh said.[2]

Exercise builds strong bones.

Bone density screening has gone high-tech and, as a result, more and more researchers can now measure the effects of various factors on the bone-building process and prevention of osteoporosis. Their research shows that exercise works better than calcium in building strong bones.

"Although calcium intake is often cited as the most important factor for healthy bones, our study suggests that exercise is really the predominant lifestyle determinant of bone strength in young women," said Tom Lloyd, PhD, an epidemiologist with the Penn State University College of Medicine, whose findings were reported in the *Journal of Pediatrics*.[3]

Exercise improves your digestion and promotes frequent bowel movements.

Exercise helps prevent constipation.[4] Studies have shown that physical activity may help to ease digestion problems and problems with the GI tract. That's the conclusion of a study in an October 2005 issue of *Clinical Gastroenterology and Hepatology*. The study of 1,801 men and women found that obese people who got some form of physical activity were less likely to suffer GI problems than inactive obese people. "It is well documented that maintaining a healthy diet and regular physical activity can benefit GI health," study author Rona L. Levy, a professor at the University of Washington in Seattle, said.[5]

Did You Know...?

If you have been watching what you eat and working out, and yet the scale isn't moving, don't be discouraged. Muscle weighs more than fat, and it increases the metabolic rate, helping to burn fat, too. So, generally speaking, the more muscle you build, the more fat you will lose.

Exercise gives you restful sleep.

One of the best ways to improve the quality of your sleep is to exercise. Researchers found that women who participated in forty-five minutes of aerobics in the morning were about 70 percent less likely to have trouble sleeping than those who exercised less.[6] You shouldn't exercise within three hours of bedtime because it can cause insomnia; however, stretching and relaxing your muscles at any time of the day help to ease stiffness and have also been shown to make people 30 percent less likely to have trouble sleeping.[7] For more information on sleep, see my book *The Bible Cure for Sleep Disorders*.

Exercise helps prevent colds and flu.

Research shows that aerobic exercise such as brisk walking, jogging, or cycling boosts the body's defenses against viruses and bacteria during the cold and flu season. Too much exercise can increase your risk of infection, but moderate amounts (thirty minutes, three to four times per week) produce positive results by increasing the circulation of immune cells from bone marrow, the lungs, and the spleen.[8]

Exercise reduces depression.

Exercise increases serotonin and dopamine levels, which helps to relieve symptoms of anxiety and depression. One study looked at aerobic exercise as a means of treating clinical depression. An aerobic exercise program was compared to standard medication in a group of older adult patients. Medication relieved symptoms of depression more rapidly at the outset, but aerobic exercise was shown to be equally effective to medication over the course of the four-month study. Since some medications for depression have adverse effects or cease to be as effective with prolonged use, this was an important finding—aerobic exercise may be a very viable long-term therapy.[9]

Exercise improves memory retention and reaction time.

Prolonged exposure of your neurons (nerve cells) to high levels of stress hormones, like cortisol, decreases your brain's ability to take up glucose, and neurons begin to atrophy and eventually die. This results in a decrease in memory retention. Regular aerobic exercise helps to lower cortisol levels, which may help to improve memory.

Exercise slows Alzheimer's disease and may help prevent Parkinson's disease.

Carl Cotman, a neuroscientist at the University of California, has conducted research with laboratory mice that suggests physical exercise can slow the progression of Alzheimer's disease. Testing has also shown that exercise may prevent Parkinson's symptoms from developing in animals predisposed with that disease.[10]

Exercise increases lung capacity.

As we age, our lung capacity diminishes. Cardiovascular activity and exercise can combat this because aerobic exercise increases lung capacity. So while our lung capacity may continue to diminish, it does so at a slower pace.[11]

Exercise alleviates pain.

It might sound crazy to suggest exercising when you are in pain, but regular exercise is a bigger pain-fighting weapon than you might think. Aerobic exercise causes the release of endorphins, which are morphine-like molecules produced by the body. In an article published by the Mayo Clinic, it was reported that regular exercise actually reduces chronic pain for many people. The article quotes Dr. Edward Laskowski of Mayo Clinic as saying, "Years ago, people who were in pain were told to rest, but now we know the exact opposite is true. When you rest, you become deconditioned—which may actually contribute to chronic pain."[12]

Exercise increases your energy level.

Aerobic exercise in your target heart rate range will actually increase your energy. Most people have the excuse that they are simply too tired to exercise; they don't realize that regular aerobic exercise can dramatically increase their energy.[13]

Hopefully, all these benefits have inspired you to start an exercise routine immediately, if you don't already have one. If you have followed the action steps for the last couple of days, then you are well on your way! Good for you! Your walking routine is a good foundation for a lifetime of exercise.

BUILDING BLOCKS TO A HEALTHY LIFE

DAY 24 DAY 24 DAY 24

POINTS TO PONDER: *Exercise tones the muscles, improves digestion, promotes frequent bowel movements, slows down the aging process, promotes mental health, and even improves the memory. Done correctly, exercise will help you sleep better.*

ACTION STEP: *Purchase a pedometer at a drug store or discount store. (A pedometer senses your body's motion and counts the number of steps you take.) You can get one for as little as ten dollars. Wear it all day today to gauge your level of normal activity.*

DAY 25: Aerobic Exercise

I can't say it enough—brisk walking is one of the best exercises I can recommend, and it's virtually free. It can give you three times the normal amount of oxygen you would otherwise get. Buy a good pair of walking shoes so you don't injure your feet, and find a soft walking surface so you don't injure your joints. Walk slow enough so that you can talk, but walk fast enough so that you can't sing. Window-shopping doesn't count. Keep a steady pace without stopping.

One of my patients started walking briskly four times a week for thirty minutes, and after one year she had lost eighty pounds. "What about your diet?" I asked her.

"I didn't change my eating habits at all," she said.

Not bad results for a regular walk around the block!

Choose your exercise location wisely. Exercising by a busy highway is almost worse than sitting at home eating bonbons. I see some people jogging by the side of the road during high traffic, and not ten feet away buses and trucks go by pumping out big plumes of diesel exhaust. Those pollutants go into every cell in your body, and it's difficult to get rid of some of them.

Walking is a form of aerobic exercise. *Aerobic* means "in the presence of air." It's the kind of exercise that gets you breathing deeply and more rapidly than normal. Aerobic exercises generally work the large muscle groups of the body in repetitive motions for a sustained period of time. Other forms of aerobic exercises include:

- Jogging
- Cycling
- Rowing
- Elliptical machine or glider
- Aerobic dance routines
- Stair stepping

Quick Quiz

A 160-pound person burns this many calories per minute while walking briskly (5 mph):

a. 8.7 calories per minute

b. 15 calories per minute

c. 2.1 calories per minute

Answer: a. 8.7 calories per minute. Slower walking (2 mph) burns only 3.4 calories per minute—less than half that of brisk walking.[1]

- Skating
- Cross-country skiing
- Singles tennis
- Racquetball
- Basketball
- Ballroom dancing or other forms of dance
- Swimming

The first thing to do before you begin any exercise program is to have your physician give you a thorough exam. Nobody should start an aerobic exercise program until they know their body can handle it. It's also a good idea to have an EKG and a stress test to ensure you have a healthy heart. Your heart is a muscle, and it must be conditioned gradually and consistently—like all your muscles—to reach its optimum performance. Don't try to run a five-mile race or a marathon tomorrow if you have been a couch potato for the last five years. It will do more harm than good! The American College of Sports Medicine recommends a medical examination and exercise testing prior to participation in vigorous exercise for all male adults over forty and females over fifty.

Once you have been examined, choose your aerobic exercise—any activity or sport that gets the heart pumping and uses major muscle groups. Obese individuals should avoid running because it jars the back, hips, ankles, and knees and eventually may predispose them to arthritis. Cycling, using the elliptical machine or glider, and brisk walking are low-intensity exercises that condition your heart without damaging or destroying joints or disks. I like for my obese patients to perspire; therefore, I usually don't start them swimming.

Watch out for high-intensity activities, where you're huffing and puffing and exceeding your target heart rate. This can result in injury to muscles, tendons, joints, or ligaments, and it usually creates many more free radicals, which may lead to heart attacks, accelerated aging, decreased immune function, and even cancer.

If you simply have no time to begin an aerobic exercise program, just begin to move more: park your car further away in the parking lot, take the stairs instead of the elevator, and take a walk after lunch or dinner. Simply moving more during the day will enable you to reap the tremendous benefits of exercise.

Exercise Targets

Once you have chosen your activity, start slow—really slow. Exercise just a few minutes a day for a few weeks. Let your body get accustomed to what you're doing. You need to gradually condition unused muscle groups. Weekend warriors injure themselves by going from no exercise to intense exercise. Not only are they more prone to sprains, strains, tendonitis, and bursitis, but also the intense exercise can trigger a heart attack or stroke. You must ease into it.

Studies show that even a few ten-minute bursts of activity per day have beneficial effects on body and mind.[2] Taking a brisk walk or climbing up and down the stairs can lower your cholesterol and blood pressure, increase your vitality, and reduce your body fat. Your goal should be to exercise four times a week for thirty minutes, or:

- Most adults: Engage in at least thirty minutes of moderate-intensity physical activity, above usual activity, at work or home on most days of the week.
- Children and adolescents: Engage in at least sixty minutes of physical activity on most, preferably all, days of the week.
- Pregnant women: In the absence of medical or obstetric complications, incorporate thirty minutes or more of moderate-intensity physical activity on most days of the week.
- Older adults: Participate in regular physical activity to reduce functional declines associated with aging.[4]

Climb Your Way to a Longer Life

One Harvard study revealed a 23 percent higher mortality risk and a 56 percent higher coronary heart disease risk in men who climbed less than twenty flights of stairs per week than those who climbed more. If you live in a two-story home, be sure to climb the stairs at least a few times per day in order to meet the minimum twenty flights per week you need to reap these benefits.[3]

Your target heart rate (or "training zone") during exercise can be figured by subtracting your age from 220. Multiply that by .6 (60 percent). Multiply the original number again times .9 (90 percent). The range between the two numbers is your target heart rate range.[5] For example, if you are forty years old:

220 - 40 = 180
180 x .6 = 108 low target
180 x .9 = 162 high target

Your target heart rate is between 108 and 162 beats per minute. If you push much higher than that, you are stressing your body too much and are probably doing more harm than good. Find your training zone, and exercise in it. Don't try to be Superman or Wonder Woman. If it has been years since you have exercised, always start out at 60 percent, which is the low target number, and gradually increase your heart rate after a few weeks to 65 percent, and then after a few more weeks to 70 percent, and so on. *Never* start at 90 percent of your target heart rate!

Dealing With Muscle Pain After Exercise

Delayed onset muscle soreness (DOMS) after exercise is normal when you begin an exercise program. You might feel stiff and sore in the hours and days after you exercise. Here are tips to treat and avoid muscle soreness:[6]

- Warm up thoroughly five minutes before activity and cool down completely three to five minutes afterward.
- Perform easy stretching after exercise.
- When beginning a new activity, start gradually and build up your time and intensity over time.
- Avoid making sudden major changes in the type of exercises you do.
- Avoid making sudden major changes in the amount of time that you exercise.
- Wait. Soreness will go away in three to seven days with no special treatment.
- Do some easy low-impact aerobic exercise—this will increase blood flow to the affected muscles, which may help diminish soreness.
- Gently stretch the affected area.
- Gently massage the affected muscles.

Whatever aerobic exercise you do, gradually increase the time and intensity, going from five minutes to ten, then eventually up to thirty or even forty minutes. Drink plenty of water to replace what you are losing through sweat and exhalation. Avoid exercising immediately after a meal because exercise triggers the body to carry blood away from your stomach and intestines to your muscles, which impairs digestion. Wait at least two hours after you eat before exercising unless you eat only a light snack.

BUILDING BLOCKS TO A HEALTHY LIFE

POINTS TO PONDER: *Walking is one of the safest and easiest forms of aerobic exercise. Walk slow enough so that you can talk, but fast enough so that you can't sing. Never exercise along a busy highway where toxic fumes and automobile exhaust can put your health at risk. When beginning an exercise program, begin with a low-intensity activity and gradually increase your level. Warm up five minutes before exercising by walking slowly and take five minutes after exercising to cool down.*

ACTION STEP: *Using the formula on page 129, find your target heart rate. If you recently started exercising, begin by exercising at the lower limit (60 percent).*

DAY 26: Anaerobic Exercise

Aerobic exercise is great for the heart and lungs, but it's also important to strengthen your bones and muscles with muscle-toning exercises. *Anaerobic*, which means "without air," refers to short, higher-intensity workouts. Working out with weights and performing calisthenics are the most effective way to do this.

Weight training and calisthenics help prevent osteoporosis—the thinning of the bones that is a major health threat to forty-four million Americans.[1] It occurs mainly in women past the age of fifty, but it can also affect men. According to the National Osteoporosis Foundation, eight million women in the United States suffer from osteoporosis, while two million men are also afflicted with the disease.[2] A person with osteoporosis may literally start shrinking in size—or develop *kyphosis*, which is a hump on their upper back.

Working With Weights

From age thirty on, everyone needs to exercise either with weights or calisthenics to keep their muscles and bones strong. Remember, low-intensity workouts are not harmful.

If you can afford it, I highly recommend that you find a certified personal trainer to train you in the correct form and technique. He or she can get you started on the right program, help you avoid injury, and teach you flexibility and stretching exercises, too. It's also helpful—and safer—to lift weights with a friend once you get going. It also keeps you accountable to someone so you are less likely to miss a workout.

Start each workout with an aerobic warm-up of five to ten minutes to get blood flowing to your muscles. This will decrease your chance of injury.

Then find a weight that you can lift for at least eight, but not more than twelve, repetitions. You will be training at about 60 percent of your maximum ability, which will prevent injury and excessive free radical formation. Perform each repetition slowly, using good control. You can perform more than one set of repetitions, but initially rest for at least a minute or two between working the same muscle group. In time, you will only need to rest thirty seconds to a minute between repetitions. Here are some of the benefits of weightlifting:[3]

- Increases muscle mass
- Elevates your metabolism, which helps burn fat
- Improves posture
- Provides better support for joints
- Reduces the risk of injury from everyday activities
- Reverses the loss of muscle tissue that normally accompanies aging
- Helps to prevent osteoporosis
- Increases levels of dopamine, serotonin, and norepinephrine, which can help to improve mood and counter feelings of depression

The heavier the weight you are lifting, the fewer repetitions you should attempt. Heavier weights with low repetitions improve muscular strength. Lighter weights with high repetitions (more than twelve repetitions) build muscular endurance and tone the muscles. Moderate weights with moderate repetitions do both.

As your strength increases over the weeks, you may increase the amount of weight you lift by no more than 5 percent each workout. I recommend training using moderate weights and moderate repetitions (eight to twelve repetitions) to avoid injury.

A certified trainer will help you exercise your eight to ten different muscle groups, including the chest, back, shoulders, arms, abdomen, upper and lower back, and legs and calves. He or she will help you to maintain proper form, work your full range of motion, and remember to exhale during the hard part of a lift.

Quick Quiz

True or false: If you don't feel pain, you're not lifting enough weight.

Answer: False. *If you feel pain, you are generally lifting too much weight and/or doing too many repetitions. You should feel resistance and should strain a bit, but pain itself is a sign you are going beyond your abilities and may injure yourself.*

Ideally you should work out with weights three days per week with a day between workouts.

Calisthenics

You can get some of the benefits of weight training by using your own body weight to build muscles. This is called calisthenics, and it includes push-ups, pull-ups, sit-ups, lunges, calf raises, and dozens more exercises. You can do these whenever you are without equipment.

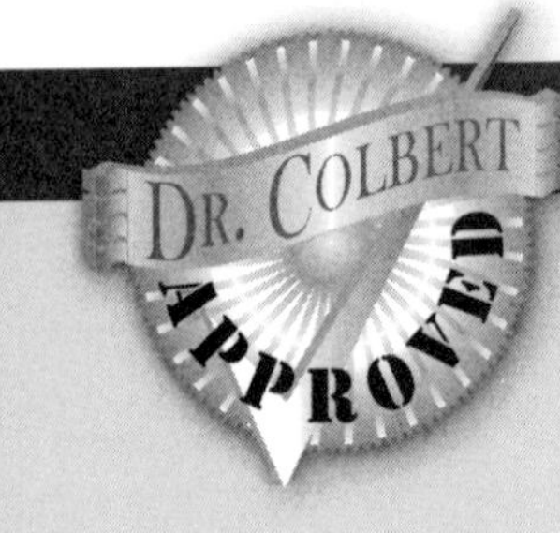

Dr. Colbert Approved Exercise Program

There are three components to a good exercise program:

1. Aerobic exercise, such as brisk walking
2. Strengthening and toning, such as weight lifting and calisthenics
3. Flexibility, such as stretching

Posture and Flexibility

Part of exercising is simply maintaining good posture. Try this throughout the day: Stand up, extend your arms straight down the side of your body, make a fist with your hands, and twist your fists backward, so that the palms of your hands face outward. Breathe slowly and deeply, in and out. Try to maintain this posture for twenty to thirty seconds.

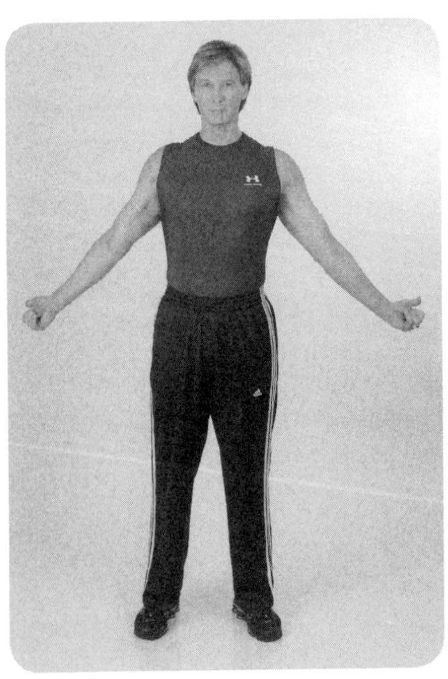

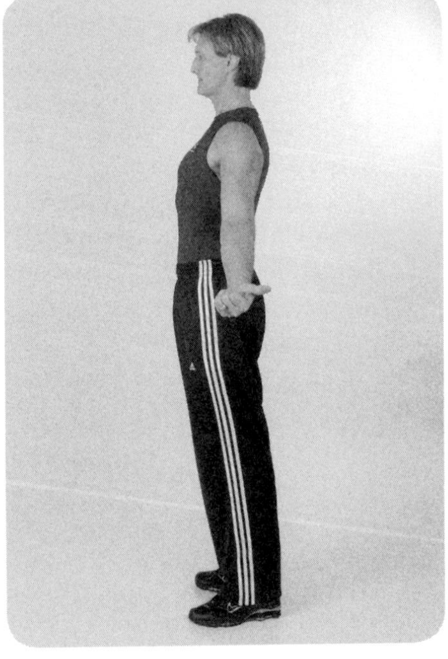

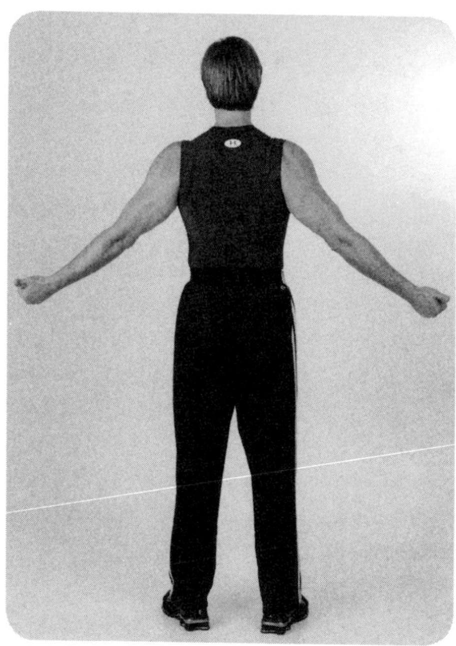

This simple exercise will usually align your spine, invigorate you, and improve your breathing. By delivering more oxygen into your lungs, you are going to have more mental clarity and energy, and you are going to feel renewed. I try to do this postural exercise at least hourly during working hours.

Anyone suffering from arthritis should begin with flexibility and stretching before starting weight training or aerobic exercises. You want to put your joints through a full range of motion.

Here are four tips for flexibility:

1. Inhale deeply before the stretch.
2. Exhale during the stretch.
3. Perform all stretching exercises slowly and without bouncing.
4. Never stretch so much that it begins to hurt.

Body Recall, Inc., is an excellent program for improving flexibility for older individuals. For more information, visit their Web site at http://www.bodyrecallinc.org.[4]

BUILDING BLOCKS TO A HEALTHY LIFE

DAY 26

POINTS TO PONDER: *Weight-training and calisthenics are part of a holistic approach to exercise, plus they help to build strong bones and muscles. Stretching promotes flexibility and can also serve as a good warm-up prior to exercise. Perform repetitions slowly using good technique.*

ACTION STEP: *Do the postural exercise a few times throughout the day today and maintain good posture. Hire a certified personal trainer and start a weight-training program, or get an exercise partner to whom you are accountable.*

DAY 27: Fun, Alternative Exercises

Many people don't enjoy traditional exercises like the ones we've been talking about, but they do enjoy alternative exercises that help stir the waters of their body with motion. Let's see some of the most helpful—and fun—alternative exercises.

Yoga

"Whoa!" you might say. "Why is a Christian doctor promoting yoga?" The answer is, I only promote *the physical exercises* of yoga, *never* its spiritual or Eastern meditative aspects. I feel that it is possible to ignore the spiritual baggage and religious associations that are often associated with yoga and still enjoy terrific, low-impact exercise that combines stretching and breathing to relax the body.

There are several types of yoga. Hatha yoga is the most popular type practiced in the United States. It concentrates on controlled breathing and posture. When I do yoga, I meditate on Christ and the names of Christ throughout the Bible. The slow breathing promotes relaxation, and the various postures of Hatha yoga promote flexibility by gently stretching the body into different positions.

Other forms of yoga include Ashtanga, or power yoga, generally preferred by athletes to develop strength and stamina. Bikram yoga is done in a hot room that is 100 degrees Fahrenheit or higher, and it is recommended only for extremely fit individuals. There are several other forms of yoga beyond these. I encourage people never to meditate on a mantra, but to meditate on the Scriptures or on the name of Jesus and His various attributes and titles in the Bible.

Yoga has been shown to decrease tension, stress, anxiety, depression, and hypertension. People who do a form of yoga called Sahaja show improvement in blood pressure, heart rate, levels of blood lactate, levels of the stress hormone epinephrine in the urine, and the galvanic skin resistance test, which indicates whether the patient is tense or relaxed.[1]

Yoga is different from most other forms of exercise in that it is not concerned with how many repetitions are performed or how well a person performs a particular exercise. Instead, yoga focuses your attention on how your body is structured and how to move without aggravating an injury or causing pain. It teaches you to breathe properly and to integrate breathing with positions of the body. You don't strain or force your body when doing yoga, but rather gently stretch various muscles. It feels terrific! It improves your strength, flexibility, and endurance. In fact, one study in the *Journal of the American Medical Association* reported that daily yoga practice could reduce the pain associated with carpal tunnel syndrome.[2]

If you are concerned with flexibility and learning to understand your various muscle groups through low-impact exercise, yoga is probably your best option. I recommend finding a Christian yoga class, and I caution you to watch for Sanskrit language that pays tribute to Hindu deities, metaphysical/New Age jargon ("negative and positive energy," "divinity within you," "focus on the third eye," etc.), and projection (emptying your mind or stepping outside your body). If you feel uncomfortable in any way, it might be God's way of telling you that a yoga class is not right for you. If that is the case, consider the next three alternatives for exercise.

Tai Chi

Tai Chi is an ancient Chinese martial art that involves slow, smooth, and fluid movements. It emphasizes diaphragmatic or abdominal breathing. It is an exceptionally good exercise for older people who have arthritis, peripheral vascular disease, chronic obstructive pulmonary disease, osteoporosis, or other physical problems. The Arthritis Foundation recommends Tai Chi for individuals with arthritis.[3]

Research has shown that Tai Chi may improve muscle mass, tone, flexibility, strength, stamina, balance, coordination, posture, and well-being. It can also give similar cardiovascular benefits to modern aerobic exercise. People who practice Tai Chi report less tension, depression, anger, fatigue, confusion, and anxiety, and feel more vigorous.[4]

Tai Chi movements are smooth, graceful, low-intensity, and accompanied by rhythmic abdominal breathing. A typical exercise session is a series of gentle, deliberate movements or postures combined into a sequential "choreography." These series of movements are called *forms*, and each form is comprised of a series of twenty to one hundred Tai Chi movements. Each form can take up to twenty minutes to complete. Tai Chi relies totally on technique rather than power or strength.

Tai Chi lowers stress hormones, increases energy, and helps clear the mind. You can do it at any age, even if you have a chronic disease or health problem. Tai Chi calms the mind, promotes flexibility, and exercises and tones the body, including the cardiovascular system. Like yoga, it includes meditation. I believe this is a great opportunity to meditate on God's Word!

Pilates

Pilates exercises were developed by Joseph Pilates in the early twentieth century. As a child, Joseph suffered from rheumatic fever, rickets, and asthma. He was determined to overcome his ailments, and he began studying anatomy at a young age. During World War II, he worked as a nurse and developed equipment to help rehabilitate the war injured. He would take bedsprings and attach them to the ceiling so that bedridden patients might exercise and gain strength. Eventually he opened an exercise studio in New York City, where he trained many great dancers.[5]

Instead of performing many repetitions of each exercise, Pilates preferred fewer, more precise movements, requiring control and form. He designed more than five hundred specific exercises. The most frequent form, called "matwork," involves a series of calisthenic motions performed without weights or apparatus on a padded mat. Pilates believed that mental health and physical health were essential to one another. He created what is claimed to be a method of total body conditioning that emphasizes proper alignment, centering, concentration, control, precision, breathing, and flowing movement (the Pilates Principles) that results in increased flexibility, strength, muscle tone, body awareness, energy, and improved mental concentration.[6] Pilates also helps to reduce tension and stress. Many health clubs now offer Pilates exercise classes.

Ballroom Dancing

Ballroom dancing is an excellent alternative for anyone who does not enjoy exercising but does enjoy dancing! It provides most benefits of aerobic exercise without the feeling that you are exercising. It is low-impact aerobic exercise that uses the large muscle groups of the body. It can be done for thirty minutes or for an entire evening.

Ballroom dancing can help you develop coordination, balance, and rhythm. It is usually associated with a very pleasant environment, with soothing music, and with an opportunity for creative expression and social interaction. Among the more common dances are the fox-trot, swing, cha-cha, tango, waltz, rumba, mambo, samba, and merengue.

People who become bored with treadmills or exercise bikes usually find ballroom dancing a fun alternative. Classes are often offered at a college, university, or private studio. The basic steps for most dances can be learned from videos, DVDs, or books. An inexpensive way to explore the possibility of doing ballroom dancing is to rent or buy a basic dance video.

Ballroom dancing is also a great way for married couples to reconnect. It's a great way to spend time together and exercise at the same time!

DAY 27 DAY 27 DAY 27

BUILDING BLOCKS TO A HEALTHY LIFE

POINTS TO PONDER: *There are many alternatives to traditional exercises. Yoga is a healthy alternative to more traditional means of exercise. It combines low-impact exercise with stretching and breathing. Tai Chi involves slow, smooth movements. It's great for older people, especially those who suffer from arthritis. Tai Chi movements help improve muscle mass, strength, and flexibility, among its other many health benefits. Pilates also involves low-intensity exercise with stretching. It helps reduce stress, increase flexibility, and tone muscles. Ballroom dancing is a fun way to exercise without feeling as if you are exercising. It's a great way for couples to reconnect and spend time together.*

ACTION STEP: *Contact your local community college, vocational school, or community activity center. Find out when the next dance class begins, join, and have fun!*

DAY 28: Exercise for Life!

Health clubs know a secret: most exercisers drop out. Clubs sign up more people than can use their facilities, knowing that many people who pay for membership won't show up. The health club pencil pushers are right. My experience as a doctor has taught me that people often start well, then quit exercising. Think about all the unused exercise equipment lying under beds, under sheets in the guest bedroom, and in garages across America. Big chains like Play-It-Again Sports thrive on good intentions that never take hold.

Quick Quiz

Walk the Dog—and Lose Weight

In a university study, people who walked their dog for twenty minutes a day, five days a week lost how many pounds after one year?

a. 4 pounds

b. 9 pounds

c. 14 pounds

d. 22 pounds

Answer: c. 14 pounds. According to a University of Missouri–Columbia study, participants, none of whom were regular walkers before the study, began by walking dogs ten minutes per day, three times each week, and worked up to twenty minutes per day, five times each week. Those who followed this program for fifty weeks lost an average of fourteen pounds. Those who walked only twenty-six weeks didn't see significant weight loss.[1]

How to Succeed at Exercising

Your body will not do the right thing without some prodding. It doesn't like being exercised at first, but after about three weeks your body will change its mind: it will desire and expect to exercise. Here are the best tips I know to bulletproof your exercise routine.

Build exercise into your schedule. Schedule it like an important doctor's appointment. Choose a time you won't waver from, and put yourself on automatic so you don't give yourself an "out."

A workout before breakfast, before lunch, or before dinner is great. Just don't exercise late at night, since you may be too charged up to sleep. Also, avoid exercise immediately after a meal. It will pull the blood from your stomach and intestines (where it's needed to help digestion) to your muscles. You are likely to start belching and to have heartburn and other digestive problems. Exercise before you eat or two hours after you eat. However, a light snack before exercising is fine.

Choose an exercise you enjoy. The best exercise is the one you'll do. If you have arthritis and walking hurts your knees, choose biking, elliptical machines, pool exercises, yoga, or Tai Chi instead. Tailor your routine to your physical condition.

Have an exercise partner. Partners keep you accountable to do the exercise and should make the exercise time more enjoyable.

Choose a location you enjoy. Walk in malls, parks, mountains, on the beach, or near a lake. Make exercise a complete sensory experience.

Change it up. Change your routine, either by location, time of day, or by the exercise you do. Make it fun.

Do occupational/transportation exercises. Seize every opportunity to increase your activity level. Park at the far end of the parking lot and walk to the store. Use stairs when you can. Default to the active option.

Below is a table of routine activities and how many calories are burned in one hour of that activity.[2]

HOW MANY CALORIES ARE BURNED DURING ACTIVITY?

Activity	Calories Burned/ Hour	Activity Level
Sleeping	55	Low
Eating	85	Low
Sewing	85	Low
Sitting	85	Low
Standing	100	Low
Driving	110	Low
Office work	140	Low
Housework, moderate	160+	Moderate
Golf, w/golf cart	180	Moderate
Golf, w/no golf cart	240	Moderate
Gardening, planting	250	Moderate

HOW MANY CALORIES ARE BURNED DURING ACTIVITY?		
Activity	**Calories Burned/ Hour**	**Activity Level**
Dancing, ballroom	260	Moderate
Walking, 3 mph	280	Moderate
Ping Pong	290	Moderate
Tennis	350+	Moderate
Water aerobics	400	Moderate
Skating/rollerblading	420+	Moderate
Dancing, aerobic	420+	Moderate
Aerobics	450+	Moderate
Bicycling, moderate	450+	Moderate
Jogging, 5 mph	500	High
Gardening, digging	500	High
Swimming, active	500+	High
Hiking	500+	High
Step aerobics	550+	High
Rowing	550+	High
Power walking	600+	High
Cycling, studio	650	High
Squash	650+	High
Skipping rope	700+	High
Running	700+	High

And if you're thinking about grabbing a snack, think again. Here are the calorie contents of popular snacks and how much exercise you would need to do to burn those calories.[3]

Snack Food	Number of calories	Amount of time to burn calories	Exercise
Chips Ahoy, 3 cookies	240 calories	30 minutes	Brisk walking
Oreos, 3 cookies	169 calories	About 20 minutes	Brisk walking
Glazed doughnut, 4 oz.	400 calories	50 minutes	Brisk walking
Ritz crackers, original, 6 oz. serving	80 calories	10 minutes	Brisk walking
Burger King Whopper	670 calories	1 hour and 30 minutes	Brisk walking
Baked Doritos Nacho Cheesier, 10 chips	8 calories each	10 minutes	Brisk walking
Lay's Classic potato chips, 10 chips	8 calories each	10 minutes	Brisk walking

Taking Cues From Your Body

Take a rest when needed. On days when you are exhausted, or after nights in which you have not slept well, don't push yourself to exercise. Listen to your body, and learn when to take a day off.

I say this from experience. For years I pushed my body very hard until I had a heat stroke and almost died. I had not allowed my body to stop when it needed to stop. Now, older and wiser, I have slowed my pace, and I listen to what my body is saying.

I have talked at length with many highly trained athletes, including marathon runners, who are compulsive exercise enthusiasts. The downside of compulsive exercise is that many of these people suffer from constant muscle soreness from overtraining and chronic fatigue. By contrast, I recommend low-intensity workouts and moderation in physical exertion, because the pressure associated with excessive exercise can undo the very thing you are trying to accomplish. It's important to get your heartbeat up to a good training rate, but exercising as hard as you can is like flooring the accelerator of your car. It's not good for the engine. When you push your body too hard, you release tremendous amounts of free radicals into your system that can damage cells, tissues, and even organs. The increase of free radicals also accelerates the aging process. Overtraining can suppress your immune system, increase your risk of injury, increase your body fat by raising cortisol levels, and interfere with your emotional and mental health. It can cause as much stress to the body as trauma, surgery, infections, and anxiety.

Examples of overtraining include:

- Spending hours on a treadmill, running off the stress of a hard day.
- Pushing yourself to lift heavier weights for more repetitions even though your strength is diminishing.
- Training at a heart rate over 90 percent of your target heart rate or starting out exercising at over 80 percent of your target heart rate.
- Lifting weights for too long, at too high intensity, at one session or for too many days in a row. It's generally best to lift weights every other day to let your muscles recuperate.

With these tips you should have everything you need to find an enjoyable way to stir the waters of life with exercise.

BUILDING BLOCKS TO A HEALTHY LIFE

POINTS TO PONDER: *Building an exercise program into your schedule doesn't have to be boring; it can be as fun as you make it. Find exercises that you enjoy doing—such as swimming or dancing. Look for opportunities throughout the day to fit in occupational/transportation or "leisure-time" activities such as gardening, walking the dog, parking your car in the space furthest away from the door to the store, taking the stairs instead of the elevator, and so on. Be creative and innovative with your exercise routine, and make it an exercise program for life!*

ACTION STEP: *Set goals for the type of exercise you will be doing and how often. Start slow, but gradually increase your activity to a level that's right for you.*

PILLAR 5

Detoxification

DAY 29: Believe It or Not—You're Probably Toxic

A few years ago a woman came into my office in great discomfort. She had been diagnosed five years ago with chronic fatigue and fibromyalgia. She had severe muscle aches in her shoulders, back, legs, and arms. She was unable to sleep at night without sleep medications. Even though she had been to numerous physicians, she was no better off. She was taking many different medications and experiencing numerous side effects from them.

During her physical exam I discovered that she had twelve large silver fillings. Realize that silver or amalgam fillings are actually about 50 percent mercury. When I performed a six-hour urine test for toxic metals, I found extremely high levels of mercury in her urine. It was also interesting to note that her symptoms began three years after she had five silver fillings replaced with five new silver fillings.

I began to slowly remove the mercury from her body with natural supplements as she saw a biological dentist, who replaced her silver fillings with porcelain crowns. After all the silver fillings were removed, I was then able to chelate (remove) the remainder of the mercury with both natural supplements and a medicine that chelates mercury. Within a few months her chronic fatigue and fibromyalgia totally resolved.

Unfortunately, it's not this simple with most of my chronically diseased patients. In most patients with chronic disease, we are dealing with numerous toxins, heavy metals, chemicals, and microbes that may be causing or exacerbating their condition. Please do not run out and have all of your silver fillings removed at once, or you may actually get sicker. But read on, and you will begin to understand that you are probably toxic.

Toxic Onslaught

Most people are toxic to some degree—and I don't mean their personalities, but their physical bodies. Everyone has toxins stored in his or her body. It's similar to forgetting to take the trash cans to the curb on trash day, and the garbage piles up in your garage. Your cans eventually overflow, and the stench worsens. You feel sick just walking near them.

After a few weeks the smell of the garbage is so bad that you can even smell it inside the house.

That's a similar picture of what happens in your body when you take in toxins but don't get rid of them. Your body has waste management systems that keep you healthy when they function properly. But, like a city that neglects its trash removal, your body can eventually become overwhelmed with toxins. That's what it means to be toxic.

Can Toxicity Be Avoided?

I'm convinced that toxicity cannot be avoided entirely. We live in a toxic world. There are about eighty thousand chemicals registered for use in the United States, and we add about two thousand more every year. These chemicals are used in food, prescription drugs, supplements, household products, personal products, and lawn care products.[1] From the moment of conception a child is exposed to a plethora of toxins in his environment, first from his mother, then from the world into which he's born. In a report by the Environmental Working Group, the American Red Cross took umbilical-cord blood samples of ten babies and tested them for contaminants. The tests showed that they had an average of 287 contaminants, including methyl mercury, fire retardants, and pesticides, including DDT and chlorine. Of these chemicals, 180 of them are carcinogenic in humans.[2]

Some of the air we breathe is toxic—more than 80,000 metric tons of carcinogens are released in the air annually in North America.[3] But we can clean our air inside our home and workplace. A significant amount of our water is polluted, with more than 2,100 chemicals in most municipal water supplies.[4] However, we can learn to choose clean, pure water. Much of the food supply also contains toxins. However, we can learn to choose living, organic foods instead of pesticide-laden foods.

Because of the way Americans eat and drink, and because of the toxicity of our environment—everything from manufacturing to agriculture—many people's bodies are backed up with microscopic garbage. It is as if their body's waste management department has gone on strike.

Thankfully, there is an answer: detoxification. There are simple things that you can start doing today to rid your body of toxins and to help your waste management systems keep them out. Decrease your exposure to toxins by:

1. Choosing more living, organic foods, free-range lean meats, and low-fat organic dairy.
2. Choose clean, pure spring or filtered water instead of tap water.
3. Breathe clean air, and do not stroll, walk, or jog along busy roads or highways. Don't wait outside airport terminals, inhaling diesel exhaust. Avoid secondhand smoke in restaurants and public buildings.
4. Wear rubber gloves if you use chemicals for cleaning. Better yet, check for natural cleaning alternatives and natural personal care products.
5. Work with your doctor to try and get yourself off of as much medication as possible. This will give your liver a break and will allow it to rid your body of built-up toxins.

BUILDING BLOCKS TO A HEALTHY LIFE

POINTS TO PONDER: *Toxicity permeates our environment, which is affecting our health, but there are some things we can change. The toxic levels in our air, water, and food supply are increasing annually. There is hope through detoxifying our waste management system.*

ACTION STEP: *Call your local waste management office and find out how you can properly dispose of toxic chemicals in your garage or shed. Get rid of old paint, unused pesticides, and used automobile oil left over from the last oil change you did.*

DAY 30: Where Toxins Come From

When you were in grade school, did you ever do an experiment where you take a celery stick and let it sit in a glass of blue- or red-colored water overnight? Remember what happened? You woke up the next morning to find a blue or red stick of celery. As the celery took in the water, it turned the color of its environment. Toxins have a similar effect on our bodies. Toxins get into our bodies through the air we breathe, the food we eat, the water we drink, and direct contact with our skin. And there are some surprising sources of toxins you need to pay attention to as well. Let's examine the main avenues by which toxins get into our bodies.

Air Pollution

Much of the planet's air is unavoidably dirty. In cities, smog is so common that people hardly notice it anymore. In rural America, pesticides, dust, and ozone contribute to the problem. Carbon monoxide from buses, cars, and airplanes; heavy metals and chemicals from factories and refineries; and smoke from agricultural fires and forest fires all contribute to the gaseous soup we breathe.

The American Lung Association State of the Air 2005 report shows that more than half of the U.S. population live in counties that have unhealthy levels of either ozone or particulate pollution. At greatest risk are people with asthma, chronic bronchitis and emphysema, cardiovascular disease, and, for the first time listed, diabetes.[1]

Smog may also harden your arteries. A study from the University of Southern California's Keck School of Medicine showed that as levels of pollution rose, so did the thickness of plaque in the carotid arteries of the study participants.[2] In other words, your commute may be killing you, and not just with frustration.

For people in agricultural areas, pesticide exposure is difficult to avoid. The most commonly used pesticides are easily absorbed into the skin and breathed into the lungs. Farmers who work with these chemicals are at greater risk to develop brain cancers, prostate cancer, leukemia, and lymphoma.[3]

The Indoor Problem

Sometimes indoor air can be just as bad as outdoor air—and is usually worse. Chemicals and bacteria get trapped and recirculated throughout heating and air conditioning systems of buildings. So do chemical compounds used in construction. New carpets and pressed wood release formaldehyde into your breathing air. Paints release unhealthy solvents.

Cigarette smoke is a major airborne health hazard. According to the American Cancer Society, about half of all Americans who continue to smoke will die because of the habit. Each year, about 438,000 people die in the United States from tobacco use. Nearly one in every five deaths is related to smoking. Cigarettes kill more Americans than alcohol, car accidents, suicide, AIDS, homicide, and illegal drugs combined.[4] Cigarette smoke contains more than forty-seven hundred chemicals, two hundred poisons, and fifty carcinogens, including benzo[a]pyrene and NNK, which cause lung cancer; nitrosamines, which cause cancer of the lung, respiratory system, and other organs; aromatic amines, which cause bladder and breast cancer; formaldehyde, which causes nasal cancer; and benzene, which causes leukemia.[6] In addition to causing emphysema, cigarette smoking increases the chance of cardiovascular disease, miscarriages, and birth defects. Smoking also increases skin wrinkles, causing smokers to look older than nonsmokers of the same age.

> **And the Winner Is . . .**
>
> Thirty percent of all cancer deaths are attributed to tobacco use, making it tied with obesity as the number one risk factor associated with the disease.[5]

Secondhand smoke is just as hazardous to the nonsmoker as the smoke inhaled by the smoker himself. One study showed that breathing in someone else's smoke for an hour is worse than smoking four cigarettes yourself.[7] As I stated in my book *Toxic Relief*, secondhand cigarette smoke contains cadmium, cyanide, lead, arsenic, tars, radioactive material, dioxin (which is a toxic pesticide), carbon monoxide, hydrogen cyanide, nitrogen oxides, nicotine, and about four thousand other chemicals.

I had a child come see me who was suffering with terrible asthma attacks. His mother smoked, but not in the house. She limited her smoking to her car, but the smoke on her clothes and hair was affecting her son's lungs. I asked her, "Do you love this child enough to stop smoking?" She quit smoking, and the child's asthma improved significantly. He has rarely had asthma attacks since then.

Although a small number of states have instituted smoking bans, many states still allow smoking sections in restaurants, but the whole idea that smoke is limited to one section is a joke. That's like using one side of your swimming pool for bathroom breaks and believing the "other" side of the pool is clean!

Here are a couple of simple solutions that you can do today to begin cleaning the air you breathe.

- Replace your air conditioner filter every month, and clean your heating and air conditioning ducts at least every five years.
- If you have pets, keep them out of your bedroom when you sleep. This applies even to short-haired pets, which cause just as many allergies as long-haired pets. It's best to keep pets outdoors if at all possible.
- Avoid air fresheners that contain pesticides or are petroleum based. Stick with fragrance jars and dried botanicals, which are widely available. As an air freshener substitute, use a lemon spray or essential oils such as lavender.

This is just to help you get started; I will offer more solutions to "clearing the air" on Day 35.

Food

Almost all non-organically grown produce may be tainted by pesticides, herbicides, parasites, and chemicals. These toxins and microbes find their way into our food supply—and into our bodies.

In 2004, perchlorate—rocket fuel—made its way into the water supply in more than twenty states and in the Colorado River—the major source of drinking and irrigation water for Southern California and Arizona.[8] Eventually that contaminated water made its way into green leaf lettuce in Arizona and bottled spring water in Texas and California.[9] Perchlorate ingestion may trigger thyroid disorders.

Pesticides are absorbed in the intestinal tract from an animal's feed, and what is not

Pesticides Linked to Alzheimer's, Parkinson's, and Cancer

In laboratory tests with rats, researchers found that pesticide exposure caused changes in the same areas of the brain involved in multiple sclerosis, epilepsy, and Alzheimer's disease.[10]

A study of 143,000 people found that those exposed to pesticides had a 70 percent higher incidence of Parkinson's disease than those not reporting exposure.[11]

Studies show that farmers who have been exposed to pesticides have increased incidence of leukemia, non-Hodgkin's lymphoma, multiple myeloma, soft-tissue sarcoma, and cancers of the skin, lip, stomach, brain, and prostate.[12]

detoxified by the animal's liver may be deposited in their fatty tissues. When you eat meat, it eventually goes into your fatty tissues—including the fatty tissues in your brain.

If you eat processed foods, you welcome a host of chemicals into your body, including synthetic dyes, flavoring agents, chemical preservatives, emulsifiers, texturizers, humectants, ripening gases, bleaching agents, and sugar substitutes like aspartame. Chemical food additives are usually made from—brace yourself—petroleum or coal tar products. Bleaching agents can be so toxic that Germany has banned their use in flour since 1958.[13] One of the most toxic bleaching agents used is chloride oxide, also known as chlorine dioxide. When this chemical agent combines with the proteins that are left after the bran and germ are removed from the wheat, it forms a substance called alloxan. Alloxan may trigger selective destruction of beta cells in the pancreas, potentially causing type 2 diabetes.[14] Despite this, the FDA still allows companies to use this bleaching agent in foods.

Quick Quiz

Tainted Breast Milk

When compared to nursing mothers who don't eat meat, how much more pesticide contamination do nursing mothers who eat meat have in their breast milk?

a. Twice as much

b. Thirty-five times as much

c. Ten times as much

Answer: b. Thirty-five times as much.[15]

Rice grown in the United States has been shown to have 1.4 to 5 times the amount of arsenic in it than rice from Europe, India, or Bangladesh. This disturbing trend happened as rice crops were grown in soils previously used to grow cotton, where arsenic was used to kill boll weevils. Arsenic-resistant rice was developed. As such the "healthy" grains accumulate more arsenic.[16]

Some extremely dangerous pesticides are banned in the United States but are still used by countries from which we import crops and foods. Those banned chemicals end up in our food supplies. Other toxic chemicals, such as DDT and PCBs, have been banned in the United States for decades, but since these chemicals remain in our water, land, and air, fish and animal products continue to be main sources of DDT and PCBs in our diets. DDT was developed as a pesticide in the 1940s, and PCBs were first created and used as cooling fluids in the late 1920s. The EPA lists DDT and PCBs as probable human carcinogens since both cause liver cancer in laboratory animals.[17]

These chemicals are stored in an animal's fat, so the best way to reduce your risk of ingesting DDT and PCBs is to choose lean cuts of organic meat and low-fat organic dairy products. Avoid sport-caught fish and shellfish, which are often high in DDT and PCBs. Commercial fish that are high in PCBs include Atlantic or farmed salmon, bluefish, wild striped bass, white and Atlantic croaker, blackback or winter flounder, summer flounder, and blue crab. Commercial fish that contain higher levels of pesticides, including DDT, are bluefish, wild striped bass, American eel, and Atlantic salmon. When preparing your meal, broil or bake your fish to allow as much fat as possible to drain from it.[18]

Parasites are another enemy of our food supply. One survey of public health laboratories reported that 15.6 percent of specimens examined contained a parasite.[19] Usually, third world countries are major exporters of food to the United States. Often the conditions in which the food is handled and shipped to the States is less than sanitary, which leaves our food supply and, ultimately, our digestive system vulnerable to parasites.[20] People who are eating more raw foods are predisposed to getting parasitic infections. Improper food handling and preparation also leave us exposed to intestinal parasites. Many times workers do not wash their hands before handling the food, which ends up on your plate.

Hydrochloric acid, which is the acid our stomach produces, is our first line of defense against these parasitic infections. Many individuals over fifty years of age as well as people who experience chronic stress will generally produce decreased amounts of hydrochloric acid as well as digestive enzymes, which predisposes them to parasitic infections, especially if they consume a lot of raw foods.

In order to maintain adequate levels of hydrochloric acid and enzymes and help prevent parasitic infections, try to learn how to relax. Doing something as simple as taking a few slow, deep breaths will enable you to unwind and secrete adequate amounts of digestive enzymes and hydrochloric acid. We will take a closer look at managing stress in Pillar 7.

There is a way to treat parasitic infections with medications and herbal remedies. People over the age of fifty may need a good digestive enzyme to help digest beans and vegetables. (See Appendix A for product information.)

Although our food and water supply may be toxic, we can detoxify our bodies by switching to an alkalinizing diet rich in fresh organic fruits and vegetables. Alkalinizing foods help to raise the pH of the tissues, enabling the body to release more toxins, whereas acidic foods cause the body to slow this process.[21] I will discuss the benefits of alkalinizing foods in detail in a couple of days.

Drink Healthy

The next step to detoxification is adequate filtered water. The most important ingredient in detoxifying the body is to drink plenty of filtered, clean water. Your body needs—minimum—two quarts of water a day.

I like to say that good water is "the ultimate detoxifier." Clean, alkaline water minus the toxins unburdens your liver and kidneys. It also gets your colon working as it should. That's why the recommendations in the first pillar of health are so important.

Like alkalinizing foods, alkaline water also helps alkalinize your tissues, another important step in detoxifying the body. Cells thrive in an alkaline environment but get constipated with metabolic waste and toxins in an acidic environment. To check the acidity of their bodies, I have my patients test their first morning urine pH, which is a good indicator of the pH of the tissues. The majority of my patients usually have a urine pH of 5.0, which is approximately 100 times more acidic than it should be. I often recommend drinking fresh, juiced organic fruits and vegetables (which are sprouts and vegetables such as wheat grass, barley grass, oat grass, spirulina, chlorella, and blue green algae) or a phytonutrient powder drink to help cleanse and alkalinize the body, as well as provide superior nutrition. We'll talk more about that in an upcoming pillar.

Soft drinks, believe it or not, are practically pesticide free. But they contain far too much sugar to have any health benefit, and diet drinks usually contain aspartame, which chemically breaks down to methanol, or wood alcohol. Some people consider aspartame to be perfectly safe, but I do not feel that drinking wood alcohol is ever safe.

Tea also contains pesticides, and that's why it's important to choose organic teas. Most green teas contain pesticides as well as fluorides. The pesticides in the green tea may be canceling out the powerful antioxidant effects of the tea. Wine is usually loaded with pesticides, and so is non-organic coffee. If you choose to drink tea, wine, and coffee, then I recommend drinking only organic teas, wines, and coffees in moderation. Organic coffee and tea are available in most health food and grocery stores. Organic wines are available in stores such as Whole Foods Markets and other health food stores that carry wines.

While outer influences can be a source of toxin for our bodies, there are also unsuspecting inner sources that can make us toxic. We need to arm ourselves with information so that we can take the necessary action to begin the detoxification process.

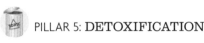

BUILDING BLOCKS TO A HEALTHY LIFE

POINT TO PONDER: *Breathing in secondhand smoke for an hour is worse than actually smoking four cigarettes yourself. Practically all non-organically grown produce is tainted with pesticides and herbicides. Our food supply may contain parasites from workers not washing their hands.*

ACTION STEP: *Change your air conditioner filter every month. If you have a permanent filter, wash it every month in a bleach solution and hose it down. If you live in a place that allows smoking in restaurants, start a petition drive to ban smoking in restaurants.*

DAY 31: Unexpected Sources of Toxins

We are being bombarded with toxins on a daily basis—and what we don't know about those products may be harmful. Think about it: How many different household products do you use to clean your home? How many personal products are sitting on your bathroom vanity right now? How many silver fillings are in your mouth? How long have those silver fillings been in your mouth? Which vaccines have you or your children received?

Toxins can enter our bodies through unexpected avenues such as vaccines. Some vaccines actually contain a mercury preservative called thimerosal. For years this toxin made it into every child's body at birth when they were immediately given a vaccine for hepatitis B, followed by up to thirty-two shots and booster shots by the age of two. Although vaccines are much safer today since the removal or reduction to trace amounts of thimerosal (the mercury preservative) from most routinely recommended vaccines for ages six and under, some may still contain this toxin. The flu vaccine and the DT booster still contain mercury. Vaccines may also contain a myriad of other toxins, heavy metals, chemicals, microbes, and animal and human by-products. For example, the MMR vaccine is considered mercury free but contains chick embryonic fluid, human diploid cells from aborted fetal tissue, neomycin, and sorbitol.[1] Other vaccines such as DTaP-HepB-IPV contain trace amounts of thimerosal.[2] In the absence of thimerosal, vaccine makers have used replacement preservatives like phenol, benzethonium chloride, and formaldehyde,[3] all of which may harm a growing child's immune system.

Avoid Heavy Metal

And I don't mean heavy metal music. I mean things like mercury, cadmium, aluminum, and lead. Some people have so much metal in their bodies that they need chelation therapy—oral, intravenous, or suppository forms of chelation to remove metals from their body. One of my patients had Lou Gehrig's, or ALS, disease. Neurologists said she had only a few months to live. She was barely able to walk into my office using a walker, and many times she needed a wheelchair. I learned she had smoked heavily for forty years, so I did a heavy metal screen on her and found off-the-charts amounts of cadmium in her urine. I started chelating this out of her body. Today she is strong enough to be back at work full time. The neurologist now says he misdiagnosed her.

Chlorophyll foods, including wheat grass, barley grass, oat grass, healthy algae, and other supplements, should be taken daily to help detoxify heavy metals. For more information, please refer to my books *What You Don't Know May Be Killing You* and *Get Healthy Through Detox and Fasting*.[4]

Another source of toxins for millions of people is in their teeth. Amalgam fillings, which are also called silver fillings, are about 50 percent mercury and also contain tin, copper, and silver. About a million people every week have amalgam fillings put in. The original fillings made from 1850 until 1974 slowly released mercury over thirty years. But the fillings made since 1974 release enough mercury into the body to cause trouble within three to five years.[5] A typical filling contains 250,000 mcg of mercury and releases 10 mcg of mercury per day.[6]

When mercury enters the membrane of a cell, the body's immune systems may identify them as an abnormal cell that must be destroyed. The immune system may then form antibodies against your body's normal cells, because they appear abnormal since they contain mercury. This can lead to rheumatoid arthritis, Hashimoto's thyroiditis, muscle pain, lupus, and other autoimmune diseases. People suffering with heavy metal toxicity, as occurs in the slow release of mercury from amalgam fillings, usually don't notice right away because symptoms build up slowly. The victims simply feel bad and say things like, "I don't know what is wrong with me—I just don't feel good, and I am very tired."

For many years the dental community maintained that mercury was tightly bound with other metal components and did not escape from amalgam fillings. But research has proven that mercury vapors do escape during chewing and brushing, and when contacted with hot or acidic food. One study found that levels of mercury vapor in the mouth after chewing were fifty-four times higher in people with amalgams than in people without amalgams.[7] We now know it is physically impossible for mercury to be "locked in" the amalgam fillings once they are placed in the teeth.

The Agency for Toxic Substances and Disease Registry lists mercury as the third most toxic substance known to mankind[8]—more toxic than lead, cadmium, and arsenic. I'm amazed that dentists still put it into people's mouths. When a dentist removes a silver filling, he is required by OSHA to put the filling in a sealed biohazard container.

Down in the Mouth

If you have silver amalgam dental fillings, you should eventually consider having them removed, but be very careful about it. Many dentists have shared horror stories about patients who had their silver fillings removed and were in worse shape afterward.

There is a proper and safe way to have amalgam fillings removed. Begin by finding a willing and cooperative biological dentist who is aware of the risks of mercury and is knowledgeable in the proper way to remove silver amalgam fillings. He may use a controlled chewing test to determine the extent of mercury being released from your dental fillings. He may conduct electrical readings on your fillings to determine the sequence for removing fillings, perhaps removing the most negatively charged fillings first or fillings that are leaking first. To find a biological dentist, call the International College of Integrative Medicine (formerly Great Lakes College of Clinical Medicine) at (866) 464-5226, or visit their Web site at www.icimed.com. Or you can visit the Web site of the International Academy of Oral Medicine and Toxicology at www.iaomt.org. Refer to my book *What You Don't Know May Be Killing You* for more information.

And if the dentist recommends silver fillings for you or your children, learn the potential dangers of mercury and refuse it. If he insists, then find another dentist. Porcelain costs more up front, but it could save your health. Be aware that if you have composite fillings placed, they should be considered to be only temporary and should not be left in long term. Please do not run out and have all your silver fillings removed, or you may actually get more sick. Instead, find a good biological dentist who can safely and slowly remove them over a period of time.

Household Products

Solvents, which are used in cleaning products to dissolve materials that are not water soluble, contain toxins that, if they come into contact with your skin, are actually absorbed into your body. Remember, pharmaceutical companies are now using transdermal (through the skin) methods to deliver hormones, some blood pressure medicines, nicotine, and other drugs. If chemicals come in contact with the skin, realize that some of the chemical will be absorbed. In some cases, most of the toxic chemical may be absorbed, especially certain solvents, cleaners, and so forth. Toxic household items include paint thinners, stain removers, varnishes, ammonia, bleach, glass cleaners, metal polish, and furniture polish.

Furniture and household items can emit toxins. For instance, formaldehyde, which is used in particleboard, carpet padding, carpet glues, upholstered furniture, curtains, and bedding, may cause fatigue and headaches.

For example, according to the Environmental Protection Agency's Web site, petroleum distillates, found in metal polishes, can cause temporary eye clouding under short-term exposure. Longer exposure can damage the nervous system, skin, kidneys, and eyes.[9]

The EPA site also says that phenol and cresol, found in disinfectants, are corrosive and can cause diarrhea, fainting, dizziness, and kidney and liver damage. Nitrobenzene, in furniture and floor polishes, can cause skin discoloration, shallow breathing, vomiting, and death, and it is associated with cancer and birth defects.[10]

Benzene is classified by the EPA as a Class A carcinogen due to its link to an increased risk of leukemia. It is used in a wide range of products many of us encounter every day—carpet cleaners, cleaning fluids, conditioners, detergents, dyes, enamel sprays, furniture, gasoline, nail polishes, paint, paint removers, paint thinners, plastics, solvents, spot removers, spray acrylics, spray paints, stains/lacquers, vinyl floorings, wood finishes, wood lighteners, wood preservatives, and many other man-made products.[12]

Don't Mix!

If you have ever mixed bleach and ammonia, you probably had an unpleasant surprise. Sodium hypochlorite, an ingredient of chlorine bleach, releases a toxic gas that if mixed with ammonia may cause mild asthmatic symptoms or more serious problems.[11]

In addition to household products, a recent study has raised questions about the benzene levels in some soft drinks, particularly those with orange, strawberry, pineapple, and cranberry flavors. Five percent of soft drinks studied had benzene levels that exceed the EPA limit for our drinking water. And buyers beware: even if a soft drink doesn't contain benzene when it is manufactured, if it contains vitamin C (ascorbic acid) and either sodium benzoate or potassium benzoate, benzene can form in it when it is exposed to heat and/or light.[13]

Perchloroethylene (also called perc, PCE, and tetrachloroethylene) and 1-1-1 trichloroethane solvents, found in spot removers and carpet cleaners, can cause liver and kidney damage if ingested. Perc, determined to be a carcinogen by the Department of Health and Human Services (DHHS), has caused liver and kidney tumors in laboratory animals.[14] Perc is commonly used in dry cleaning. To avoid adverse reactions from perc, be sure to remove the plastic wrapping from your dry-cleaned items and allow them to air out for several days before wearing or ironing them.

Switch to Natural Products

Most people may not realize that they have an option. They don't have to purchase products containing harmful chemicals in order to clean their homes. Below are a couple of natural products most people have in their pantry that can be used as household cleaners.

- **Lemon juice**, which contains citric acid, is a deodorizer and can be used to clean glass and remove stains from aluminum, clothes, and porcelain. It is a mild lightener or bleach if used with sunlight.
- **Vinegar** contains about 5 percent acetic acid, which makes it a mild acid. Vinegar can dissolve mineral deposits and grease, remove traces of soap, remove mildew or wax buildup, polish some metals, and deodorize. Vinegar can clean brick or stone, and it is an ingredient in some natural carpet cleaning recipes. Use vinegar to clean out the metallic taste in coffeepots and to shine windows without streaking. Vinegar is normally used in a solution with water, but it can be used straight. Make an all-purpose cleaner from a vinegar-and-salt mixture or from four tablespoons baking soda dissolved in one quart of warm water.

If you do use chemical cleaners, I encourage you to wear rubber gloves. This will keep chemicals away from your skin so they are not absorbed into your body. Use cleaning agents in well-ventilated areas so that the fumes do not affect your lungs.

Personal Care Products

Every day you apply personal products—spraying, brushing, patting them on your body—all of which may contain chemicals from sources you never consider. We are rubbing chemicals on our faces, applying them to our skin, and spraying them on our hair.

Chemicals such as ammonia, formaldehyde, triclosan, and aluminum chlorohydrate are in antiperspirants and deodorants. The chemical triclosan, which is found in some deodorants, has been found to cause liver damage in laboratory rats.[15]

However, there are some safe alternatives. Some companies have pledged not to use chemicals that are harmful to humans. Visit the Web site www.safecosmetics.org for a list of companies. This Web site will also help you see which of your products are safe or not safe, in their "skin deep report."

Toluene (a solvent similar to benzene), a common ingredient in perfumes and colognes, may contribute to arrhythmias of the heart as well as nerve damage. One way to avoid this is to apply perfume or cologne to your clothes instead of your skin.

A compound called p-Phenylenediamine (PPD) is used in almost every hair dye on the market—even so-called "natural" and "herbal" products. Usually, the darker the color, the higher the concentration of PPD. People can be exposed to PPD through inhalation, skin absorption, ingestion, and skin and/or eye contact. Some studies have suggested a connection between hair dyes and myelodysplasia, multiple myeloma, leukemia and preleukemia, non-Hodgkin's lymphoma, and Hodgkin's disease.[16] To reduce your risk of PPD exposure, I recommend sticking to lighter hair colors, and if you must use a darker hair color, please use semi-permanent or nonpermanent coloring.

Although we may be exposed to unsuspected toxins, another method we can use to detoxify is to exercise regularly. Remember on Day 23, under the "Benefits of Exercise, Part I," one of the benefits of exercise is that it helps the lymphatic system remove cellular waste. Aerobic exercise can increase lymphatic flow threefold, which means that the body can release three times the amount of toxins with regular aerobic exercise.

Tomorrow we will see what toxins do to our bodies.

BUILDING BLOCKS TO A HEALTHY LIFE

POINTS TO PONDER: *Mercury, found in most dental fillings, is one of the most toxic elements on the planet. Some vaccinations, such as the DT booster and flu vaccine, still contain mercury. Silver fillings are composed of about 50 percent mercury. A common ingredient used in perfumes and colognes is toluene, which may cause heart arrhythmias and nerve damage. Armed with the correct knowledge, you can begin to reclaim your health from unexpected sources of toxins.*

ACTION STEP: *Next time you purchase personal care products, visit your nearest health food store and substitute a natural personal care product for one of yours.*

DAY 32: What Toxins Do to the Body

A few years ago, I had a patient who complained of some of the worst body odor. She would shower and still smell like body odor, even after using soap.

One day, a few weeks after seeing this patient, I was on an airplane. The flight attendant recognized me, so she began talking to me about the changes she had made in her diet and lifestyle.

The flight attendant said, "I used to have the worst body odor, until I became a vegetarian. Now I have no body odor whatsoever. I don't even need to wear deodorant."

I then realized that I had not told my patient with body odor to stop eating all meat. When I got back in town, I called this patient back and learned that she was eating red meat and pork at least three times a week. As soon as she quit eating red meat and pork, the body odor went away. She was ecstatic.

I have since seen this problem time and again in other patients. One man I treated had terrible body odor, and his T-shirts were stained yellow. He said he would scrub under his arms and get out of the shower and still smell the same. He also said he would load bacon on his plate six inches high at buffets. I put him on a meat fast, and he quit stinking.

Deadly Toxification

I wish toxicity were only a matter of bad body odor, but it's much more serious than that. When your body can't break down a toxin or dispose of it properly, it usually stores it in fatty tissues, which include the brain, breasts, and prostate gland. Those "love handles" around your waist may actually be toxin-storage sites! Toxins may also trigger inflammation, which is the main cause of heart disease, Alzheimer's, arthritis, asthma, and many other diseases. Inflammation, we are finding, is strongly related to the foods we eat, like red meats.

Highly toxic people open themselves up to many more problems, including:

- Chronic fatigue
- Heart disease
- Memory loss
- Premature aging

- Skin disorders
- Arthritis
- Hormone imbalances
- Anxiety
- Headaches
- Emotional disorders
- Cancers
- Autoimmune diseases

What the Toxins Do

When toxins build up in your body and the liver and elimination systems can't process and eliminate them all, you then develop toxic overload. You usually lack energy, experience environmental allergies and food sensitivities, and develop excessive mucus production. You may also develop recurrent sinus problems, bronchitis, and eventually degenerative diseases. Some people complain of forgetfulness, foggy thinking, mood changes, sallow and saggy skin, respiratory problems, joint aches, arthritis, acne, eczema, psoriasis, and poor immune function.

But what do these toxins do? Sampling just some of the research gives us all the information we need. For example, pesticides have been linked to a lower sperm count in men and to higher amounts of xenoestrogen in men and women. Xenoestrogens are chemical counterfeits that fool the body into accepting them as genuine estrogen. When this occurs, it throws a woman's hormones out of balance, leading to symptoms of PMS, fibrocystic breast diseases, and potentially endometriosis. It can even stimulate breast cancer and endometrial cancer.[1]

> **Working With Paints and Woods**
>
> Mineral spirits in oil-based paints are a skin, eye, nose, throat, and lung irritant. High air concentrations can cause nervous system damage, unconsciousness, and even death. Ketones and toluene in wood putty are highly toxic and may cause skin, kidney, liver, and central nervous system damage as well as damage to the reproductive system.[2]

In the book *Our Stolen Future*, Theo Colborn recorded the effects of a pesticide spill on Lake Apopka, just outside Orlando, Florida, in 1980. Following the spill, the alligator and turtle populations were affected. The female alligators showed ovarian abnormalities in their eggs and egg follicles. The males showed structural abnormalities in their testes and penises and had elevated levels of estrogen and lower levels of testosterone. After the spill there was a striking absence of male turtles. There were many female turtles in the lake and many turtles that were neither male nor female. These turtles were unable to reproduce.[3]

Solvents used in common products like cleansers, glues, typewriter correction fluids, and more can injure your kidneys and liver. They can suppress your central nervous system, dissolve into the membranes of your cells, especially your fat cells, and accumulate there. Like pesticides, solvents are fat soluble and are stored in the fatty tissues of the body, including the brain, breasts, and prostate gland. Could pesticides and solvents be the reasons why one in seven women in the United States develop breast cancer and one in six men in the United States develop prostate cancer?[4] Long-term exposure to these solvents may cause leukemia, heart arrhythmias, and nerve damage.[5] Unfortunately, children have learned that many of these chemicals give them a "high," and they are huffing them. They are damaging their brains, livers, and many other organs.

One way to detoxify the body from solvents and pesticides is through fasting. During fasting, our cells, tissues, and organs begin to dump out accumulated waste products of cellular metabolism as well as chemical solvents, pesticides, and other toxins. Sauna therapy is also very effective at removing solvent and pesticide toxins from the body. I'll talk more about sauna therapy on Day 34 and fasting on Day 35, but if you want a detailed plan on how to detoxify your body through fasting, refer to my books *Fasting Made Easy*[6] and *Get Healthy Through Detox and Fasting.*

As you help your body take out the trash, your body will begin to heal itself. We will see how in the next couple of days.

BUILDING BLOCKS TO A HEALTHY LIFE

POINTS TO PONDER: *Toxins may trigger most degenerative diseases, including cancer and heart disease. Body odor is sometimes a sign of a toxic body. Pesticides and solvents, such as cleansers, are fat soluble and are stored in fatty tissues, including tissues in the brain, breasts, and prostate gland.*

ACTION STEP: *Mix one scoop of Divine Health Living Food with eight ounces of water, and drink every three to four hours, along with two quarts of pure water. Do this for one day.*

DAY 33: It's Time to Get Rid of Toxic Trash

Your body is designed with an incredible defense system that keeps you healthy even under extreme circumstances—and you never have to give it a second thought. God built your body with a waste management team designed to take out its own trash and to detoxify your body. This team includes your:

- Colon
- Lungs
- Skin
- Urinary tract
- Lymphatics
- Liver

Your body is created to heal itself! Ideally, these organs dispense with toxic trash quickly and efficiently. We have already discussed the colon, lungs, skin, and lymphatics. The urinary tract is also important to your body's defense system. When we drink clean, alkaline water, the urinary tract helps to flush the toxins of our system. Our liver also is our body's best defense for getting rid of toxins.

What Causes Cirrhosis of the Liver?

While the most common cause of cirrhosis of the liver is usually alcoholism, this liver disease can also be caused by contracting the hepatitis C virus (HCV). HCV may result from a blood transfusion. Also, a fatty liver from a poor diet may eventually lead to cirrhosis. Nonalcoholic fatty liver disease leads to nonalcoholic steatohepatis, in which 15 to 30 percent of cases result in cirrhosis.[1]

The Liver—Our Body's Detox Filter

The liver is the most important organ for detoxification. A properly functioning liver protects you from environmental and metabolic toxins. The liver is able to detoxify toxins through the coordinated effort of two families of enzymes, which are called the cytochrome p450s and conjugative enzymes. However, both types of enzymes require activation, and their levels must be kept in proper balance, or even more free radicals may be formed. The cytochrome p450s generate free radicals while performing their job. The conjugative enzymes catch these free radicals, inactivate them, and get them ready for excretion.

The liver needs to be fueled properly to perform its detoxification duties and to maintain adequate levels of antioxidants, including glutathione, to continue the detoxification process.

Certain foods increase the capacity of the liver to detoxify harmful toxins—foods like wasabi, broccoli, cabbage, brussels sprouts, kale, and cauliflower. (Wasabi is the green spicy paste usually served with sushi.) Green foods including cereal grasses, micro algae, plant greens, green vegetables, sea vegetables/seaweed, and aqua greens are also great detoxifiers.

Supplements that are important for liver detoxification include a comprehensive multivitamin, milk thistle extract, grape seed extract, green tea, N-acetylcysteine (NAC), R-form alpha-lipoic acid or DHLA, and curcumin. For more information this subject, please refer to my books *Toxic Relief* and *Get Healthy Through Detox and Fasting*.

An Apple a Day Keeps the Doctor Away

There's a measure of truth in this old adage. Quercetin, an antioxidant that contains flavonoids, appears to help fight a host of disorders, from asthma to cancer to heart disease. As an antioxidant, it combats the destructive "free radical" molecules that play a part in many diseases. Quercetin is found primarily in onions and—you guessed it—apples.

There are some things we can do to help our waste removal systems do their jobs. Here are a few suggestions.

Eat Fiber

The colon is the body's most important toxin disposal system. It receives toxins from our diet and from the liver, which dumps them into the bile and sends them to the small intestines, then into the large intestines.

Unfortunately, many Americans are constipated. When your home septic tank backs up, it stinks up the house. Likewise, when waste matter sits in your colon for too long, some of that putrefying, rotting material is absorbed into your body. Patients I treat for severe body odor are often excreting toxins through the skin because they are severely constipated or clogged.

One woman came into my office recently and told me she had just undergone an abdominal X-ray. The radiologist had brought her X-rays in and asked her, "Are you feeling OK? Your colon is entirely impacted." She had clogged her colon with her beloved low-fiber Italian foods and white breads.

Practically every week in my practice, at least one person tells me they have a bowel movement only once a week. They think that's normal. They are shocked when I tell them people should have a bowel movement three times a day, especially after every meal. The colon should experience peristalsis when you eat food, which is the gastrocolic reflex that propels food through. For some people, once the colon gets moving, weight loss happens as if by magic. It also helps you avoid hemorrhoids, colorectal disease, irritable bowel syndrome, diverticulosis, colon polyps, and even cancer.

You need twenty-five to thirty grams of fiber a day to keep the colon moving those toxins along. Many fruits are a good source of fiber—apples, pears, and citrus fruits. Carrots, beans, lentils, legumes, and peas are good vegetable sources of fiber. Whole-grain products are a terrific source of fiber.

Remember that fiber and water work together to stimulate the colon. When you eat more fiber, you need to drink more water. Your goal should be to have one or more bowel movements a day. Your regularity is timed to the meals you had one or two days earlier. The average time for the bowel to excrete a meal is about twenty-four hours. Patients eating a lot of white bread and low-fiber foods can delay that another twenty-four or forty-eight hours.

Eat Chemical-Free Foods

When choosing toxin-free produce, here's the rule to remember: generally, the thicker the peel, usually the safer the fruit. For example, bananas have a thick peel and have fewer pesticides. Oranges, tangerines, lemons, grapefruit, pineapples, watermelons, and figs also have a thick peel. However, some fruits with a thick peel, such as cantaloupes, have a very porous peel, which absorbs pesticides.

The following produce have been known to carry much higher levels of pesticide residue than others: apples, bell peppers, celery, cherries, imported grapes, nectarines, peaches, pears, potatoes, red raspberries, spinach, and strawberries. Among fruits, nectarines followed by pears and peaches had the highest percentage of pesticide residues, according to researchers at Environmental Working Group. Among vegetables, spinach, celery, and potatoes had the highest percentage.[2]

It's best to buy organic if possible.

Enjoy your salads, but peel off the first two or three layers of lettuce leaves to remove any pesticide-tainted leaves if you do not purchase organic lettuce. Some broccoli can contain higher levels of pesticides, so if you are eating a lot of broccoli, you may want to purchase an organically grown variety or wash it well. The two vegetables with the highest levels of pesticides are spinach and celery. Spinach grows near the ground, and its leaves have no protective covering, which is why it tends to have high concentrations of pesticides. Make sure you wash your vegetables thoroughly.

Your mother may have taught you that the best vitamins are found in the skin of the potato—but so are the pesticides. Because potatoes grow in the dirt, they absorb pesticides from the surrounding soil. So don't eat the potato skins unless you use organically grown potatoes.

Limit your intake of meat and dairy products that have been chemically exposed. We already learned that the riskiest foods are fatty cuts of meat. Switch to a leaner cut of meat, and eat free-range or organic meats from cattle grazed on lands not sprayed with pesticides. As I recommended in Pillar 3, avoid organ meats, like livers and kidneys, since these organs are higher in chemicals and toxic residues. Also avoid cold cuts or any packaged meats such as bologna, salami, and processed ham because of the high amounts of nitrates and nitrites they contain. Limit pork products since they harbor significant amounts of toxins in the fatty cuts of meat. Wild Pacific or Alaskan salmon is vastly better than farmed salmon. Farmed fish are fed pellets of concentrated fish products, which contain high concentrations of toxins. (These pellets are made by drying and grinding up other fish that are caught in fishing nets but don't have market value.[3]) One wide-ranging study of farmed salmon vs. wild salmon recommended that people eat farmed salmon no more than once a month because of the high toxin content.[4] On average, farmed salmon have 16 times the dioxin-like PCBs found in wild salmon, 4 times the levels in beef, and 3.4 times the dioxin-like PCBs found in other seafood.[5] I recommend avoiding farmed fish altogether; stay on the "wild" side with wild salmon. Free-range organic chicken and turkey are also, for the most part, pesticide- and hormone-free.

Other foods may surprise you with their toxin content. The heaviest concentrations of pesticide residues are found in peanuts and raisins. That means that peanut butter and cereals with raisins may not be the best choices for your family. Buy organically grown peanuts and organically grown raisins. Even if you choose organic peanuts, it's best to limit peanut butter servings to once per week because it may contain a cancer-causing chemical called aflatoxin. If you choose to eat peanut butter, check for nut butters made with peanuts from New Mexico where the dry air prevents the growth of the aflatoxin. Almond butter is a better choice, as aflatoxin is not an issue. Look for "certified aflatoxin free" products on the label of peanut butters when shopping.

Acid- and Alkaline-Forming Foods

Your diet should probably consist of 50 percent (or higher) alkaline-forming foods and 50 percent (or less) acid-forming foods. That's about one serving of vegetables and one of fruit or other alkalinizing foods for every serving of acidic foods (meats or grains). As I mentioned in Pillar 1, a pH below 7.0 is acidic. A pH above 7.0 is alkaline. A healthy urine pH is from 7.0 to 7.5.

Alkaline-forming foods include most fruits, green vegetables, lentils, spices, herbs and seasonings, and seeds and nuts. Acid-forming foods include meat, fish, poultry, chicken eggs, most grains, legumes, and especially desserts, processed foods, and fast foods. Below are two charts to help simplify it.[6]

ALKALIZING FOODS	
Vegetables	Alfalfa • Barley grass • Beets • Broccoli • Cabbage • Carrots • Cauliflower • Celery • Chlorella • Collard greens • Cucumber • Eggplant • Garlic • Green beans • Green peas • Kale • Lettuce • Mushrooms • Mustard greens • Nightshade veggies • Onions • Peas • Peppers • Pumpkin • Radishes • Rutabaga • Spinach, green • Sprouts • Sweet potatoes • Tomatoes • Watercress • Wild greens • Wheat grass
Fruits	Apple • Apricot • Avocado • Banana • Berries • Blackberries • Blueberries • Cantaloupe • Cherries, sour • Coconut, fresh • Cranberries • Currants • Dates, dried • Figs, dried • Grapes • Grapefruit • Honeydew melon • Lemon • Lime • Muskmelons • Nectarine • Orange • Peach • Pear • Pineapple • Raisins • Raspberries • Strawberries • Tangerine • Tomato • Tropical fruits • Watermelon
Grains	Millet
Nuts	Almonds • Chestnuts
Sweeteners	Stevia
Spices and Seasonings	Chili pepper • Cinnamon • Curry • Ginger • Herbs (all) • Mustard • Sea salt

ALKALIZING FOODS	
Other	Alkaline antioxidant water • Apple cider vinegar • Duck eggs Fresh, squeezed fruit juice • Ghee (clarified butter) • Green juices Mineral water • Quail eggs • Soured dairy products • Veggie juices
Minerals	Calcium: pH 12 • Cesium: pH 14 • Magnesium: pH 9 Potassium: pH 14 • Sodium: pH 14

ACIDIFYING FOODS	
Vegetables	Corn • Olives • Winter squash
Fruits	Pickled fruits • Cranberries
Grains, Grain Products	Barley • Bran, oat • Bran, wheat • Bread • Corn • Cornstarch Crackers, soda • Flour, wheat • Flour, white • Macaroni • Noodles Rice (all) • Rice cakes • Rye • Spaghetti • Spelt Wheat germ • Wheat
Beans and Legumes	Black beans • Chick peas • Kidney beans • Lima beans Pinto beans • Soybeans • White beans
Dairy	Butter • Cheese • Cheese, processed Ice cream • Ice milk
Nuts and Butters	Brazil nuts • Hazelnuts • Legumes • Peanut butter Peanuts • Pecans • Pine nuts • Walnuts
Animal Protein	Bacon • Beef • Carp • Clams • Cod • Corned beef Fish • Haddock • Lamb • Lobster • Mussels • Organ meats Oyster • Pike • Pork • Rabbit • Salmon • Sardines Sausage • Scallops • Shellfish • Shrimp Tuna • Turkey • Veal • Venison
Fats and Oils	Almond oil • Butter • Canola oil • Corn oil Safflower oil • Sesame oil • Sunflower oil • All fried foods
Sweeteners	Corn syrup • Sugar
Other Foods	Catsup • Cocoa • Coffee • Mustard Pepper • Soft drinks • Vinegar
Drugs and Chemicals	Aspirin • Chemicals • Drugs, medicinal • Drugs, psychedelic Herbicides • Pesticides • Tobacco

BUILDING BLOCKS TO A HEALTHY LIFE

POINTS TO PONDER: *Your body's waste management system was designed to take out the toxic trash on a daily basis, not once a week. Get adequate amounts of fiber on a daily basis (about twenty-five to thirty grams a day). Limit your intake of meat and dairy; always choose the leanest cuts of meat and fat-free or low-fat organic dairy products. Eat organic foods as often as possible, and remember, the thicker the peel in non-organic produce, the safer it is, generally speaking.*

ACTION STEP: *Highlight all alkaline foods from the list that you will eat. Then plan to eat at least 50 percent of your diet in alkaline foods.*

DAY 34: Detoxing Through the Skin

There was a time when I was young and actually believed that I was healthy because I had stopped sweating. I thought my body was in such good shape that I had less need to perspire. How wrong I was! The truth was exactly the opposite. I had stopped sweating because my body was becoming dangerously toxic, to the point where I put myself on a detoxification regimen that I believed helped to save my life. I tell the full story in my book *What You Don't Know May Be Killing You.*

Now I know that by sweating and taking care of your skin you help your body get rid of toxins. Years ago a painter came to see me at my office. He had developed Parkinson's disease. During our interview something interesting came up. He said he had stopped sweating a few years before he had developed the disease. I believe his perspiring had detoxified his body, but when he stopped perspiring, the toxins accumulated, and Parkinson's was the manifestation of this toxic buildup.

Go Ahead and Sweat It!

Here in the United States we live in air-conditioned homes, work in air-conditioned offices, drive in air-conditioned cars, shop in air-conditioned malls, and exercise in air-conditioned gyms. We avoid heat, avoid sweating, and wear antiperspirants to keep us from perspiring. The result is a buildup of toxins in our bodies.

I often say that summer was created by God to be our "sweat season," when our bodies expel toxins through the skin. God actually told Adam he would work by the sweat of his brow. The skin has been called "the third kidney" by some in the medical field because it is able to release so many toxins such as pesticides, solvents, heavy metals, urea, and lactic acid from the body. It as also called this because the consistency of the sweat is similar to our urine.[2] Approximately 99 percent of perspiration is water; the remaining 1 percent is toxic waste.[3] But because of air conditioning, antiperspirants, and a general bias against sweating, much of the U.S. population never really sweats.

Did You Know...?

You have about two to three million sweat glands in your skin. Sweat glands keep you cool and prevent you from drying out. So go ahead and let 'em see you sweat![1]

If you don't sweat, you are not fully healthy. The skin is one of your main toxin-excreting organs. A colleague of mine told me of a patient, a painter, who on one occasion, after undergoing infrared sauna therapy, actually sweated out mineral spirits, which took the paint off the wall of the room where the sauna was located, at the exact spot where he was leaning against it! For years he had washed his hands with mineral spirits, and after having infrared sauna therapy for a few weeks, his sweat began to carry out those mineral spirits.

Don't be afraid to perspire when you exercise; it means you are healthy! Exercise also improves circulation to the skin, which brings nutrients to the skin and removes cellular waste. Also remember that aerobic exercise can increase lymphatic flow threefold, which means the body can release three times the amount of toxins.

Here are some other suggestions for detoxifying your body through the skin.

Quick Quiz

What is the maximum volume of sweat a person who is not adapted to a hot climate can produce in one hour?

a. One liter per hour
b. Half a liter per hour
c. An eighth of a liter per hour

Answer: a. One liter per hour. But if you move to a hot climate, your body trains itself to produce two to three liters per hour within about six weeks. This appears to be the maximum amount that you can produce.[4]

Hop in the Sauna

If you don't work outdoors in the heat, or if for some reason you cannot exercise, consider sauna therapy.

An infrared sauna is especially effective. Infrared saunas use an infrared radiant heat source that causes your body to eliminate up to three times more toxins in the perspiration than do conventional saunas. An infrared sauna stimulates the cellular metabolism and breaks up water molecules that hold toxins within the body, thus allowing the body to sweat out these toxins. This natural process may also burn up to 300 calories during a twenty- to thirty-minute session. (See Appendix A.)

I have an infrared sauna at home and in my office that my patients, as well as myself, use to sweat out toxins. I usually place the temperature between 130 to 150 degrees, and I stay in it for at least thirty minutes. I prefer to take my sauna after an aerobic workout, and I always drink plenty of alkaline water while in the sauna.

I would advise you to consult your doctor before doing any kind of sauna therapy.

Brush Your Skin

You are now aware that your body excretes toxins and waste through your skin every day. Therefore, taking proper care of your skin is extremely important. If the pores of your skin become clogged with dead skin cells, the toxins may remain locked inside your body, putting more stress on your liver and kidneys.

Dry-skin brushing is an excellent way to keep the pores of your skin open and clear so that your skin is allowed to breathe and excrete the toxins. Brushing the skin also stimulates blood and lymphatic flow throughout the body, leading to a more efficient removal of waste and toxins.

I strongly recommend investing in a loofah sponge or a natural soft-bristle brush. To brush your skin, start with the soles of your feet, working up your legs, torso, and arms until you have brushed the majority of your body, avoiding only your face. Use firm, hard strokes, brushing toward your heart to increase blood flow. The entire process should take about five minutes. It usually makes your skin feel warm due to increased circulation. I recommend dry-skin brushing prior to taking a shower.

In short, sweating, brushing your skin, and sauna therapy can help you detoxify through your skin.

BUILDING BLOCKS TO A HEALTHY LIFE

POINTS TO PONDER: *Perspiration is another way to rid the body of toxins. Sweating is actually a sign of being healthy. Don't be afraid to perspire when you exercise; it generally means you are healthy!*

ACTION STEP: *Try using an infrared sauna or a regular sauna, or buy a loofah sponge and do the dry-skin brushing technique to detox through the skin.*

DAY 35: Other Important Detoxifiers

Some years ago I suffered from a severe case of chronic fatigue and barely had enough energy to work. My skin looked sallow and sickly. I felt exhausted all the time. Almost every evening when I came home from work I would go straight to bed.

After much searching to determine the cause of my fatigue, hair and urine analyses revealed I had elevated mercury levels. I put myself through a special mercury detoxification regimen to begin binding and removing the mercury and to strengthen my immune system by using vitamins, minerals, and other supplements. Then I had eight large amalgam fillings in my mouth taken out and replaced with porcelain by a biological dentist. The detoxification program and the removal of the fillings made a significant difference. My skin color returned to normal, and my renewed energy level was astounding. I had also stopped sweating due to mercury toxicity, but on this regimen I started perspiring again.

Here a few suggestions for detoxifying your body.

Clean the Air

A woman came into my office complaining of headaches and foggy thinking. It turned out she was remodeling her home, and workers were painting the walls with oil-based paints and putting in new flooring. I had her open her windows during the day to air it out, buy an air filter for her bedroom, and place plants around the home—like philodendron and spider plants—to help clean the air.

Air is probably the most difficult pollutant to control, and so your lungs are exposed to many different environmental toxins. You have no choice but to breathe, and sometimes you can't avoid secondhand cigarette smoke, smog, car and diesel exhaust, dust, and other airborne trash. Your lungs use mucus to both excrete and trap the toxins. A "runny nose" or cough usually means the body is getting rid of toxins. Mucus also traps incoming toxins, and the lungs destroy them with enzymes.

On Day 30, I gave you a couple of suggestions for "clearing the air"; here are a few more on how to clean your air.

Open a door or window and turn on a fan, provided you don't live next to a busy highway or street. But when pollen counts are high in your area, keep the windows closed and use the air conditioner.

Buy an air purifier for your bedroom. Hepa filters remove air particles with almost 100 percent efficiency.[1] Other air purifiers like ionizers are good at this also. According to *Consumer Reports*, the best room air purifiers are made by Friedrich, Kenmore, and Whirlpool.[2] There are even air purifiers for your car.

Buy indoor plants, which create oxygen in the air and can neutralize toxins. The best plants to fight indoor pollution and the easiest to grow include the attractive white peace lily (*Spathiphyllum*), weeping fig, Boston fern, spider plant, mother-in-law tongue, and dracaena. Plus, they create a peaceful, pleasant environment.

Sleep Tight

The average bed contains approximately two million dust mites![3]

Get encasements for your pillows, mattresses, and box springs to prevent dust mites, the most common cause of allergies. Dust mites love fabric and humid environments. One way to combat dust mite allergies is simply to purchase a hypoallergenic encasement for your mattress and pillows. If you have persistent allergies to dust, consider replacing your carpets with hardwood floors or tile; take down the drapes and buy non-fabric furniture. If you live in a humid environment, buy a dehumidifier. Replace down pillows with pillows made of hypoallergenic fibers. Avoid feather-filled comforters. Wash bedcovers in hot water weekly. And, in general, get rid of your clutter where dust mites thrive—piles of extra clothes, stuffed toys, couch pillows, throw rugs, and so on.

Guard against mold in your home by watching for leaks in plumbing and the roof, hunting down moldy smells, and by keeping vegetation from touching your home. Homes with ivy growing on them or shrubs right up against the house are much more susceptible to mold problems. Trim your bushes and trees a foot or two away from your walls, and patch that roof before the next rainy season.

Fast

Another good way to detox your body is by giving your GI tract a break now and then. Many religions practice fasting, which provides a way for people to refocus their thoughts on something or someone greater than themselves.

As a doctor, I witness the benefits of fasting all the time. Fasting cleanses the body from built-up chemicals, metals, and other toxins. When you fast, your cells, tissues, and organs dump out the accumulated waste products of cellular metabolism as well as chemicals, heavy metals, pesticides, and solvents. Fasting revitalizes you in every way: mentally, physically, and spiritually. It also allows the overburdened liver to "catch up" on its detoxification work.

The fast I recommend most often is a fresh, juiced organic vegetable and fruit fast as opposed to a water-only fast. A juice fast creates an alkaline environment for your body's cells and tissues so they can begin to release toxins on a cellular level and eliminate them through the body's channels of elimination. Even the blood and lymphatic system can be cleansed of toxic buildup through fasting or a phytonutrient powder. (See Appendix A.) The fiber that is present in juiced fruits and vegetables keeps the colon working to detox the body.

When you fast, don't be surprised if you feel light-headed or "foggy." People who diet or fast experience this because they may experience low blood sugar and also because their fat cells shrink and begin to release the chemicals they've been storing.

Don't go overboard. I recommend fasting just one day a month to only a few days a month. If you fast too much, such as one or two weeks every month, you may interfere with your body's natural metabolic processes. You may lose muscle mass, which slows down your metabolic rate, and your immune system may become compromised. However, a three-week juice fast once a year may be very beneficial. I offer specific fasting programs in my books *Get Healthy Through Detox and Fasting, Fasting Made Easy,* and *Toxic Relief.*

Organic Cleansers

Finally, use non-chemical solvents and cleaners like white distilled vinegar, borax, baking soda, lemon juice, or peroxide. Use natural pesticides, not poisons. Here are a few suggestions, taken from an excellent fact sheet published by the EPA.[4]

Can't Get Rid of Musty Odors?

Combine 1 tsp. of tea tree oil and 1 cup of water in a spritzer bottle. Spray the area, but don't wipe it off. In a couple of days the smell should be gone and the tea tree oil will have dissipated. If not, repeat the spraying.

Baking soda can scrub shiny materials without scratching, extinguish grease fires, and be used as a deodorizer in the refrigerator, on smelly carpets, on upholstery, and on vinyl. It softens fabrics and removes certain stains. It can be used as an underarm deodorant and as toothpaste.

Borax, a naturally occurring mineral that is water soluble, can deodorize, inhibit the growth of mildew and mold, boost the cleaning power of soap or detergent, and remove stains.

Cornstarch can be used to clean windows, polish furniture, shampoo carpets and rugs, and starch clothes. If you have mildew in books, sprinkle a little onto the pages lightly. Let it sit for a while, then shake the cornstarch out of the book.

Isopropyl alcohol is an excellent disinfectant. Lemon juice is a deodorizer and can be used to clean glass and remove stains from aluminum, clothes, and porcelain.

Mineral oil, derived from seeds, is an ingredient in several furniture polish and floor wax recipes. Use steel wool as a strong abrasive to remove rust and stubborn food residues and to scour barbecue grills.

As you can see, a number of detoxification methods, like periodic juice fasting, drinking alkaline water and eating alkaline foods, taking an infrared sauna, taking nutritional supplements, and keeping a regular aerobic exercise program, will mobilize and eliminate a vast array of toxins. Many other detoxification measures beyond the scope of this book exist as well, such as chelation therapy for heavy metal detox, specific mud packs to remove localized toxins, ionic footbaths, homeopathy, EAV, light beam generators and other lymphatic drainage techniques, and laser-assisted detox.

Our world is toxic, but you don't have to be. You can decrease your exposure and risk by making choices that help your body's elimination systems take out the toxic trash.

BUILDING BLOCKS TO A HEALTHY LIFE

POINTS TO PONDER: *Periodic fasting is one of the most powerful ways to detoxify the body. Consider having indoor plants or an air purifier for your home. Choose natural cleansers instead of chemical boxed cleansers.*

ACTION STEP: *Visit your local garden center or nursery, and buy a few indoor plants, such as the ones listed above—some for the office and some for home.*

PILLAR 6

Nutritional Supplements

DAY 36: Your Nutritional Deficit

In 2002, the *Journal of the American Medical Association*, one of the leading medical journals in the United States, shocked the medical community by publishing a study that recommended that all adults should take a multivitamin supplement to help prevent chronic diseases.[1] For decades most of the medical establishment had insisted multivitamins were not necessary, that people got all the vitamins and minerals they needed from the foods. Some doctors actually said that multivitamins only gave people "expensive urine."

But the authors' findings went directly against conventional medical wisdom. They reviewed studies of the relationships between vitamin intake and various diseases published between 1966 and 2002 and concluded that when people did not take in enough vitamins, they were at increased risk of a variety of chronic diseases, including heart disease and cancer. The best course, said the authors, was for all adults to take nutritional supplements.[2]

The medical community was flabbergasted by this study, but the bias against multivitamins and supplements remains so strong that some doctors still won't recommend them. They insist that multivitamin supplements, and most other supplements, are "alternative therapy" or should only be recommended for sick and elderly patients who are more vulnerable to vitamin deficiency. Unfortunately, these doctors don't appreciate the extensiveness of vitamin deficiencies and the problems these deficiencies create for people's health.

Why Diet Alone Isn't Enough

In a perfect world, the human body would indeed get all the nutrients it needs from food. The vitamins and minerals our bodies need to thrive should come through the foods we eat. However, processed foods have been stripped of much of their nutrient content. Cooking and storage are also reasons why our food loses more nutrients. Our toxic environment and toxins in our food, water, and air, as well as our overstressed lifestyles, have increased our nutrient requirements. Even if we were to eat adequate fruits and vegetables, the nutrient content in them has decreased due to our depleted soils.

But few, if any, people get the nutrients they need from food alone, even if they eat a completely healthy diet. That's why the sixth pillar of health is nutritional supplements, because supplements give you the nutrients you are likely missing from your normal diet. Those nutrients are the building blocks of health, and they will protect you against disease. Without them, you are likely to have nutrient deficiencies.

It's extremely difficult to get all the nutrition your body needs from your diet alone. Admittedly, I do have a very few patients who are incredibly meticulous about their diets. They pay attention to everything they eat, keeping diet logs to monitor what they will eat and when they will eat. Some are vegetarians, and many insist on eating only foods made and prepared according to healthy standards. They end up spending much of their time planning what to eat, shopping for food, and preparing their food. For a few, the time and energy it takes to plan can consume their life.

God's Bible Cure for Depleted Soil

In biblical times, God told His people to work the land for six years, and on the seventh year, the land was given a "Sabbath rest." (Read Leviticus 25:1–7.) In so doing, this gave the soil time to regenerate its nutrients.

As I stated previously, one of the biggest reasons diet alone is not enough is because today's soil has fewer nutrients in it than ever before. When soil has fewer nutrients, so do the things that grow in it. Today's soil has suffered massively at the hands of agribusinesses, which plant and harvest produce on a large scale, aiming not for nutritious crops, but for crops that look good and last a long time on store shelves. Unfortunately, nutrition has been sacrificed along the way. Long gone are the days when farmers rotated crops or mulched their fields, all of which preserved minerals in the soil. Now, agribusinesses overwork the fields and add back a narrow range of minerals instead of letting the land naturally regenerate its nutrients.

According to the 1992 Earth Summit, North America has the worst soil in the world—85 percent of vital minerals have been depleted from it.[3] People noticed this trend as far back as 1936, when the U.S. Senate issued Document 246, which said that impoverished soil in the United States no longer provided plant foods with minerals needed for human nourishment.[4]

Modern farmers fertilize the soil with a limited number of nutrients—mainly nitrogen, phosphorus, and potassium. These three nutrients have been found to grow big, beautiful crops, but they are just a few of the dozens of nutrients our bodies need to be healthy. Apples or lettuce bunches on store shelves may look beautiful, but the beauty is only skin deep. They are usually poor in many nutrients because they were grown in depleted soil.

Many studies show how depleted soil has affected the mineral content of vegetables and fruits. One observer compared the data from the USDA handbook from 1972 to the USDA food tables of today and found dramatic reductions in nutrient content. For example, nearly half the calcium and vitamin A in broccoli have disappeared. The vitamin A content in collard greens has fallen to nearly half its previous levels. Potassium dropped from 400 mg to 170 mg, and magnesium fell from 57 mg to only 9 mg. Cauliflower lost almost half of its vitamin C along with its thiamine and riboflavin. The calcium in pineapple went from 17 mg to 7 mg. Those astonishing losses in nutrients eventually will have a significant impact on your health.[5]

Acid rain is another culprit in soil degradation. Even a modest amount of acid rain causes soil to lose nutrients. One thirty-year study showed that acid rain steadily depleted the soils of the forest by 38 percent at one site in South Carolina and made the soil more acidic.[6]

I believe the depletion of our soil is part of the curse God placed on the land after Adam and Eve were forced to leave the Garden of Eden. But I also believe that as we come under God's grace, He has blessed us with the tools and the knowledge that will make our land—and our food—rich in nutrients again.

Good Grains—How They Rank

It's almost impossible to rank grains because we need to consider all the different elements involved (size, soil, and so on). These grains have unique and wonderful flavors and textures, not to mention a broad range of nutrients, including fiber, B vitamins, and trace minerals that refined grain products do not contain. Among the world's healthiest grains are barley, oats, millet, rye, and brown rice.[7]

Poor Digestion

Another reason people need nutritional supplements is because of poor digestion. I will occasionally do a blood test to check intracellular nutrient levels for certain patients, and very often they are deficient in several nutrients, even if they eat a healthy diet and take supplements. This is because it's not just what you eat but what you assimilate and absorb into your body. Your GI tract acts as a barrier as well as an absorber of nutrients. If it detects something it deems toxic, it blocks it from entering. That's one reason why people get diarrhea. Your intestine is flushing out what it thinks is harmful.

An estimated 100 million Americans have some type of digestive disorder.[8] This means that even if they put nutritious foods in their mouths, the nutrients may not be adequately absorbed by their bodies. One reason for poor digestion is lack of enzymes in the diet. As we saw earlier, enzymes are essential to the body's digestion, assimilation, and absorption of food. But many adults do not have enough enzymes that are essential for normal digestion. This could be for a number of reasons:

1. They choose highly processed food that is void of enzymes.
2. They chew poorly, making it difficult for enzymes to break down the food.
3. They cook food at high temperatures, destroying the enzymes in the food.
4. They consume excessive amounts of fluids with their meals, which washes out their enzymes.

Also, as we grow older, our capacity to make enzymes diminishes. Stress also hinders digestive enzymes from being produced.

We saw earlier that many people, especially individuals over fifty years of age, have low levels of hydrochloric acid, which is needed for proper digestion. Also millions of Americans are consuming antacids, Pepcid, Mylanta, Zantac 75, Prilosec, and other medications that reduce hydrochloric acid. Other people have poor digestion because they are stressed or are on birth control pills or other medications that affect how well vitamins are absorbed. Each of these may contribute to vitamin and mineral deficiencies.

Quick Quiz

Most digestion takes place in the:

a. Stomach

b. Small intestine

c. Large intestine

Answer: b. Small intestine.

The bottom line is that to be healthy you almost certainly need to start taking nutritional supplements. Which ones to take, and in what quantities, will be the subject of the rest of this section. Let's start by taking a look at which deficiencies are most common and which ones you might be suffering from.

BUILDING BLOCKS TO A HEALTHY LIFE

POINTS TO PONDER: *Whole grains such as barley, millet, oats, and brown rice contain more of the nutrients we need than their refined counterparts, such as white rice or white bread. Proper digestion is essential to helping the body absorb the nutrients our bodies need. However, even the healthiest diet needs to be supplemented with nutrients.*

ACTION STEP: *Consider taking a daily multivitamin. (See Appendix A.) Please consult with your physician if you are on the medication Coumadin before you begin taking any supplement.*

DAY 37: The Most Common Nutrient Deficiencies

Today's reading may get a little technical, but bear with me. Remember, I wrote this book for the enrichment of your life and the vitality of your years. Although there's lots of information to get through today, I also provide lots of practical tips and suggestions to help you get all the nutrients you need.

Most people have the misconception that vitamins will give them instant energy. Vitamins are not pep pills. *Vitamin* literally means "vital amine," and they are indeed needed for many biological processes, including growth, digestion, mental alertness, and resistance to infection. Vitamins enable your body to use carbohydrates, fats, and proteins, and they speed up chemical reactions. Vitamins and minerals *are not optional* for your health. They are at the *very foundation* of your health.

What Happens When You Don't Get Enough Nutrients

Most Americans don't get even basic amounts of recommended vitamins and minerals. Here are the fast facts on the vitamins and minerals most Americans lack, what those nutrients do, where they are found, and what happens when you don't get enough of them.

Vitamin E

Research shows that 93 percent of Americans have inadequate intakes of *vitamin E*,[1] which decreases free-radical damage of lipid membranes and protects the heart, blood vessels, and tissues of the breast, liver, eyes, skin, and testes. Vitamin E decreases blood clotting, which further reduces the risk of heart disease. Most people get vitamin E from vegetable oil products like salad dressings, though cold-pressed vegetable oils (such as extra-virgin olive oil) are generally highest in vitamin E. (Most vegetable oils are heat processed.) You can also get vitamin E from dark green leafy vegetables, legumes, nuts, seeds, whole grains, brown rice, corn meal, eggs, milk, oatmeal, and wheat germ. Common sources include the following:[2]

Food	Amount of Vitamin E
Wheat germ oil, 1 Tbsp.	20.3 mg (about 30 IU*)
Almonds, dried, 1 oz.	6.72 mg (about 10 IU)
Sweet potato, 1 medium	5.93 mg (about 9 IU)

* An IU (International Unit) is a unit of measurement used in pharmacology based on the biological activity of the substance being measured.

I recommend the natural vitamin E, which contains all eight forms of vitamin E: alpha-, beta-, delta-, and gamma-tocopherol, and alpha-, beta-, delta-, and gamma-tocotrienol. The names of all types of vitamin E begin with either "d" or "dl." The "d" is the natural form, and the "dl" is the synthetic form, which comes from petroleum. The synthetic form has only about 50 percent of the activity of natural vitamin E.[3] But tremendous confusion and even controversy have surrounded vitamin E since its discovery in 1922. One recent study concluded that in patients with vascular disease or diabetes, the long-term supplementation with the natural source vitamin E (400 IU) does not prevent cancer or cardiovascular events and may actually increase the risk for heart failure.[4] That conclusion had unfortunate consequences, because most Americans already lack sufficient amounts of this important nutrient. Some doctors warned their patients not to take vitamin E in a supplement.

The study also ignored the benefits of vitamin E. A different study showed that men who take 50 IU a day, as opposed to the recommended daily value of 30 IU, had 41 percent fewer deaths from prostate cancer than those who did not receive supplemental vitamin E.[5] That's a significant benefit.

One form of vitamin E, gamma-tocopherol, is extremely important. One study found that men with the highest concentration of gamma-tocopherol had a fivefold lower risk of developing prostate cancer than men with the lowest levels.[6] Gamma-tocopherol may also protect one from developing colorectal cancer and Alzheimer's disease.

Prolonged vitamin E deficiency may eventually cause severe neurological complications, including unsteady gait, loss of muscle coordination, muscle weakness, peripheral neuropathy, and diminished reflexes. It can also cause infertility, menstrual problems, miscarriages, and shortened red blood cell lifespan. I'll talk more about how much vitamin E and what type to take in the next couple of days.

Magnesium

Magnesium is needed for protein, fatty acid, and bone formation, but 56 percent of Americans aren't consuming enough.[7] Magnesium is used in making new cells, in relaxing muscles, and in the clotting of blood. It helps form ATP, which gives us energy. It assists with over three hundred different enzyme reactions in the body; helps prevent muscle spasm, heart attacks, and heart disease; aids in lowering blood pressure; and eases asthma. It also helps prevent osteoporosis and helps regulate the colon and bowels. The recommended daily amount for the average person from fifteen to fifty years old is 400 mg. Magnesium is found in nuts, seeds, dark green leafy vegetables, grains, and legumes. It is easy to see why many Americans are deficient in this important mineral, because many are eating fast foods and junk foods instead of "living foods." Common sources of magnesium include:[8]

Magnesium and Regularity

Your colon needs magnesium to help it undergo peristalsis, which propels food through and out. Most Americans don't take adequate amounts of fiber, magnesium, and water.

Food	Amount of Magnesium
Halibut, 3 oz., cooked serving	90 mg
Almonds, 1 oz., dry roasted	80 mg
Cashews, 1 oz., dry roasted	75 mg
Spinach, organic, frozen, ½ cup, cooked	75 mg
Black-eyed peas, ½ cup, cooked	45 mg

In order to get your reference daily intake (RDI), you would have to eat about five ounces of almonds every day. If you don't get enough magnesium, you may experience loss of appetite, nausea, and fatigue. If the deficiency worsens, patients may develop muscle weakness, muscle twitches, irregular heartbeat, leg cramps, insomnia, and eye twitches. Symptoms of deficiency also include constipation, headaches, personality changes, and coronary spasms. Magnesium is a building block of your health.

Calcium

Calcium is also required by your body in relatively large amounts. About 99 percent of your calcium resides in your bones and teeth. The remaining 1 percent circulates in your blood and carries out the critical function of regulating muscle contraction, heart contraction, and nerve function. Calcium gives you strong bones and prevents osteoporosis. It even lowers blood pressure. Some studies suggest that when you get adequate calcium in dietary and supplemental form, you decrease your risk of colon cancer.[9]

Calcium is found in higher amounts in these foods:[10]

Food	Amount of Calcium
Yogurt, plain, low-fat, 8 oz.	415 mg
Calcium-fortified soy or rice milk, 8 oz.	80–500 mg
Turnip greens, 4 cups, boiled	396 mg
Kale, cooked, 4 cups	376 mg
Milk, nonfat, 8 fl. oz.	302 mg
Cheddar cheese, 1.5 oz.	206 mg
Tofu, firm, made with calcium sulfate, ½ cup	204 mg
Cottage cheese, 1% milkfat, 1 cup unpacked	138 mg
Spinach, ½ cup, cooked	120 mg

Children and teens age nine to eighteen need 1,300 mg a day, persons age nineteen to fifty need 1,000 mg a day, and individuals over age fifty-one need 1,200 mg a day.[11] The problem is, if you don't consume enough dietary calcium, your body will eventually cannibalize the calcium from the bones to maintain calcium levels in the blood. This can quietly lead to osteopenia and osteoporosis, which literally means "porous bones"—or bones lacking in minerals and mass. Very few women get all the calcium they need from diet, and in old age their skeletons shrink. The first bones to go are the jawbone and the vertebra in the back, which is why older people lose their teeth and height. Calcium deficiencies can also result in leg cramps, muscle cramps, and even hemorrhage (since calcium is essential to blood clotting).

Studies show that more than 75 percent of Americans do not meet the current recommendations for calcium intake.[12] Low calcium intake has become a major public health problem in the United States.

Vitamin A

An estimated 44 percent of Americans are lacking adequate intake of *vitamin A*,[13] which protects us against cancer and heart disease, prevents night blindness and other eye problems, helps the skin repair itself, and helps in the formation of bones and teeth. Vitamin A is important for the immune system, protecting us against colds, the flu, and infections of the kidneys, bladder, lungs, and mucous membranes.

Beta-carotene is converted in the body to vitamin A and is found in carrots, apricots, leafy greens, garlic, kale, papayas, peaches, red peppers, and sweet potatoes.[14] The recommended daily intake for most adults is 2,300 to 3,000 IU daily. Lactating women need 4,000 IU a day. Children need only 1,000 to 2,000 IU daily.[15]

Be careful not to go overboard when taking vitamin A. Excessive amounts of vitamin A may lead to liver damage.[16] Dosages greater than 10,000 IU a day of vitamin A were reported in the *New England Journal of Medicine* to have probably been responsible for one out of fifty-seven birth defects in the United States. However, this does not refer to beta-carotene or other caretonoids.[17] Women who are at risk for becoming pregnant should keep their supplemental vitamin A levels below 5,000 IU or choose carotenoids instead of vitamin A.[18] Also, carotenoids, such as beta-carotene, are safer than vitamin A because the body will convert beta-carotene to vitamin A without producing vitamin A in toxic amounts.[19]

The chart below gives some food sources for vitamin A and beta-carotene:[20]

Sources of Vitamin A		**Sources of Beta-Carotene**	
Food	**Amount of Vitamin A**	**Food**	**Amount of Beta-Carotene**
Cod liver oil, 1 tsp.	2,000 IU	Carrots, boiled, ½ cup slices	13,418 IU
Milk, fortified skim, 1 cup	500 IU	Carrot, raw, 7 inches	8,666 IU
Cheese, cheddar, 1 oz.	249 IU	Cantaloupe, cubed, 1 cup	5,411 IU
		Spinach, raw, 1 cup	2,813 IU
		Mango, sliced, 1 cup	1,262 IU
		Peach, 1 medium	319 IU

Lack of vitamin A in your body can cause dry hair and skin, dry eyes, poor growth, frequent colds, skin disorders, sinusitis, insomnia, fatigue, and respiratory infections.[21]

Vitamin C

Vitamin C helps form collagen, a protein that gives structure to—and maintains—bones, cartilage, muscle, and blood vessels. It also plays a role in wound healing. The adequate intake is 90 mg per day for adult men and 75 mg for adult women, but studies show that 31 percent of Americans don't get enough.[22] Common sources include:[23]

Food	Amount of Vitamin C
Guava, 1 medium	165 mg
Red bell pepper, ½ cup	95 mg
Papaya, 1 medium	95 mg
Orange, 1 medium	60 mg
Broccoli, ½ cup, steamed	60 mg
Strawberries, ½ cup	45 mg
Cantaloupe, ½ cup	35 mg

I recommend a four-ounce glass of fresh-squeezed orange juice every day with the pulp added to it. Vitamin C deficiency causes weakness, fatigue, swollen gums, nosebleeds, and, in extreme cases, scurvy.[24] During stress there are higher requirements for vitamin C. It is also reported to reduce the risk of cataracts and retinal damage, increase immune function, and decrease heavy metal toxicity. Increased intake of vitamin C is linked to a reduced risk of cancer of the cervix, stomach, colon, and lungs. It also reduces LDL oxidation, which causes plaque buildup in arteries, and it supports healthy blood pressure.[25]

It's a Fact!

According to the USDA, just over one in four Americans meet their adequate intake of vitamin K.

Vitamin K

Studies suggest that 73 percent of Americans do not get adequate intake of *vitamin K*,[26] which is important in blood clotting, for bone mineralization, and in helping to regulate cellular growth.[27] The daily reference intake for vitamin K for men age nineteen and above is 120 mcg. For women in that age bracket it is 90 mcg.[28] Vitamin K is found in:[29]

Food	Amount of Vitamin K
Brussels sprouts, 1 cup, cooked	460 mcg
Broccoli, 1 cup, cooked	248 mcg
Cauliflower, 1 cup, cooked	150 mcg
Swiss chard, 1 cup, cooked	123 mcg
Spinach, 1 cup, raw	120 mcg
Beef, 3.5 oz.	104 mcg

Most of your body's supply of vitamin K is synthesized by the friendly bacteria in your intestines. But when you take antibiotics, you increase your need for vitamin K. The antibiotics kill many of the good bacteria, and as a result, the remaining good bacteria cannot produce adequate amounts of vitamin K.[30]

Vitamin K deficiency is associated with easy bruising and bleeding and increased risk of osteoporosis. Vitamin K has been shown to be supportive in preventing calcification or hardening in the arteries.[31] The presence of vitamin K in green leafy vegetables may be one reason vegetarians have a lower incidence of kidney stones.[32]

Dietary fiber

Dietary fiber, as we saw on Day 19 in the pillar on living foods, is vital to your health. Insoluble fiber helps to prevent gallstones and control irritable bowel syndrome, constipation, and almost any GI disorder. Soluble fiber helps control cholesterol and blood sugar. Insoluble fiber generally does not cause excessive gas, whereas soluble fiber does. For more on this topic, refer to my book *What Would Jesus Eat?*

"Lettuce" Eat Fiber?

Less than 5 percent eat more than their adequate intake of dietary fiber. Contrary to popular belief, lettuce is not the best source of fiber. Lettuce is actually very low in fiber. For instance, 1 cup of romaine lettuce has only 0.7 grams of fiber, 1 cup of iceberg lettuce has only 1 gram of fiber, and 1 cup of butterhead lettuce has 1.3 grams of fiber.

Dietary fiber is simply nondigestible polysaccharides, which are found in plant cell walls.[33] Most people get fiber from whole-grain cereals, nuts, seeds, dried beans, fruits, and vegetables; however, studies show that 96 percent of Americans do not have an adequate intake of fiber.[34] Some other good sources include:[35]

Food	Amount of Dietary Fiber
Pinto beans, ½ cup, cooked	7.4 grams
Artichoke, 1 medium, cooked	6.5 grams
Kidney beans, ½ cup, cooked	5.8 grams
Navy beans, ½ cup,cooked	5.8 grams
Apple, 3-inch diameter	5.7 grams
Figs, 3 small	5.3 grams
Orange, 3-inch diameter	4.4 grams
Green peas, ½ cup, cooked	4.3 grams
Raspberries, ½ cup	4.2 grams
Barley, ½ cup, cooked	4.2 grams

Food	Amount of Dietary Fiber
Blackberries, ½ cup	3.8 grams
Mango, medium	3.7 grams
Banana, 7 inches long	2.8 grams
Whole-wheat noodles, ½ cup	2.3 grams
Whole-wheat bread, 1 medium slice	1.9 grams
Brown rice, ½ cup, cooked	1.7 grams

Inadequate intake of fiber is associated with increased constipation, hemorrhoids, diverticulosis, diverticulitis, bowel irregularities, and colorectal cancer. It is also associated with elevated cholesterol, irritable bowel syndrome, toxin buildup, and poor blood sugar control in diabetics. Most Americans eat an estimated twelve grams or less of fiber daily. But the recommended goal is twenty-five to thirty grams a day.[36]

Switch Slowly

When switching from a low-fiber diet to a high-fiber diet, do it in increments. If you do it too suddenly, you might experience bloating or gas.[37]

Vitamin B_6

Vitamin B_6 performs many functions in your body, but studies show that 28 percent of women nineteen years of age and older do not have adequate intake of this vitamin.[38] It is needed for more than one hundred enzymes involved in protein metabolism; it is also essential for red blood cell metabolism. The nervous and immune systems need it to function efficiently. It helps increase the amount of oxygen carried to your tissues, and it helps to keep your blood sugar level in a normal range. It is very important in the synthesis of neurotransmitters—serotonin and dopamine.[39]

Vitamin B_6 is found in fortified cereals, fish, poultry, red meat, and some produce. Recommended intake for adults age nineteen to fifty is 1.3 mg a day, and around 1.6 mg for people over fifty.[40]

Food	Amount of Vitamin B_6
Potato, medium, baked	0.70 mg
Banana, medium	0.68 mg
Chicken, ½ breast, cooked	0.52 mg
Garlic, 1 oz.	0.35 mg
Brussels sprouts, 1 cup, boiled	0.28 mg

Food	Amount of Vitamin B_6
Collard greens, 1 cup, drained, boiled	0.24 mg
Sunflower seeds, kernels only, 1 oz., dry roasted	0.23 mg
Red bell peppers, 1 cup, sliced, raw	0.23 mg
Broccoli pieces, 1 cup, steamed	0.22 mg
Watermelon, 1 cup	0.22 mg
Tomato juice, 6 oz.	0.20 mg
Avocado, raw, ½ cup, sliced	0.20 mg

Signs of vitamin B_6 deficiency include skin irritation, headaches, sore tongue, depression, confusion, convulsions, anemia, and PMS. If you are deficient in vitamin B_6, B_{12}, or folic acid, then levels of homocysteine, a toxic amino acid, may rise in the blood. Homocysteine has a toxic effect on the cells lining the arteries, causing plaque to form on the artery lining. High levels of homocysteine in the blood are associated with increased risk of cardiovascular disease as well as Alzheimer's disease.[41]

Did You Know...?

Fourteen percent of Americans have inadequate intake of vitamin B_6 from food.

Vitamin D

Research indicates that 20 percent of children and adults up to age fifty and 95 percent of adults over fifty do not have adequate intake of *vitamin D*,[42] which is required for your body to absorb calcium and phosphorus. It is critically important for growth and for the normal development of bones and teeth.[43] It may protect against prostate and breast cancer. The higher the vitamin D levels in the blood, the lower the risk for colon and colorectal cancers.[44]

But vitamin D deficiency is common among young women (only 20 to 40 percent get the amounts they need) and in people over fifty, particularly women, for whom vitamin D deficiency is epidemic.[45] Very few people overall get enough vitamin D (400 IU) from their diet alone.[46]

Sun exposure is the most important source of vitamin D, because the skin synthesizes vitamin D in response to UV rays. Most people need only ten to fifteen minutes of direct sun exposure, twice a week, without sunscreen, to meet their vitamin D requirement.[47] However, few doctors recommend this since it may increase the risk of skin cancer for some individuals.

There are few good food sources of vitamin D. Cod liver oil offers a whopping 1,360 IU per tablespoon. I don't recommend cod liver oil because it has so many toxins. It also has to be over processed, thus rendering it unstable, and it contains a high percentage of oxidized fats. Three and one-half ounces of cooked salmon give 360 IUs. And a cup of milk fortified with vitamin D gives about 100 IU.[48]

Vitamin D_3 is the active form of vitamin D. In its active form, vitamin D enhances the absorption of calcium from the small intestines. Even though the recommended dose of vitamin D for adults over fifty is 400–600 IU a day, the National Osteoporosis Foundation recommends 800 IU for those at risk. [49]

Vitamin D deficiency is associated with osteoporosis and hip fractures. In a review of women with osteoporosis, hospitalized for hip fractures, 50 percent were found to have signs of vitamin D deficiency.[50]

Potassium

Potassium is a mineral that helps muscles contract, maintains fluid balance, sends nerve impulses, and releases energy from food. Potassium is needed to regulate blood pressure, neuromuscular function, and levels of acidity. Your body needs sodium and potassium to maintain good health. They both help regulate fluids in and out of your body cells. According to a new report, most adults consume excessive amounts of sodium, and many don't consume enough potassium. The reason is that processed and fast foods are high in sodium, and fruits and most vegetables are high in potassium. The average American diet is lacking in fruits and vegetables. The Institute of Medicine of the National Academies of Science recently issued recommendations for sodium and potassium intake levels, saying healthy adults between nineteen and fifty should consume about 1,500 mg of sodium per day and 4,700 mg of potassium.

Did You Know . . . ?

Less than 5 percent of the population eat more than their adequate intake of potassium.[51]

Potassium is one of the main electrolytes in the body, along with sodium and chloride. These three electrolytes play a key chemical role in every function of the body. The RDI (reference daily intake) of potassium for anyone ten years old and above is 2,000 mg.[52]

Reach your recommended daily intake of potassium by adding these foods to your daily menu: fish, potatoes, avocadoes, dried apricots, bananas, citrus juices, dairy products, and whole grains are wonderful sources of potassium. The top foods are:[53]

Food	Amount of Potassium
Sweet potato, baked	694 mg
Tomato paste, ¼ cup	664 mg
Beet greens, ½ cup, cooked	655 mg
Yogurt, plain, nonfat, 8 oz.	579 mg
Prune juice, ¾ cup	530 mg
Carrot juice, ¾ cup	517 mg
Halibut, 3 oz., cooked	490 mg
Soybeans, green, ½ cup, cooked	485 mg
Banana, medium	422 mg
Peaches, dried, ¼ cup	398 mg
Milk, nonfat, 1 cup	382 mg
Cantaloupe, ¼ medium	368 mg
Kidney beans, ½ cup, cooked	358 mg
Orange juice, ¾ cup	355 mg

That means the average adult would have to eat the equivalent of three baked sweet potatoes every day to get the RDI. Not many people eat sweet potatoes or other foods high in potassium each day, which is why we need supplements.

Eating too much salt may lower your body's store of potassium. Low potassium intake is associated with high blood pressure, irregular heartbeat, wheezing and asthma, weakness, nausea, loss of appetite, altered mental states including nervousness and depression, dry skin, insomnia, and fatigue.

Iodine

Iodine is essential for proper thyroid function. Without adequate iodine intake, the thyroid gland is unable to make adequate amounts of thyroid hormones. An iodine deficiency can cause hypothyroidism, developmental brain disorders, and goiter (thyroid enlargement). In children, hypothyroidism as a result of iodine deficiency can cause stunted growth, mental retardation, and speech and hearing problems.

Even though iodine is not yet recognized as a major deficiency in America, I have found that many of my patients are iodine deficient. Some researchers believe that iodine deficiency is on the rise in the United States. The October 1998 issue of the *Journal of Clinical Endocrinology and Metabolism* reported that the percentage of Americans who don't consume enough iodine has more than quadrupled in the past twenty years.[54]

Americans are consuming less iodine because our soil is deficient in it, especially in inland and mountainous areas. Also, approximately 50 percent of people use salt without iodine. Breads and pastas no longer contain iodine but instead contain bromide, which behaves like a goitrogen and inhibits iodine binding. Fluoride and chlorine, found in much of our tap water, also inhibit iodine binding.

In addition to the conditions listed above, low iodine is linked to fibrocystic breast disease and polycystic ovaries, making women more likely to suffer from physical problems as a result of iodine deficiency.[55] Evidence shows that adequate intake of iodine makes a difference in warding off these conditions.

These vitamins and minerals, and many others, are absolutely essential to good health and long life. Maintaining long-term deficiencies of any of them is like asking your car to do its job without the proper fuel. I will give specific recommendations about vitamin and mineral supplementation, but first let's look at antioxidants and phytonutrients, two fascinating food ingredients that boost your health immensely.

BUILDING BLOCKS TO A HEALTHY LIFE

POINTS TO PONDER: *A healthy diet will rarely supply all the nutrients you need. In fact, most Americans don't get even basic amounts of recommended vitamins and minerals. Nutrients that are commonly lacking in the American diet include vitamins A, B_6, C, D, E, and K, magnesium, calcium, fiber, and potassium.*

ACTION STEP: *If you don't have a history of skin or pre-skin cancer, consider spending five to ten minutes a day in sunlight without sunblock. This enables your body to produce adequate amounts of vitamin D. Don't forget to wear sunglasses.*

DAY 38: Your Need for Antioxidants

Let's say that you eat five to thirteen servings of fruits and vegetables a day and that you take a multivitamin that contains adequate amounts of vitamin E, vitamin C, selenium, and beta-carotene every day. You believe that you are consuming all the antioxidants you will need to prevent disease. However, you are most likely not taking the correct antioxidants.

Before discussing antioxidants, it is critically important to understand free radicals—how they start and how we can protect ourselves from them. Let's begin by discussing the process of oxidation, which is a chemical process. When metals such as iron are oxidized, rust is produced. When oxidation occurs on painted surfaces, the paint begins to flake off. When you cut an apple in half, it begins to turn brown within a few minutes due to oxidation. Oxidation also occurs when food spoils, meat rots, and fats rancidify. Free radicals cause oxidation.

Want to Live to Be 100?

Blood levels of antioxidants generally decrease with age. However, Italian researchers discovered that centenarians (individuals one hundred years of age or older) needed significantly higher blood levels of vitamins A and E than their counterparts who were younger. The Italian researchers concluded, "It is evident that healthy centenarians show a particular profile in which high levels of vitamin A and vitamin E seem to be important in guaranteeing their extreme longevity."[1]

So, exactly what is a free radical? Picture, if you will, an atom that has a nucleus with electrons around it. As electrons circle the nucleus, they are usually paired. When an electron becomes unpaired, it tries to pull an electron from another atom or molecule in order to return to a state of equilibrium. Free radicals are simply atoms with unpaired electrons. Free radicals are very aggressive, and as they steal electrons from other atoms, they damage cells in the process. They damage cell membranes and nuclear membranes, and eventually may damage the DNA in the nucleus of the cell. Also, when free radicals steal electrons from other atoms, these atoms become free radicals themselves, leading to a chain reaction. A vicious cycle can be created, leading to damage and destruction of cells and eventually to chronic diseases.

Now, free radicals are generated in our bodies simply by breathing. Normal metabolism creates free radicals referred to as reactive oxygen species (ROS). Just as smoke comes from a fire, free radicals come from the normal metabolism and production of energy in the mitochondria of our bodies. Foods—including hydrogenated and partially hydrogenated fats; excessive intake of highly processed foods, excessive sugar, fried foods, excessive amounts of polyunsaturated fats found in salad dressings, cooking oils, sauces, gravies, and so on—will also create excessive free radicals.

Many diseases are inflammatory and are creating tremendous amounts of free radicals, including most cancers, arthritis, coronary artery disease, asthma, Alzheimer's disease, Parkinson's disease, multiple sclerosis, lupus, and colitis. Frequent colds, flu, sinus infections, bronchitis, and bladder and yeast infections create more free radicals. Trauma from sprains, strains, muscle aches, and even excessive exercise creates a tremendous amount of free radicals. This is why those who over-train, as well as long-distance runners and marathoners, appear to actually age faster.

Super-Antioxidant Drinks

Which of the following beverages is highest in antioxidants?

a. Green tea

b. Coffee

c. Hot chocolate

Answer: c. Hot chocolate. Dark chocolate extracted from organic cocoa beans has the highest level of antioxidants. So drink up (in moderation, of course), but hold the sugar and choose low-fat dairy.

And finally there is our toxic exposure. Unfortunately, no one is exempt. There are pesticides and other toxins in our food, water, and air, and these toxins create an added burden on the liver. In the detoxification process by the liver, more free radicals are produced, and the toxic burden may be so great that the liver is unable to keep up with detoxification. These toxins increase in the body, which causes the production of more free radicals. Inhaling sidestream smoke and car exhaust, drinking tap water with chlorine and all the other chemicals, eating the standard American diet laced with chemicals and inflammatory foods—these all are producing a flood of free radicals that are causing diseases, which create even more free radicals. It becomes a vicious cycle of ever-increasing free radicals. Unfortunately, Americans are running to their doctors who are prescribing medicines that turn off symptoms yet create a greater burden on the liver and actually cause more free radicals to be produced.

The answer to free radicals is simple: antioxidants. Antioxidants have the ability to neutralize free radicals. Antioxidants are to free radicals what water is to a raging forest fire burning out of control. Of course, it also involves choosing more living foods, detoxification, and the other pillars of health. But antioxidants are the most important key for the free-radical riddle.

Just think about what happens when you squeeze lemon juice on an exposed slice of apple. The vitamin C and bioflavonoid antioxidants in the lemon quench free radicals, slowing down the oxidation process, which means it takes *much* longer for the apple slice to turn brown. That's why antioxidants are usually added to processed food—to prevent oxygen from combining with different food components. Without them, many processed foods would become stale, rancid, or inedible.

Researchers have known for years that there are literally thousands of different compounds that function as antioxidants. Many are found in foods and supplements, and others are actually produced by our bodies. That's right, our bodies have developed a powerful army of antioxidants that neutralize free radicals. By consuming living foods containing powerful antioxidants and phytonutrients, taking specific antioxidant supplements, and supporting our own antioxidants produced by our bodies, we will be able to quench many free-radical reactions.

Different antioxidants are able to neutralize free radicals in every part of the body. I believe that it's important to have adequate amounts of three key antioxidants produced by the body and five key antioxidants from supplements. Instead of discussing all the antioxidants, I'll focus on the key antioxidants and a few others.

The key antioxidants that our bodies produce include glutathione, superoxide dismutase (SOD), and catalase.

Glutathione

Glutathione is a powerful antioxidant that is produced in the liver and works throughout the body in cells, tissues, and fluids to detoxify free radicals created from oxygen known as reactive oxygen species (ROS). It simply acts as a powerful detoxifier and free-radical quencher. When one is exposed to a high level of toxins, glutathione is depleted faster than it can be produced, setting the stage for toxin-induced diseases, including cancer. Glutathione can be synthesized from three amino acids: cysteine, glutamic acid, and glycine. It can also be obtained in the diet by consuming fresh fruits and vegetables, cooked fish, and meats.

> **It's a Fact!**
>
> Ninety to 95 percent of your body's 60 to 100 trillion cells are replaced every year.

Vitamin C and N-acetyl-cysteine (NAC) increase the rate of synthesis of glutathione. However, high doses of NAC can increase free-radical formation. I recommend between 250 to 800 mg of NAC a day. The herb milk thistle helps prevent the depletion of glutathione and can actually raise the level of glutathione in the liver by up to 35 percent. To raise glutathione levels, NAC, vitamin C, and milk thistle are important supplements to consider. Also, there is one oral glutathione supplement that has been clinically proven to be absorbed intact and effective.[2] (See Appendix A for more information on Recancostat.)

Superoxide Dismatase (SOD)

SOD is an antioxidant that also works to detoxify the free radical superoxide to hydrogen peroxide, which is also a free radical. SOD then works with another antioxidant, catalase, to break down peroxide to water. It also works with glutathione to inactivate both peroxide and lipid peroxides. SOD is made from three basic minerals: copper, zinc, and manganese. Copper and manganese come from whole grains and nuts, and zinc comes from egg yolks, milk, oatmeal, nuts, legumes, and meat. Supplements of SOD are generally ineffective. Simply taking a good multivitamin that contains adequate amounts of copper, zinc, and manganese will usually help to supply adequate amounts of SOD in most non-diseased states. However, in elderly individuals—and especially those with disease—supplementation with copper, zinc, and manganese may not be enough. They will probably need a combination of powerful antioxidant herbs, which increase the production of catalase in the body. Read on to learn more about these herbs.

Catalase

Catalase is a powerful antioxidant and is an iron-dependent enzyme. It is designed to prevent a buildup of hydrogen peroxide, another free radical, in the body. Catalase in the skin converts hydrogen peroxide to water. It also oxygenates the epidermis to form smooth, younger skin.

I remember a few years ago when I was working on my book *Toxic Relief*. I experimented with different types of fasts, including water fasts, juice fasts, and partial fasts. On a seven-day water fast, I noticed little white spots that began forming on my arms and legs, and I broke the fast immediately. It looked like tiny drops of bleach had splashed on my skin. But what had happened was that my system had formed a lot of free radicals and hydrogen peroxide. During the fast I had exhausted my catalase, and I did not have enough catalase antioxidant to convert the peroxide to water. I have since noticed many patients with these tiny white spots who have been helped with supplements. SOD and catalase are actually metabolic enzymes that work together and are the body's first line of defense against oxidative stress. Supplements of SOD and catalase, however, are generally ineffective since they are broken down during digestion.

Unfortunately, aging is associated with increased levels of free radicals and decreased production of SOD and catalase. However, a unique combination of antioxidant herbs is able to increase production of these powerful antioxidants.[3] Catalase and SOD are referred to as catalytic antioxidants. A catalyst simply promotes a reaction and isn't consumed in the reaction. In other words, these powerful antioxidants can quench millions of free radicals and are not spent in the process, but they can continue to destroy more free radicals at another time. These antioxidant enzymes work inside the cell. The herbs that make up this powerful antioxidant combination include green tea, Ashwagandha, turmeric, bacopa, and milk thistle. Another excellent antioxidant supplement contains turmeric and synergistic herbs. (See Appendix A for information on Protandim.)

Other Antioxidants

Lester Packer, PhD, is professor of molecular and cell biology at the University of California–Berkeley; he is also a leading researcher in antioxidants and author of the book *The Antioxidant Miracle*.[4] Dr. Packer has identified five specific antioxidants that he claims are the key antioxidants to protect against heart disease, cancer, Alzheimer's disease, cataracts, and other diseases associated with aging. He believes that the body is best protected by a blend of antioxidants working in synergy. He theorizes that antioxidants are more effective and able to prevent cellular damage when they are present in a balanced combination. Simply put, they work best as a team. The five most important antioxidants, according to Dr. Packer, include vitamin C, vitamin E, coenzyme Q_{10}, alpha-lipoic acid, and glutathione (which we have already discussed).

Antioxidants work by protecting different parts of the cell; therefore, a team of antioxidants will provide free-radical protection for the entire cell. Vitamin C protects the water-soluble interior of the cell, and fat-soluble vitamin E protects specific areas of the cell's fatty outer membrane. Also, there are eight different forms of vitamin E (as I mentioned in Day 37)—alpha-, beta-, delta-, and gamma-tocopherol, and alpha-, beta-, delta-, and gamma-tocotrienol. Alpha-lipoic acid protects both the inside of the cell and the outside cell membrane.

Most multivitamins will contain vitamin C and only one form of vitamin E (d-alpha-tocopherol). In addition, most individuals are not getting lipoic acid, coenzyme Q_{10}, or glutathione or a supplement that increases glutathione. As I stated in Day 37, avoid the synthetic form of vitamin E that is derived from petroleum. It is called "dl-alpha-tocopherol" or "dl-alpha-tocopheryl."

Lipoic acid

Alpha-lipoic acid is a naturally occurring compound that is synthesized by plants and animals, even humans.[5] In its reduced form (R-dihydrolipoic acid, or R-DHLA) it functions as a powerful antioxidant to protect the liver and help detoxify the body from the effects of medication and radiation. It binds metal ions and prevents them from generating free radicals. It neutralizes free radicals in both the water-soluble and fat-soluble parts of the body. DHLA also helps the body "recycle" and extend the life span of vitamin C, glutathione, coenzyme Q_{10}, and vitamin E. Lipoic acid has been shown to elevate intracellular glutathione levels. It improves insulin metabolism in type 2 diabetes and has been used to treat diabetic neuropathy in Germany for more than twenty years. The R-form alpha-lipoic acid is also an excellent form of lipoic acid. The two most powerful forms of lipoic acid are R-DHLA and R-form alpha-lipoic acid. (See Appendix A.)

Coenzyme Q_{10}

Coenzyme Q_{10} (CoQ_{10}) is a powerful antioxidant that is concentrated in heart cells. It plays a critical role in the production of energy in every cell in the body. Deficiencies are commonly seen in periodontal disease, heart disease, diabetes, HIV, and AIDS. The amount of coenzyme Q_{10} produced by the body declines with age, so I strongly recommend it be supplemented by individuals over fifty. However, you should definitely supplement coenzyme Q_{10} if you are taking cholesterol-lowering drugs such as Mevacor, Pravachol, Lipitor, and Zocor. Not all coenzyme Q_{10} is equal. Many forms are synthetic and don't have studies showing that the CoQ_{10} is actually absorbed into the cell. There is also a better form of coenzyme Q_{10} that is actually absorbed into the brain and is able to protect the brain cells.[6] A reduced form of CoQ_{10} was recently developed. This reduced form is a more powerful antioxidant than regular CoQ_{10}. Realize as many as 30 percent of the population may not be able to convert and equate amounts of CoQ_{10} to its active form ubiquinol or reduced CoQ_{10}. (See Appendix A.) Coenzyme Q_{10} is found in sardines, spinach, peanuts, and beef.

Carnosine

Carnosine is a new and exciting—and most unusual—nutrient considered by many to be a powerful antioxidant and by others to be a powerful chelating agent of copper-zinc. Carnosine inhibits lipid peroxidation and the formation and protein cross-linking of AGEs. Remember that on Day 18 we learned that AGEs are advanced glycation endproducts formed by a reaction between sugars and proteins. They are associated with cataracts, Alzheimer's disease, cancer, and arterial plaque. Carnosine is a great source for fighting the production of these dangerous free radicals.

Oddly enough, carnosine is mainly found in red meat, and vegetarians have higher levels of AGEs than meat-eaters. Realize excessive intake of red meat, however, is linked to both cancer and heart disease. Therefore, exercise moderation.

There are just a few more important antioxidants that need to be briefly mentioned. Grape seed and pine bark extracts are proanthocyanidins that are approximately twenty times more powerful than vitamin E and fifty times more powerful than vitamin C. These are often recommended for vascular disorders.

It's also important to remember that living foods are a powerful source of antioxidants. You can get plenty of antioxidants from the following foods: blueberries, cranberries, blackberries, raspberries, strawberries, red beans, kidney beans, pinto beans, black beans, artichokes, apples, pecans, cherries, black and red plums, cruciferous vegetables, broccoli, cabbage, cauliflower, tomatoes, watermelon, carrots, canteloupes, sweet potatoes, oranges, tangerines, lemons, limes, grapefruits, spinach, romaine lettuce, onions, garlic, soy, and green tea.

As you can see, there are three main antioxidants produced by the body and five major antioxidants that need to be supplemented. Later this week you will learn the dosages needed for these powerful antioxidants. Now let's look at the phytonutrients.

BUILDING BLOCKS TO A HEALTHY LIFE

POINTS TO PONDER: *Antioxidants are to free radicals what water is to a raging forest fire burning out of control. The key antioxidants that our bodies produce include glutathione, superoxide dismutase, and catalase. Five antioxidants that work as a team include vitamin C, vitamin E (all eight forms), coenzyme Q_{10}, lipoic acid, and glutathione. Carnosine is a nutrient that can also act as a powerful antioxidant.*

ACTION STEP: *If you are over fifty years of age, begin to plan your antioxidant defense system to help prevent disease and to slow down the aging process. However, you may want to start doing this even as early as age forty, especially if you are suffering from chronic disease.*

DAY 39: The Power of Phytonutrients

The other major ingredients for optimum health are called phytonutrients (also called phytochemicals). Phytonutrients are biologically active substances that give fruits and vegetables their color, flavor, smell, and natural disease resistance. They can have major health benefits for your body.

Phytonutrients play perhaps the most important part in preventing cancer and heart disease. Some researchers estimate forty thousand phytonutrients will one day be cataloged and understood.[1] At the present time there are over two thousand known phytonutrients. These compounds protect plants from pests, excessive amounts of ultraviolet radiation, and disease. Each plant has thousands of different phytonutrients that provide protection from free radicals because they contain natural antioxidants.

In humans, phytonutrient consumption is associated with reduced rates of many different cancers. They also protect against heart disease and protect or slow the progression of dementia and age-related cognitive decline. They increase longevity, are associated with reduced rates of chronic disease, and protect us against cataracts and macular degeneration. Regular consumption of phytonutrients is the best natural health insurance policy that I can recommend to protect a person from all degenerative diseases, including cancer and heart disease.

Phytonutrients are hard at work in your body, saving you from various threats you probably were never even aware of. For example, saponins, found in kidney beans, lentils, chickpeas, and soybeans, may prevent cancer cells from multiplying. A phytonutrient found in tomatoes interferes with the chemical process that creates carcinogens. The list of wonderful things phytonutrients do goes on.[2]

The Healing Power of Plants

Approximately two-thirds of all drugs are derived from plants.[3]

As of 2005, the USDA and U.S. Department of Health and Human Services recommend that Americans consume five to thirteen servings of fruits and veggies a day, but most Americans do not consume even the minimum of five servings. The CDC, in a nationwide survey in 2002, reported that 82 percent of men and 72 percent of women are falling short of eating five servings of fruits and vegetables per day.[4] Unfortunately, this also means that most Americans are missing out on the great benefits provided by the phytonutrients found in fruits and vegetables.

Rainbow of Health

Fruits and vegetables can be grouped according to color. Each group has its own set of phytonutrients that provide unique protective benefits.

Typically, phytonutrients are classified by their chemical structures. This is an extensive classification, and it is also quite confusing, since many phytonutrients provide similar protection. The main classifications include:

- *Organo-sulfurs,* such as cruciferous vegetables and the sulfur compound in garlic
- *Terpenoids,* such as limonene in citrus as well as carotenoids, tocopherols, tocotrienols, etc.
- *Flavonoids,* including certain red/purple pigmented fruits and vegetables
- *Isoflavonoids* and *lignans* found in soy foods and flaxseeds
- *Organic acids* found in whole grains, parsley, licorice, and citrus fruits

Since there are so many different phytonutrients, they are also classified in families, and this depends on the similarities in their structure. As you can see, it can be quite confusing! That's why I like to simply group them by color.

Our goal should be to include as many colors as possible in our daily diet. Approximately half of all Americans don't even eat one piece of fruit all day, and most others will eat the same fruit or vegetable day after day. We need to try and consume all seven colors of the phytonutrient rainbow every day to receive the protection we need. To do this, we need to eat a variety of foods. Eating a colorful salad every day and/or taking a powerful phytonutrient powder are two easy ways to make sure you are consuming all seven phytonutrient color groups. (See Appendix A.)

Think of phytonutrients as a "rainbow of health," God's promise to you to keep you healthy. Let's look at each group.

Red

Tomatoes, watermelon, guava, and red grapefruit contain a powerful carotenoid called *lycopene,* which is about twice as powerful as beta-carotene. Lycopene is the main pigment responsible for the red color. Lycopene is the most abundant carotenoid in the prostate, and high blood levels of lycopene are linked to prevention of heart disease and prostate cancer. A study conducted by Harvard researchers examined the relationship between carotenoids and the risk of prostate cancer. Only the carotenoid lycopene was associated with protection. Men who ate more than ten servings of tomato-based food a week had a 35 percent decreased risk of prostate cancer compared to those eating less than 1.5 servings a week. In this study, the only tomato-based food that didn't correlate with protection was tomato juice. The men in this study with the greatest protection against prostate cancer consumed at least 6.5 mg a day of lycopene from tomato products.[5] Men over forty should especially begin eating more organic tomatoes and organic tomato sauce cooked with organic extra-virgin olive oil to get the protection against prostate cancer. About one man in six may develop prostate cancer during his lifetime.[6]

You Say "Tomatoe," I Say "Tomato"

Did you know that tomatoes are really a fruit and not a vegetable? That's because, botanically speaking, a tomato is the ovary, along with its seed, of a flowering plant—hence, it is a fruit. But back in the late 1800s, when U.S. tariff laws imposed a duty on vegetables but not fruits, the truth about tomatoes got called in question. The U.S. Supreme Court settled this controversy in 1893, declaring that the tomato is a vegetable, along with cucumbers, squashes, beans, and peas, using the popular definition that classifies vegetables by use, that they are generally served with dinner and not dessert. The case is known as Nix v. Hedden.[7]

Red/purple

Blueberries, blackberries, hawthorn berries, raspberries, grapes, eggplants, red cabbage, and red wine contain a powerful flavonoid called anthocyanidin, which is the pigment responsible for the brilliant, beautiful red/blue and purple colors. These colors actually draw us to these attractive fruits and vegetables, which in turn protect us from a host of diseases. Anthocyanidins protect cells from free-radical damage in water-soluble and fat-soluble compartments of the body. They have approximately fifty times the antioxidant activity of vitamin C and are twenty times more powerful than vitamin E. They also may help prevent arthritis and atherosclerosis.

Pine bark, grape seeds and skins, bilberry, and cranberry contain another flavonoid called proanthocyanidin, which is a significant source of antioxidants. These powerful phytonutrients—anthocyanidin and proanthocyanidin—strengthen and repair connective tissue and stimulate the synthesis of collagen. They help to strengthen capillaries and to maintain elastin, which assists in maintaining the elasticity in our skin and blood vessels, thus aiding in preventing wrinkles, spider veins, and varicose veins.

Resveratrol is found in red grape skins and seeds, purple grape juice, and red wine; it is a phenolic compound that inhibits the development of cancer in animals and also helps prevent the progression of cancer. It decreases the stickiness of platelets, preventing blood clots, and it helps blood vessels remain open and flexible. This powerful phytonutrient also raises the HDL or "good" cholesterol.

Strawberries and cranberries also contain powerful flavonoids. There are over four thousand unique flavonoids, but the fruits and vegetables listed above are some of the best sources of them. Flavonoids have anti-inflammatory, anticarcinogenic, antitumor, and antiviral activity. They are powerful antioxidants and metal chelators. They are also important dietary supplements to prevent both cancer and heart disease.

Orange

Orange-colored fruits and vegetables, including carrots, mangoes, cantaloupes, pumpkin, sweet potatoes, yams, squash, and apricots, have high amounts of carotenoids. Typically, the more orange the fruit or vegetable is, the higher the concentration of provitamin A carotenoids. There are more than six hundred carotenoids, with about fifty that can be transformed into vitamin A. Orange fruits and vegetables generally are high in beta-carotene.

Lobster and salmon are pink because they have ingested plants containing carotenoids, which has colored their tissues. Even egg yolks get their yellow color from carotenoids eaten by the hen.

Carotenoids quench singlet oxygen, which is a reactive oxygen species (free radical) that damages cells and tissues. They also help prevent cancer and heart disease. The antioxidants vitamin E, vitamin C, lipoic acid, and coenzyme Q_{10} help to replenish carotenoids in tissues. The body converts beta-carotene into vitamin A as needed. Beta-carotene that is left over is able to quench free-radical reactions and prevents cholesterol from oxidizing, helping to prevent plaque formation in arteries. A diet high in carotenoids, especially alpha-carotene, is protective against cancer. Eating just one small carrot every day may help protect you from cancer.[8]

However, synthetic beta-carotene supplements actually increase the risk of lung cancer in smokers! In one study of 29,000 men in Finland who smoked and drank alcohol, the men were given beta-carotene (20 mg a day) and/or vitamin E. There was an 18 percent increase in lung cancer in the beta-carotene group.[9]

Beta-carotene used in supplements is mainly the synthetic, trans form. Foods such as carrots supply mixed carotenoids and include the natural forms, which are better than synthetic antioxidants. Instead of taking only beta-carotene, consider organic orange fruits and veggies that have mixed carotenoids, which work together to protect the body. The synthetic beta-carotene supplements may trigger cancer in smokers, and for that reason I recommend orange foods high in carotenoids over beta-carotene supplements.

Orange/yellow

Oranges, tangerines, lemons, limes, yellow grapefruit, papaya, pineapple, and nectarines are rich in vitamin C and citrus bioflavonoids and protect us against free-radical damage since they are powerful antioxidants. Citrus bioflavonoids include rutin, quercetin, hesperidin, and naringin. They are able to increase intracellular levels of vitamin C. Citrus bioflavonoids strengthen blood vessels by supporting the collagen and strengthening the cells that form the inner lining of blood vessels. They also maintain the collagen that forms tendons, cartilage, and ligaments. They prevent the release and production of compounds that promote allergies and inflammation. They have also been used both to prevent and treat bruising, hemorrhoids, varicose veins, and spider veins.

Yellow/green

Spinach, kale, collard greens, mustard greens, turnip greens, romaine lettuce, leeks, and peas are typically rich in lutein and zeaxanthin. *Lutein* is the main carotenoid present in the central portion of the retina of the eye called the *macula*. Lutein is able to reduce the risk of macular degeneration, which is the leading cause of blindness in older adults.

A study found that adults with the highest dietary intake of lutein had a 57 percent lower risk of macular degeneration compared with those individuals with the lowest intake. Also, of all the different carotenoids, lutein and zeaxanthin were the most strongly associated with this protection.[11] Lutein may also protect the lens of the eye from sunlight damage, slowing down the development of cataracts.

Did You Know...?

Elderly men who eat lots of dark green and deep yellow vegetables have a 46 percent decrease in heart disease risk compared to men who eat few of these vegetables.[10]

Dark green leafy vegetables contain two pigments, lutein and zeaxanthin, which protect the eye from damage.

Many people don't understand why dark green vegetables are rich in these powerful carotenoids—lutein and zeaxanthin. Carotenoids also occur in dark green leafy vegetables where their color is concealed by the green pigment called *chlorophyll,* which also protects us against cancer.

Green

Broccoli, cabbage, brussels sprouts, cauliflower, watercress, bok choy, kale, collard greens, and mustard greens are considered cruciferous vegetables. These cancer fighters contain more phytonutrients with anticancer properties than any other family of vegetables. The word *cruciferous* comes from the same word root as *crucifying,* which means "to place one on a cross." The flowers of cruciferous vegetables contain two components that appear similar to the shape of a cross. The powerful cancer-fighting phytonutrients in the cruciferous vegetable family include indoles, isothiocyanates, and sulforaphanes, which are sulfur-containing compounds. They also contain phenols, coumarins, dithiolthiones, and other phytonutrients yet to be discovered. Indoles, including DIM and indole-3-carbinol, are powerful anticancer phytonutrients that are able to suppress cancer growth and induce programmed cell death in a variety of cancers, including breast cancer, prostate cancer, colon cancer, endometrial cancer, and leukemia.[12] They stimulate detoxifying enzymes in the GI tract and the liver. They protect us against carcinogens, which are cancer-causing agents. Indole-3-carbinol supports a healthy estrogen balance and decreases the risk of female related cancers. Sulforaphanes stimulate liver detoxification enzymes. Isothiocyanates inhibit enzymes that activate carcinogens and stimulate enzymes that remove cancer-causing agents.

Did You Know...?

When abnormal cells are formed, these cells are designed in a healthy body to undergo programmed cell death, or apoptosis, so that cancer is not formed. Cancer cells do not die but continue to grow and spread.

Studies have correlated a high intake of cruciferous vegetables, especially cabbage, with lower rates of cancers, especially cancers of the breast, prostate, and colon. Broccoli sprouts have some of the highest concentration of protective phytonutrients. Young broccoli sprouts that are about three days old contain twenty to fifty times more sulforaphane than mature broccoli.

DIM

A powerful new phytonutrient has recently been discovered in cruciferous vegetables. DIM, or diindolylmethane, is found in cruciferous vegetables such as broccoli and cauliflower. DIM is vitally important in estrogen balance and may help prevent female-related cancers such as breast, uterine, ovarian, and cervical dysplasia—a precancerous condition marked by changes in the cells of the cervix.[13]

Eating vegetables only will not supply you with adequate amounts of DIM. You would have to eat about two pounds of broccoli each day to get adequate amounts of DIM. That's why I recommend a supplement. (See Appendix A.)

White/green

Onions and garlic contain powerful phytonutrients. Onions contain the flavonoid quercetin, which has anti-inflammatory properties, antiviral activity, and anticancer properties. Quercetin is often recommended by nutritionists to treat both allergies and asthma. Apples, red wine, and black tea also contain quercetin. In fact, quercetin is the reason why people say, "An apple a day keeps the doctor away." Onions and garlic also contain organic sulfur compounds, which can be used for detoxification by the liver.

Several of the components in garlic have significant anticancer effects. Garlic also inhibits the formation of nitrosamines, which are cancer-causing compounds formed during digestion. Garlic has significant antimicrobial activity against bacteria, viruses, fungi, and even parasites. It also has cholesterol-lowering activities and can even lower blood pressure as well as help prevent blood clots.

Powerful phytonutrients that also need to be mentioned include green tea, curcumin, and soy.

Green tea's active constituents are polyphenols, especially the catechin called *epigallocatechin gallate* (EGCG). The polyphenols in green tea have been shown to reduce the risk of gastrointestinal cancers, including cancers of the stomach, small intestines, colon, and pancreas, as well as lung and breast cancers. As an antioxidant, green tea is two hundred times more powerful than vitamin E and five hundred times more powerful than vitamin C. It provides powerful antioxidants to help repair damaged DNA. It also activates detoxification enzymes in the liver, which helps defend your body against cancer. The normal amount of green tea consumed by the Japanese is about three cups a day. I recommend organic green tea in dioxin-free tea bags.

Curcumin

Curcumin is the substance that gives turmeric its bright yellow color. Turmeric is the main ingredient of curry powder. It is an herb of the ginger family. Turmeric has significant antioxidant activity, and curcumin is its most powerful component. Both turmeric and curcumin have anticancer effects at all steps of cancer formation. Curcumin has powerful anti-inflammatory properties, especially with acute inflammation such as sprains, muscle strains, and inflamed joints. It also may help individuals with Alzheimer's disease and especially in prevention of Alzheimer's disease by reducing inflammation.[14] It also helps lower cholesterol and prevent blood clots.[15]

Soy

Soybeans and soy products such as tofu, tempeh, soy flour, and soy milk contain powerful phytonutrients called *isoflavones* and protease inhibitors. Soy products need to be non-GMO (genetically modified organisms). The isoflavones genistein and daidzein may help to block tumor growth by preventing the growth of new blood vessels that feed the tumor. This may be effective against prostate cancer and breast cancer. The isoflavones also appear to offer protection against other cancers, heart disease, and osteoporosis.[16] However, the use of isoflavones in cancer patients is controversial and should be discussed with your oncologist.

I find it fascinating and lovely that our bodies are designed to eat produce from across the color spectrum. Each gives you unique phytonutrients with the ability to protect you from illnesses such as cancer and heart disease. These can also be taken in supplement form, as I will explain later.

Rating the Produce

Another way to judge the benefits of each fruit and vegetable is by their Oxygen Radical Absorbance Capacity, or *ORAC*. This is a standard tool used by nutritionists to measure foods' antioxidant capacity. The higher the ORAC, the higher the concentration of antioxidants in that food, and the greater protection it provides against free radicals.

In studies of animal and human blood at the Agricultural Research Service's Human Nutrition Research Center on Aging (the chief scientific agency of the U.S. Department of Agriculture), eating plenty of high-ORAC foods raised the antioxidant power of human blood 10 to 25 percent.[17] Based on these findings, we can see that the first step in raising our antioxidant levels is to increase our intake of high-ORAC foods. Although there is no standard established yet, 3,000–5,000 ORAC units per day from a variety of antioxidant sources is thought to be a good intake level.[18]

A terrific study in the June 2004 issue of the *Journal of Agriculture and Food Chemistry* tested the antioxidant power of more than one hundred different kinds of fruits, vegetables, nuts, and spices. They came up with a list of the top antioxidant foods. The top twenty are:[19]

1. Mexican red beans (dried)
2. Wild blueberries
3. Red kidney beans
4. Pinto beans
5. Cultivated blueberries
6. Cranberries
7. Artichokes (cooked)
8. Blackberries
9. Prunes
10. Raspberries
11. Strawberries
12. Red Delicious apples
13. Granny Smith apples
14. Pecans
15. Cherries
16. Black plums
17. Russet potatoes (cooked)
18. Black beans (dried)
19. Red plums
20. Gala apples

Blueberries contain polyphenols that protect the brain from inflammation and oxidative stress, which in turn may protect the brain from the degenerative effects of aging and from injury from ischemic stroke.[20] Blueberries may even help prevent Alzheimer's disease and Parkinson's disease. When rats suffering from Alzheimer's-like symptoms were supplemented with blueberries in their diets, they were able to perform normally on tests involving memory and motor behavior.[21] I recommend a serving of organic blueberries every day.

The more we learn about phytonutrients and antioxidants, the more we understand how amazingly beneficial they are. There are tens of thousands of them, many yet undiscovered. In addition to eating high-ORAC foods and varied and brightly colored foods, I recommend taking antioxidants and phytonutrients in supplement form since we are usually unable to eat all the colors of the phytonutrient rainbow. Realize that consuming these powerful phytonutrients on a daily basis protects us from developing heart disease, cancer, macular degeneration, and practically all degenerative diseases. I'm just about to get to my recommendations, but first let me clear up some of the major confusion that often surrounds the subject of supplements, multivitamins, and more.

BUILDING BLOCKS TO A HEALTHY LIFE

POINTS TO PONDER: *Phytonutrients give fruits and vegetables their color. Fruits and vegetables can be grouped according to color and provide a rainbow of health, protecting us from cancer and heart disease. Red—tomatoes, watermelon—contain lycopene. Red/purple—blueberries, grapes—contain a powerful flavonoid called anthocyanidin. Orange—carrots, cantaloupes, sweet potatoes—contain carotenoids. Orange/yellow—oranges, tangerines—contain bioflavonoids. Yellow/green—spinach, mustard greens—contain lutein. Green—broccoli, cabbage—are cruciferous vegetables containing multiple powerful phytonutrients, especially DIM and indole-3-carbinole. White/green—onions, garlic—contain quercetin.*

ACTION STEP: *Each day plan to eat a salad that contains all of the colors of the phytonutrient rainbow.*

DAY 40: Vitamin Confusion

If you have ever walked into a health food store, you probably felt the same way many people do: overwhelmed by shelf after shelf crammed with thousands of multivitamins and minerals and individual supplements, each claiming to be the key to your health. Nutritional supplements have become big business, and confusion reigns for the poor consumer.

Supplements are no longer a niche market as it used to be. Americans now spend more than $17 billion a year on supplements for health and wellness.[1] And yet most chronic diseases continue to rise. For example, in 2002, coronary heart disease produced one out of every five deaths, and one person in four had some form of cardiovascular disease.[2] In 2005, men in the United States had slightly less than a one in two lifetime risk of developing cancer (meaning the probability of developing or dying from cancer over a lifetime); for women the risk was a little more than one in three.[3] Apparently, nutritional supplements are not helping as they should. Why? There are several important reasons.

Disagreement Over What Nutrients We Need

There is great confusion among consumers about how much of certain nutrients they need. Some scientists say the human body needs forty essential nutrients; some say fifty. Every decade or so the list of essential nutrients changes, which is why I believe in a conservative approach to supplements. Well-informed scientists disagree about the health benefits of phytonutrients, certain antioxidants, certain vitamins, and so on. Some consider them central to good health; others believe they are peripheral. The list of controversies goes on.

But health experts don't help by creating an alphabet soup of recommended intakes—reference daily intake (RDI), recommended daily allowance (RDA), daily value (DV), daily reference value (DRV), adequate intake (AI), and tolerable upper limit (UL). Few people know what these things mean, how they compare to each other, or how they are measured. And yet people still rely too heavily on the percentages they read on nutrition labels, thinking these percentages represent healthy amounts. In fact, these recommended amounts don't tell you how much you need to be healthy—only how much you need to avoid the most egregious deficiency diseases, such as rickets (caused by lack of vitamin D), beriberi (lack of vitamin B_1), or scurvy (lack of vitamin C). If you get 100 percent of your RDA for every nutrient every day, you will avoid these uncommon diseases, but you won't necessarily be healthy. You will have, at best, marginal health, and you will still be exposed to the ravages of degenerative diseases and possibly cancer and heart disease. These recommended daily intakes are often well below the ideal level required for your optimal health.[4]

It's important for consumers to understand that as knowledge of nutrition increases, recommendations change. Nutrients that we now call nonessential may one day be viewed as essential. RDAs and RDIs are imperfect but helpful guides. It is each person's job to gain knowledge by reading books such as this one, doing research, and taking charge of their health.

Hidden Hazards in Supplements

Now that nutritional supplements have become big business, many pharmaceutical companies have jumped on the bandwagon and are manufacturing multivitamins, omega-3 fats (fish oil pills), and many others that are sold in huge quantities at discount stores and supermarkets. But many companies are more concerned about their profits than your health, and they choose the cheapest option rather than the healthiest one. The evidence is in the pills themselves.

Most mass-produced nutritional supplements contain poor quality synthetic nutrients, which are not nearly as healthy for you as are natural nutrients and may, in fact, be harmful.[5] These man-made multivitamin and mineral supplements are usually made from mineral salts, which are poorly absorbed by your body and therefore vastly less effective but very inexpensive. The manufacturers seem to believe that they can standardize, process, and manufacture vitamins in the same way they manufacture prescription drugs, which, by the way, is not a natural process. The result is an inferior quality of supplements—and usually toxic excipients (fillers) that you didn't expect to make it into your daily tablets.[6] Some big pharmaceutical companies even use ingredients such as toxic partially hydrogenated soybean oil as fillers for their soft gels containing fish oils, vitamin E, and so on. They also add artificial colors, which may have been extracted from coal tar, and put them in their tablets and capsules. A friend of mine calls these "toxic tagalongs."

More than 7 percent of the U.S. population has some sensitivity to these chemicals, so in these cases the supplement is having a dual effect, causing unhealthy side effects while it delivers inferior vitamins and minerals.[7] The larger the tablet, typically the more binding agents and fillers they contain.

Rancid Oils

One of the worst offenders is in fish oil supplements. At my request, many patients come into my office and bring me their fish oil capsules. I stick a needle in and pull out a drop, put it on their finger, and have them taste it. They typically grimace and say, "Why did you make me taste that? It's awful." And yet they swallow those pills daily without thinking about what's inside!

Fish oils and omega-3 supplements can be good for you, but much of the fish oils in supplement form are rancid. Taste it and see for yourself. The fats oxidize quickly and become toxic, causing even more free-radical damage to your body. They do more harm than good. Some fish oils will not even have a rancid odor and taste, yet still contain high amounts of lipid peroxides.[8] See Appendix A for more information on omega-3 supplements.

Also, fish oil is a highly unstable product. As soon as it is extracted from the fish and exposed to oxygen, light, heat, or metals, it begins to oxidize or rancidify. Fish oil at this late stage of oxidation will smell rancid or fishy. In early stages of oxidation, most fish oil products won't smell yet, but will still be harmful. Not only that, but also many fish oils aren't tested for PCBs, mercury, or other toxins that can make it into your body through your supplement.[9]

Certain companies add forms of vitamin E and lemon oil, which help keep fish oil from turning rancid.[10] But be aware of what you are taking! Fish oils are very healthy, but if you take the wrong ones, you could invite more inflammation and toxins into your body.

If you have been blindly taking supplements on a neighbor's advice or because of something you heard on the radio, it's time to dig deeper and discover what is in that round of pills you consume each day. Supplementation should never be random, but well researched, thought out, and tailored to your specific condition and needs. Otherwise you may be getting things you never wanted in your pills.

BUILDING BLOCKS TO A HEALTHY LIFE

POINTS TO PONDER: *Do any of the supplements you are currently taking contain the toxic fillers or agents mentioned in today's entry? Supplements, like prescription medications, have become a multibillion-dollar business. Recommended amounts of nutrients don't tell you how much you need to be healthy, but how much you need to prevent disease.* Caveat emptor—*let the buyer beware: there are supplements that may be harming you, such as rancid fish oils.*

ACTION STEP: *Sample your fish oil supplement by sticking a needle in it and smelling or tasting a small drop. If it smells and tastes really "fishy," you can bet it's rancid.*

DAY 41: Mega-Dosing

One day a man came into my office with a huge suitcase; he even brought it into the exam room.

"What's that?" I asked him.

"These are my supplements," he said, and opened the suitcase to reveal dozens of nutritional supplements, probably worth thousands of dollars. He said he took some for his arthritis, some for high blood pressure, others for diabetes, and still others for digestion problems. Simply the tremendous number of gelatin capsules and fillers that he was taking would give most people digestive problems.

Some people get so excited about taking vitamin supplements that they go overboard and begin mega-dosing. I see it often in my practice. People come in complaining of skin problems, digestion problems, and various other things. It sometimes turns out they are taking too many vitamins, minerals, and other supplements, and they are actually hurting themselves.

This may shock you, but the unhealthiest people I see are the ones who are mega-dosing on supplements. This has to do with their mind-set toward supplements. They have a problem and want to treat the symptoms with a supplement, just as other people treat problems with medications. They are using supplements the way doctors use some drugs—to treat symptoms but not the cause. Sometimes these patients don't want to make other lifestyle and dietary changes, so they rely on pills from the health food store.

But taking pills in high doses can harm you. There is the simple fact that pills are made of much more than the vitamin or mineral or extract you are hoping to consume. As we learned yesterday, these pills often contain all sorts of binding agents, fillers, gels, toxic fats, and dyes.[1] Some of my patients tell me they take hundreds of pills every day. (Yes, literally. They are the exception to the rule, though.) They get good deals on supplements at the health food store or through vitamin catalogs, but then they complain to me of fatigue, diarrhea, breakouts, terrible indigestion, belching, and gas. Their supplements have stopped being the cure and are now causing their problems. People sometimes don't produce enough hydrochloric acid in their stomachs and pancreatic enzymes from their pancreas to digest all that gelatin and other fillers in their supplements.

Their pills then get passed into their stool because of poor digestion. Mega-dosing can also create sensitivities and allergies to their supplements.

Too Much of a Good Thing

Like anything else in life, too much of a good thing may eventually harm your body. Mega-dosing on one type of vitamin or mineral is no different. For example, mega-doses of vitamin B_6 can lead to neuropathy or damage to nerves in your arms and legs.[2] Too much vitamin A will promote liver disease.[3] Too much selenium promotes liver impairment,[4] and too much vitamin E is associated with possible heart disease.[5] Taking massive amounts of vitamin C, as was the fad in past decades, may cause kidney stones.[6] Also, nutrients work synergistically; simply supplementing with large doses of one vitamin or one mineral may cause imbalances in another vitamin or mineral. For example, a proper balance of copper and zinc is a one-to-ten ratio, and mega-dosing with zinc will dramatically affect that ratio. For adequate intake, see the tables listed in Appendix B of this book.

Did You Know...?

Taking too much vitamin D can cause:

- Nausea
- Constipation
- Weight loss
- Confusion[7]

In the revolutionary *Journal of the American Medical Association* article I cited at the beginning of this pillar, both authors warned that excessive dosage levels may have toxic effects.[8] One such proof came from the ATBC trial, which tried to determine the long-term effects from vitamin supplements in smokers. The researchers followed the participants for an additional eight years after the trial ended to ensure the accuracy of their results. The study tested the effects of alpha-tocopherol (a form of vitamin E) and beta-carotene on cancer prevention.[9]

The ATBC study concluded that men who smoked and took beta-carotene had an 18 percent greater incidence of lung cancer and an 8 percent increased overall mortality rate. They hypothesized that excessive beta-carotene was somehow worsening the lung cell proliferation induced by smoke. Participants taking vitamin E had 32 percent fewer cases of prostate cancer and 41 percent fewer deaths from prostate cancer, but the risk of death from hemorrhagic stroke increased by 50 percent in men taking alpha-tocopherol supplements. The increase occurred primarily among men with high blood pressure.[10] This information shows that if you have a specific disease like hypertension or lung cancer, mega-dosing on supplements can actually kill you.

If you are taking high doses of any single vitamin, mineral, or supplement, or high doses of a combination of these, you may be putting yourself in harm's way. You must stop what you are doing and change your mind-set toward supplements. They are not a cure-all. When it comes to supplements, more is not necessarily better. You must remember that supplements are just that—to supplement a healthy diet. They are not the diet itself. As long as you eat a healthy diet, you don't have to meet all your nutritional needs with supplements. Pills should not be your first source of nutrition; a healthy diet is your foundation, and supplements are simply to complement your diet to ensure you receive adequate vitamins, minerals, antioxidants, and phytonutrients.

When one of my patients is mega-dosing, I often have him take a one- or two-week break from supplements. After a week or two with no supplements, the symptoms often go away. After that I may have him take one day off a week without any supplements. I generally limit his supplements to a good whole-food multivitamin, antioxidant, phytonutrient, omega-3 supplement, and perhaps a digestive enzyme, and for women, the same with extra calcium.

In your zeal for health, don't mega-dose. Don't treat supplements like drugs or medications. Rather, learn to choose the healthiest kinds of supplements, and avoid impostors. I'll give you advice on how in the next chapter.

BUILDING BLOCKS TO A HEALTHY LIFE

POINTS TO PONDER: *Supplements do not exist to replace a healthy diet; they exist to complement it. Taking supplements in high doses or taking an excessive amount of supplements can actually harm you. Generally, the unhealthiest patients that I see are the ones who are mega-dosing.*

ACTION STEP: *If you have been mega-dosing on supplements, take a break from them for one to two weeks. The results may surprise you.*

DAY 42: How to Pick the Right Supplements

What constitutes a good multivitamin? The answer is the same things that make living food healthy. As we saw earlier in the week, most multivitamins are made of synthetic ingredients and toxic fillers. They may have all the vitamins you need, but the vitamins are typically in sub-optimal amounts and in a cheap form made of mineral salts, which are poorly absorbed. People who take these pills usually don't get the nutrition they need.

These chemical-based supplements also lack that vital combination of nutrients that characterize living foods. Nature never produces nutrients in isolation. Oranges, for example, contain much more than vitamin C. Carrots contain much more than beta-carotene. When you eat them, you get a myriad of vitamins, phytonutrients, flavonoids, and more that interact in ways that are not fully understood, but that we recognize to be healthy.

When you isolate one of these nutrients and take it in high doses, especially in synthetic form, your body may treat it like a foreign substance, and why not? When only synthetic vitamins are consumed, there is generally no synergy or balance. It's similar to taking a drug or medication. It ignores the complexity of nutrition.

It's a Fact!

Most multivitamins contain mineral salts instead of chelated minerals. Chelated minerals are minerals attached to amino acids, which improve the absorption of minerals.

For example, pharmaceutical companies are now jumping onto the phytonutrients bandwagon, realizing that these have a certain appeal to consumers. But the manufacturers usually strip out a single phytonutrient and put it into capsules and supplements. The problem is that phytonutrients were almost certainly not meant to be consumed one at a time. There is not a single fruit or vegetable in the world that contains only one kind of phytonutrient, vitamin, or mineral. Nutrients can be isolated, but I am not sure if it will have a healthy effect when it is taken in high doses. Rather, the healthiest supplements combine the enzymes, coenzymes, trace elements, antioxidants, activators, phytonutrients, vitamins

Dr. Colbert Approved

I usually recommend supplementation with both pancreatic enzymes and/or HCL, especially for patients over fifty years of age. I prefer that nutritional supplements be in vegetable capsules, be excipient (filler) free, and nonirradiated. See Appendix A, "Recommended Products," for additional information.

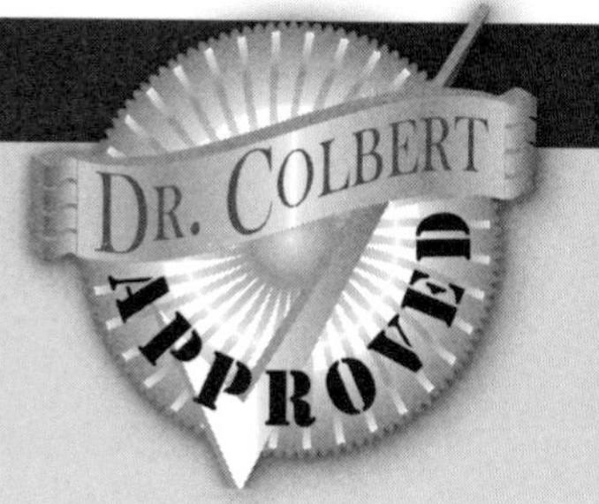

and minerals, and many other elements, which all work together synergistically. These supplements are called whole-food supplements and are generally what I recommend.

Nutritionist Paavo Airola, MD, PhD, in his book *How to Get Well,* stated, "When you take natural vitamins, as for instance in the form of rose hips, brewer's yeast, or vegetable oil, you get all the vitamins and vitamin-like factors that naturally occur in these foods. That is, all those that are already discovered as well as those that are not discovered yet."[1] In other words, whole-food vitamins are able to provide nutritional balance and synergy, whereas synthetic vitamins typically do not.

Whole-food supplements combine portions of the plants we know are healthy and those portions we have not yet discovered to be healthy. I believe it's wise to do this because medical knowledge is expanding so quickly that it gets outdated practically every few years. A nutrient we hadn't heard of a year ago can suddenly be discovered to protect against certain kinds of cancer or disease.

You need a comprehensive multivitamin, made from living ingredients and combined with living nutrition.

How to Choose a Supplement

The reason we have so many vitamin and mineral deficiencies is because most Americans have embraced fast foods and processed foods, rarely consuming adequate amounts of whole grains, fresh fruits, vegetables, and nuts and seeds, which are excellent sources of these nutrients. (For more information, read my book *What Would Jesus Eat?*) So we do need supplements, preferably whole-food supplements.

My goal is to simplify your life, not complicate it. When choosing a supplement, you should look for a multivitamin that contains all thirteen vitamins and seventeen to twenty-two minerals with 100 percent of daily values. Also, you need omega-3 fats and a phytonutrient powder. *That's it!* To see what the daily values are according to your age and sex, please refer to the charts located in Appendix B. Realize if you consume a healthy diet, you will probably get at least 50 percent of the daily values of vitamins and minerals.

If you are over fifty years of age, you will probably need extra antioxidants, extra calcium and vitamin D, sublingual B_{12}, and maybe digestive enzymes. If you already have a disease or simply want more protection, start taking extra antioxidants after the age of forty.

Basics for everyone

When choosing a supplement (see Appendix A), here is what I recommend for everyone, regardless of age:

1. Choose a comprehensive multivitamin that has at least 100 percent of the daily value (DV) or reference daily intake (RDI). (See the chart below.) Start slowly because they may upset your stomach. Start with half the recommended amount and space them out during the day after meals. You may increase the amount as tolerated, but do not take over 100 percent of the daily value.

COMPONENTS OF A COMPREHENSIVE MULTIVITAMIN	
Vitamins	Vitamin A, vitamin B_1 (thiamine), vitamin B_2 (riboflavin), vitamin B_3 (niacin), vitamin B_5 (pantothenic acid), vitamin B_6 (pyridoxine), vitamin B_{12}, biotin, folic acid, vitamin C, vitamin D, vitamin E, vitamin K
Minerals	Boron, calcium, chromium, cobalt, copper, iodine, iron, magnesium, manganese, molybdenum, phosphorus, potassium, selenium, silicon, sodium, sulfur, vanadium, zinc

2. Choose a high-quality omega-3 fat to take daily. Start slowly with one a day and increase as tolerated.
3. Choose a phytonutrient powder. This powder should contain a combination of colorful organic fruits and vegetables such as red, yellow, green, orange, and purple. Start slowly with just a teaspoon a day, and increase the amount as tolerated. Living foods may cause gas and bloating as your body adjusts to them.

For those fifty and older

If you are fifty years of age or older, you should take a multivitamin, a phytonutrient powder, and omega-3 fats; also make sure you get extra antioxidants, calcium, vitamin D, digestive enzymes, and a sublingual B_{12}. (See Appendix A for recommended products.)

1. Vitamin E (mixed tocopherols and tocotrienols), 200 to 400 IU a day (may be present in a multivitamin). Be careful not to take over 400 IU of vitamin E a day.
2. Vitamin C, 250 mg twice a day (may be present in a multivitamin)
3. Coenzyme Q_{10}, 100 mg a day
4. R-form alpha-lipoic acid or R-DHLA, 100 mg a day
5. N-acetyl-cysteine (NAC), 250 to 500 mg a day, or Recancostat (glutathione), one capsule once or twice a day
6. Turmeric and synergistic herbs (such as Protandim), one a day
7. Calcium and vitamin D: calcium, 400 mg three times a day, and vitamin D, 400 IU or higher a day. Men generally only need 400 mg of calcium twice a day.
8. Digestive enzymes and/or HCL, one after each meal
9. Sublingual B_{12}, 1,000 mcg a day

I recommend a sublingual B_{12} supplement for patients over fifty years of age. After age fifty many Americans do not produce adequate amounts of hydrochloric acid, which is required for binding B_{12} to intrinsic factor for absorption in the ileum, which is the last part of the small intestines.[2]

Appendix B contains tables that categorize each of these essential nutrients according to age and sex. Use this as a guideline to determine the amount that is right for you.

Supplements in a vegetable-based capsule are far less likely to contain toxic components. Some gelatin capsules are made from animal by-products, and with the concern over mad cow disease, it's best, if possible, to make sure the supplement is in a vegetable-based capsule made from herbal and vegetable concentrates.

The Importance of Omega-3 Fats

High-quality fish oils, or omega-3 fats, are vitally important for good health. Realize that many deadly degenerative diseases are inflammatory, such as cancer, heart disease, Alzheimer's disease, arthritis, autoimmune disease, and so on. Fish oil is able to decrease inflammation significantly. I believe omega-3 fats are special fats the body needs as much as it needs vitamins. Much of the research on these powerful fats was done in the 1980s after realizing the Inuit Indians, who are Eskimos, rarely developed heart attacks or rheumatoid arthritis, yet their diet contained an enormous amount of fat from fish, seals, and whales, which are all high in omega-3 fats.

By decreasing inflammation, fish oil is able to help treat and prevent conditions such as cancer, heart disease, rheumatoid arthritis, psoriasis, migraine headaches, allergies, Alzheimer's disease, and even diabetes. Fish oil also helps balance and stabilize neurotransmitters in the brain, which may be helpful in patients with attention deficit disorder, depression, and bipolar disorder.

Realize that we change the oil in our cars every three thousand to five thousand miles. Shouldn't we also begin to give ourselves an "oil change" regularly so that we can prevent a host of diseases?

Phytonutrients

We have seen the importance of these powerful plant pigments in preventing heart disease and cancer. I firmly believe that *everyone* needs these supplements on a daily basis, and multivitamins simply do not provide them. Unfortunately, most of us, as well as our children, are also falling way short of the USDA-recommended servings of fruits and vegetables each day, and we are falling prey to disease as a result of that shortage. A phytonutrient powder should provide a combination of colorful organic fruits and vegetables such as red, yellow, green, orange, and purple, as well as fiber in order to have phytonutrient protection on a daily basis.

Living in Divine Health

Opinions will always differ on what vitamins and minerals to take and on the amounts necessary. Before making any dramatic changes in the amount of vitamins or minerals you add to your daily diet, always consult your personal physician. There are other nutritional supplements that are important, including carnosine, glucosamine sulfate, gingko biloba, and supplements for prostate health. However, the ones discussed today are the *foundation* for good health. Also, natural, bioidentical hormone replacement therapy is extremely important for women and men, especially over the age of fifty. Refer to Appendix A for guidance on how to find physicians who are trained in natural hormone replacement in your area.

As more research is done on nutritional supplements, we will find that some supplements may be healthier than we thought and others may be less healthy. It is impossible to banish all confusion regarding supplements, so we must do the best we can with the information we are given for the moment. This pillar of health represents the latest, most proven research on nutritional supplements to give you a great start to living in divine health. (See Appendix A for recommended products.)

BUILDING BLOCKS TO A HEALTHY LIFE

POINTS TO PONDER: *Everyone needs a good multivitamin and a phytonutrient supplement. Most everyone needs essential fats in the form of high-grade fish oil. If you are over fifty years of age, you will also need extra antioxidants, extra calcium and vitamin D, a sublingual* B_{12}, *and maybe a digestive enzyme and/or HCL.*

ACTION STEP: *If you are under fifty years of age, start to take a good whole-food multivitamin, a phytonutrient powder, and an omega-3 supplement. If you are over fifty years of age, add to this list extra antioxidants, extra calcium and vitamin D, and a sublingual* B_{12}, *and take a digestive enzyme after each meal.*

PILLAR 7

Coping With Stress

DAY 43: Stress and Your Health

Many years ago my pastor would sometimes ask me to address the church on health topics. By the time I walked onto the platform I would be drenched in sweat, feeling as if I wanted to run out the nearest exit door and disappear into the night so I wouldn't have to face the few hundred people in the audience. I was terrified of public speaking. I remember my pastor putting his hand on my shoulder one time and saying, "You're perspiring terribly. Is it that hot in here?" I didn't have the guts to tell him I was scared to death to be under the spotlight with him. Those moments of stress and plenty of other hard-earned stress lessons from my own life have taught me a lot about the subject.

Some people go through life stressed. Just driving in heavy traffic stresses them out; so does saying hello to a neighbor or calling to inquire about a bill. That stress reaction, so useful in moments of actual emergency, becomes a self-destruct switch that eventually can lead to exhaustion and disease.

Stress Can Be Good

Good stress is healthy, such as a wedding or a promotion. Stress is also our body's natural reaction to a threat or perceived threat. It causes a sudden release of adrenaline and other hormones that cause your blood pressure to go up, your heart to beat faster, and your lungs to take in more air among other physiologic events. These stress hormones give you extra strength and mental acuity for a few moments, and they empower you to either fight or flee.

But when the stress response occurs too frequently or goes on long term, those stress hormones that were meant to save your life begin to actually harm you. They can leave you feeling depressed, anxious, angry, with low sex drive, and predisposed to obesity, type 2 diabetes, high cholesterol, hypertension, and all kinds of illnesses. The same hormones that save your life in an emergency can actually begin to destroy your health.

The Consequences of Stress

In June 2005, the *Wall Street Journal* devoted an entire section of their newspaper to how to live longer. The front-page article of the section said, "Increasingly, researchers are viewing stress—how much stress we face in a lifetime, and how well we cope with it—as one of the most significant factors for predicting how well we age."[1] The article concluded that stress "kills" people as much or more than poor health habits like smoking, drinking alcohol, or not exercising.

Stress is not just a mental problem; it's the cause of many of the diseases and maladies I treat in my practice. Many recent studies have demonstrated this. The renowned Nun Study has shown that elevated stress levels inhibit and deteriorate the hippocampus, the part of the brain associated with memory and learning. A smaller hippocampus is a sign of Alzheimer's disease.[2]

Final Exam

Students in one study were shown to be more prone to catch a cold, develop cold sores, or get infections when stressed during final-exam week.[3]

A long-term study at the University of London showed that chronic unmanaged mental stress was six times more predictive of cancer and heart disease than cigarette smoking, high cholesterol levels, and elevated blood pressure.[4] In a Mayo Clinic study of people with heart disease, psychological stress was the strongest predictor of future cardiac events.[5]

In a ten-year study, people who were not able to manage their stress effectively had a 40 percent higher death rate than those who were "unstressed."[6]

Stress, Strokes, and Sickness

Excessive stress long term can make you obese and unhealthy. In response to long-term stress, the hormone cortisol rises, which can cause the blood pressure to rise, can cause the release of fats and sugar in the bloodstream, and may cause weight gain, elevated triglycerides, high cholesterol, and blood sugar. Cortisol will save your life if you are a POW or experiencing famine, because it slows your metabolic rate and helps to preserve your fat stores. But most of us aren't POWs or experiencing famine, and so the high cortisol levels usually lead to weight gain.

Stressed-out people also tend to develop brown marks under their eyes and frown lines on their foreheads, around the eyes, and around the mouth. Some even get bulging eyes, a tight jaw, and flared nostrils. Plastic surgeons are cashing in on the stress epidemic, performing face-lifts and offering Botox injections and more.

Cortisol affects the "control loop" that regulates the sex hormones. Elevated cortisol is associated with a drop in DHEA and testosterone, which can lead to a decreased sex drive and erectile dysfunction. In women, elevated cortisol is associated with lower levels of progesterone and testosterone. During periods of chronic stress, progesterone is actually converted to cortisol in the body, which can lead to a progesterone deficiency. This, in turn, can lead to menstrual problems and PMS, as well as significant menopausal symptoms such as hot flashes and night sweats. Levels of estrogen become imbalanced in the presence of high cortisol.

Chronic stress also has commonly been associated with depression. Elevated cortisol levels cause an imbalance of neurotransmitters in the brain, notably serotonin and dopamine. In one scientific study, as many as seven out of every ten patients with depression had enlarged adrenal glands, some with glands that were 1.7 times the size of a normal gland in a person who is not depressed.[7] In other words, the adrenal gland had enlarged in response to the demand for more cortisol. The cortisol, in turn, causes an imbalance of these important neurotransmitters.

Excessive stress can predispose a person to develop or aggravate every conceivable affliction. Clearly, disease and illness are often the shrapnel wounds from stress. If you want to manage your stress, you must first learn to identify causes of stress.

Causes of Stress

The causes of stress are all too familiar to most Americans. Trouble with finances, relationships, job problems, health, or sudden traumatic events head the list, followed by a myriad of minor stressors like computer trouble, traffic, poor customer service, dirty laundry stacking up, cleaning house, driving children to extracurricular activities, ongoing conflict with friends or family members, loneliness, or even aggravating lights or noise near your home.

Stress comes in two categories:

1. Things we can and should control
2. Things we cannot control

In the rest of this section I will help you learn to cope with stress by winning on those two battlefields. Let me illustrate with two examples.

For a long time I was the king of stress clutter in my home office. I received so much "important" material—books, articles, magazines, journals, videos, and more—that I felt I had to read it all. I couldn't bring myself to throw any of it away. I had stacks everywhere of "indispensable" stuff. A normal desk wouldn't accommodate it, so I had to get a huge table to use for a desk. Then my clutter migrated like "the blob" to the kitchen table. I piled books and articles around the house, even in my bedroom, creating knee-high stacks wherever I went. My wife, Mary, or I would walk into the kitchen, my office, or our bedroom and immediately feel stressed out. Neither of us could stand to be in those places.

But the clutter problem was within my realm of control. One day, I took responsibility for my messy domain and tossed out as much stuff as I could bear. What I kept, I filed. I have stuck to that system to this day, and my office, kitchen, and even our bedroom are organized and pleasant. I took action and reduced my stress.

What a Headache!

Americans consume sixteen tons of aspirin every year, much of it due to headaches and pains caused by stress.[8]

But there are also problems that we can't control. In 2004, we went through three major hurricanes within a period of two months, and I was very stressed out. We were without electricity for days, and the weather was extremely hot. My office was closed for a few days after each hurricane.

My roof leaked, and rain poured into our living room. Our beach condo was flooded and most of the carpet destroyed. The stench of the garbage piling up was terrible because the garbage trucks couldn't get through due to fallen trees and tree limbs blocking the roads. I would lie in bed thinking, *What if we don't have electricity for weeks and I'm not able to open my office or pay my bills, and then end up in extreme debt? What if it costs a lot to repair the roof and fix the condo? What if I can't find a roofing contractor since so many roofs are damaged?*

After each hurricane these thoughts were running through my mind, and I was actually creating more stress for myself than the hurricanes caused.

Although each hurricane lasted no longer than a day and left a lot of debris that took a few days to clean up, I continued to stress for weeks afterward. My perceptions were at the root of my stress, and they determined how I saw the situation—positive or negative. Instead of having a grateful attitude, I had a "worrywart" attitude. This emotional habit was triggering a continued release of stress hormones. You see, even though the traumatic hurricanes had passed, I was reliving the stress in my mind over and over, and spewing out stress hormones in the process.

Everybody has to deal with unwanted, uncontrollable stress in their lives—natural disasters, unexpected job loss, the death of a loved one, an accident, or an illness. All of these lie mostly outside of our realm of control. They require us to change our perceptions and change our reactions.

When I began to practice mindfulness by enjoying the present moment and to reframe the situations by practicing gratitude, my perceptions and reactions changed. I was able to accept my circumstances.

You will learn these powerful stress reduction techniques in the following days.

The seventh pillar of health—coping with stress—is so important that I have written an entire book on it called *Stress Less.*[9] I encourage you to purchase it if stress is a problem for you or someone you love. For the next week we will focus on simple, proven techniques each day to help you relax and deal with stress.

BUILDING BLOCKS TO A HEALTHY LIFE

POINTS TO PONDER: *Stress can be bad (like experiencing a financial setback), but it can also be good (like getting married). Stress generally falls into two categories: situations that we can control, and situations that are uncontrollable and beyond our skill or knowledge. If we don't learn to manage stress well, it eventually affects every part of us, from the inside out.*

ACTION STEP: *The first step toward stressing less is to identify what things you can control and what things are beyond your control.*

DAY 44: Practicing Mindfulness

Dan was a colleague of mine and one of the most goal-oriented men I have ever known. When he was a teenager, he couldn't wait to graduate from high school and go to college. He worked hard and graduated from college a year early. Then he entered medical school and finished near the top of his class. His next goal was to finish his surgery residency, which he did in five years. Then he entered a group practice where he was on call every second night, which meant he was usually up all night. By that time he had driven himself so hard for so long that he had forgotten how to enjoy his life.

Dan was fun-loving on vacation, but the majority of the year he was simply driven. He rarely spent quality time or had fun with his spouse and children. He divorced and remarried three times and had one child with each of these three wives. His children became rebellious.

Every time Dan reached a goal, he quickly set a new one. Over the years, "vacation" became his top goal. Dan seemed to live and work for his two-week vacation each year. He focused his attention on that future and regretted his past. He lived in constant mental stress.

Enjoying the Present Moment

Dan needed to learn "mindfulness." This concept, studied and explained best by Herbert Benson, MD, is the practice of learning to pay attention to what is happening to you from moment to moment. To be mindful, according to Benson, you must slow down, do one activity at a time, and bring your full awareness to both the activity at hand and to your inner experience of it.[1] Mindfulness provides a potentially powerful antidote to the common causes of daily stress.

Benson's definition of mindfulness reminds me of the words of Jesus: "Therefore do not worry about tomorrow, for tomorrow will worry about its own things. Sufficient for the day is its own trouble" (Matt. 6:34, NKJV). Jesus taught us to be mindful of the present, not of the future. The apostle Paul likewise taught us to forget "those things which are behind," meaning the past. Mindfulness means letting go of any thought that is unrelated to the present moment and finding something to enjoy in the present moment.

But like my colleague Dan, most people do not live in the present moment. They are wishing for a different moment—either past or future. They go through the motions required to function in the present moment, but they are thinking things like: "I'll be happy when..."

- "I get a bigger place to live."
- "I get that promotion."
- "My kids are out of school."
- "I pay off these bills."
- "I get a new car."

Mindfulness works differently. It trains your mind to let go of any thought that is unrelated to the present moment and to find something to enjoy in the present—continually. When you walk or drive, pay attention to the beautiful scenery, the chirping of the birds and crickets, and the feel of the warm sunshine or the chill in the air. Focus on the way your body feels as you go through routine motions of driving, opening the door, walking to your destination. During work breaks and in the evening, refuse to think about goals, projects, or tasks that are not part of the present moment. If a stressful thought comes to mind, choose to move on to a thought that is related to what you are presently seeing, hearing, smelling, or feeling.

If you have to stop at a red light while driving to work, don't get frustrated, but consider it a welcome opportunity to be thankful for your car, your job, your boss, and so on. The majority of people in third world countries would love to have your car, your job, and your boss. Quit complaining about what you don't have, and start practicing gratitude for what you do have. You can practice gratitude by enjoying the music, the sights around you, the fact that you have air conditioning or heating for your car—and the fact that you have a car and are well enough to drive.

Quick Quiz

According to one survey, how many American workers describe their jobs as very stressful?

- 40 percent
- 60 percent
- 20 percent

Answer: *Forty (40) percent of American workers describe their jobs as very stressful.*[2]

As you practice mindfulness, your muscles will relax, your body unwinds, and your stress is relieved. I encourage my patients to take a drive in the country, take a walk, smell the flowers, or go to the zoo and look at the animals. This teaches them to get absorbed in the present moment so their minds can de-stress naturally.

To have complete mental and physical health, mindfulness must become a way of life, a continual pattern for practicing relaxation during your day. Make mindfulness a habit by practicing it daily.

Thankfulness and Gratitude

Nothing exemplifies mindfulness better than thankfulness and gratitude. The Book of Psalms is filled with the poetry of thanksgiving, such as this one:

> Bless the LORD, O my soul;
> And all that is within me, bless His holy name!
> Bless the LORD, O my soul,
> And forget not all His benefits:
> Who forgives all your iniquities,
> *Who heals all your diseases,*
> *Who redeems your life from destruction,*
> *Who crowns you with lovingkindness and tender mercies,*
> Who satisfies your mouth with good things,
> So that your youth is renewed like the eagle's.
>
> —PSALM 103:1–5, NKJV, EMPHASIS ADDED

It's interesting that the Bible says you enter His gates with thanksgiving, because an "attitude of gratitude" helps you take the focus off your situation and shifts it to the One who can work everything out for you. Hebrews 13 tells us to give the sacrifice of praise continually, not just when we feel like it, "the fruit of our lips giving thanks to his name" (verse 15). Paul said, "In every thing give thanks [even in the midst of trials and tribulations]: for this is the will of God in Christ Jesus concerning you" (1 Thessalonians 5:18).

Gratitude and thanksgiving go hand in hand. I recommend that you start each day by identifying at least twenty or thirty specific things, great and small, for which you are grateful. Do this with your family at the breakfast table and alone in the shower. Make it part of your running mental dialogue wherever you go.

Thankfulness and mindfulness will go a long way toward erasing the stress in your life.

One day I discussed these things with my colleague Dan. I explained that it wasn't mentally healthy to entertain every thought that popped into his head and that he had the ability to choose what he was going to think about. Even though Dan was a brilliant physician and surgeon, he had never considered these ideas.

Dan began to learn how to live in the present moment by practicing gratitude. He replaced his old thought patterns and perceptions with new ones as he practiced mindfulness. He is now happily married and enjoys spending time with his children, who come to visit him regularly and who turned from all of their rebellious ways once their father began to show genuine love and gratitude toward them and expressed a desire to spend time with them. He no longer lives for vacation, but he enjoys each day of his life. His tension and stress levels are greatly reduced.

You will have similar benefits as you begin to live in the present moment instead of the past or future and as you give praise and thanksgiving to God every moment of every day.

BUILDING BLOCKS TO A HEALTHY LIFE

POINTS TO PONDER: *Mindfulness is training your thoughts to let go of anything other than the present moment. Instead of constantly focusing on getting bigger, better, or more expensive things, be thankful about what you have at the moment, and resist comparing yourself or your possessions with others. Learn to quickly take in what benefits and blessings you have before you, and show (or express) your gratitude regularly.*

ACTION STEP: *Go back to the "appreciation list" you compiled on Day 11 (under the pillar on sleep). Take some time to update it and write down ten things for which you are grateful. Then post the list where you can see it throughout the day (like on your bathroom mirror or on the refrigerator door).*

DAY 45: Reframing

A forty-seven-year-old woman came into my practice. She had suffered from breast cancer that went to her bones. Both breasts had been removed, and now she had cancer throughout her spine. She was about to have radiation of her spine, and she faced more surgery. I performed a comprehensive physical and nutritional exam to detect the source of recurring illness in her body. Then I checked her belief system, and that's where I found the major problem.

This woman didn't believe she deserved to be healed. She felt responsible for her husband's happiness, and because her husband was a miserable person, she felt this was her fault. She believed he deserved another wife, and she wanted to die so he could be happy.

I told this woman that her autopilot was set on one destination: death. "You could wrestle with that autopilot like an airplane captain wrestling with a yoke, but as soon as you let it go, it will go right back to autopilot," I said. "Your belief system is set on disease and death. There's not much I can do until you change that."

Thankfully, she took my advice, and I helped her change her autopilot with a list of scriptures, affirmations, and a de-stressing technique called *reframing.*

Change Your Perspective

Mindfulness is learning to live in the present moment. Reframing is learning to see the past, present, and future in a positive light. Reframing calls upon a person to shift his focus away from his present point of view in order to "see" another person or a situation from a new perspective.

Here's a simple example of the concept of reframing. We had a beautiful painting in our living room, but it was never noticed because the picture frame didn't do the painting justice. My wife finally decided to reframe it with a beautiful new frame. The result was amazing. It was as if the painting almost came alive, and practically everyone noticed it immediately upon entering the room. People who had been in my house dozens of times and never noticed it were now awestruck by its beauty. They would ask where we had purchased the remarkable new painting. I replied that we had the painting hanging there all along, but no one had ever noticed it until we changed the frame.

Yes, it's true that you cannot control everything that happens to you, but you can control your perceptions and interpretations of what happens. Any psychologist will tell you that your perceptions and reactions are more important to your mental and physical health than the event itself.

Every thought you have ripples throughout your entire being—your physical body and emotions. Stressful thoughts do damage to your body and mind, like a grenade going off. Proverbs 16:22 states that the mind is the wellspring of life. We know from stress studies that the mind can also be a source of death. That means we must learn to reframe every event in our lives that we perceived as tragic, painful, traumatic, or in any way negative.

I knew one woman who had witnessed her father kill her mother with a gun. This woman spent many years trapped in anxiety and panic attacks, dwelling on the fact that her mother was killed in front of her. My wife finally told her, "Look at what God protected you from instead of what the enemy was successful at doing. You weren't killed that day. You were spared." That woman began to reframe her past and see it in a better light and, as a result, eventually overcame both the anxiety and the panic attacks.

Unfortunately, many people choose to relive the painful past experience. When their expectations are not met, even on small matters, they consider it a crisis of epic proportions. Because of the way they have been "programmed" to think either by their upbringing or by choice, they never break free and never begin to reframe events by God's standard of truth. But to cope with stress, we must recognize and "cast down" any perception that is contrary to the truth. His stress management program is much better than what has been programmed into us in childhood.

Reframing is a concept pioneered by psychologist Albert Ellis, whose Rational Emotive Therapy sought to help people replace irrational beliefs and perceptions with rational, realistic statements. When negative thoughts pop up spontaneously, Ellis said, you should challenge and assess them. Don't just accept them automatically.[1]

This is exactly what the apostle Paul meant by "casting down every imagination" and "being transformed by the renewing of your mind."

> *Casting down imaginations,* and every high thing that exalteth itself against the knowledge of God, and bringing into captivity every thought to the obedience of Christ.
>
> —2 Corinthians 10:5, emphasis added

> Do not be conformed to this world, but *be transformed by the renewing of your mind*, that you may prove what is that good and acceptable and perfect will of God.
>
> —Romans 12:2, NKJV, emphasis added

Jesus said in John 16:33, "In the world ye shall have tribulation: but be of good cheer; I have overcome the world." James, the brother of Jesus, taught us the meaning of reframing when we face trials:

> My brethren, count it all joy when you fall into various trials, knowing that the testing of your faith produces patience.
>
> —James 1:2–3, NKJV

James was giving us God's perspective. Scriptural reframing is one of the most powerful ways to relieve stress. It is simply replacing our fears, worries, failures, grief, sorrows, and shame with God's promises.

One woman I treated had been carjacked while at a phone booth at a service station. Two thugs almost raped her, but they didn't. They stole her brand-new car, which had her purse. This woman had panic attacks because she knew the men had her identification that told them where she lived. She lived in fear that they would come back and rape her.

But the fact was they did not rape her, and they never came back for her. All she lost was her car and her purse, and the car was insured. She lost no money other than what was in her purse, but she lost her peace. I told her to reframe the event in her mind. Instead of reliving the traumatic experience, I told her to start being grateful that she was protected from any harm.

I told her, "Let this be a lesson that angels encamp around you and stand guard to protect you."

She said, "I've never seen it that way." As she reframed the event, the fear and anxiety resolved. In reframing, see your trials as your teacher. I have found that practically all traumatic events can be reframed so that a lesson is learned and gratitude expressed.

The story of one Holocaust survivor, Dr. Viktor Frankl, a Jewish psychiatrist, is a powerful example of reframing. One day he was naked and alone in a small room, and it suddenly dawned on him the "last of human freedom"—his inner identity—was the very freedom that his Nazi captors could not take away. This freedom was the power to choose a response. Frankl also encouraged his fellow prisoners to tell at least one funny story every day about something that they intended to do after they were freed. Frankl was reframing his thoughts as well as helping his fellow prisoners reframe their thoughts. He understood the healing power of laughter and eventually went on to develop a school of psychotherapy called *logo think-*

ing, which incorporates humor as a major component of therapy. He also gave them a vision of being free since the funny story was about something they intended to do after they were freed.[2] Proverbs 29:18 says that where there is no vision, the people perish.

Help Your Heart

Reframing your thoughts can have a very real effect on your body, beginning with your heart. The heart, unlike your other major organs, has an extensive communication system with the brain and exerts a unique and far-reaching influence on your emotions and body. The heart is much more than a pump; it also functions as a hormonal gland, a sensory organ, and an information-encoding and -processing center. The heart also contains approximately forty thousand neurons or nerve cells. With every beat, the heart transmits complex patterns of neurological, hormonal, pressure, and electromagnetic information to the brain and throughout the body that play a major part in determining your emotions or how you feel.

Your heart beat is not monotonously regular, but it varies from moment to moment. Heart rate variability is the measure of the beat-to-beat changes in the heart rate as the heart speeds up and slows down in different patterns. These changes are especially influenced by a person's emotions and attitudes. When you experience stress and negative emotions such as anger, frustration, fear, and anxiety, your heart rate variability pattern becomes more erratic and disordered, and it sends chaotic signals to the brain. This causes your system to get "out of sync." The result is excessive stress with toxic emotions, energy drain, and added wear and tear on your mind and body. In contrast, sustained positive emotions, such as appreciation, love, joy, and compassion, are associated with highly ordered patterns on the heart rate variability tracing and a significant reduction of stress.

In other words, toxic emotions such as anger, resentment, fear, anxiety, grief, and depression create excessive stress, whereas positive emotions such as gratitude, joy, love, and peace actually relieve stress. This can now be measured by an instrument called "heart rate variability."

The heart has a magnetic field that is approximately five thousand times stronger than the brain and an electrical field that's forty to sixty times stronger than the brain. To illustrate this point, consider this story.

Christian Huygens was a seventeenth-century clock maker who invented the pendulum clock. One night, while lying in bed admiring his clock collection, he noticed that all his pendulum clocks were swinging in unison with one another. He knew he didn't set them that way, so he got out of bed and reset all the pendulums so that they were all out of sync with one another. However, after a short period of time all the pendulum clocks were back swinging in unison with one another. He never understood why. Years later it was discovered that the largest clock with the strongest rhythm was able to pull all other nearby pendulums in sync with itself. This was called *entrainment.*[3]

The largest clock pendulum with the strongest rhythm pulls all other nearby pendulums in sync with itself. The heart, by practicing gratitude and thanksgiving, is able, with its powerful magnetic field five thousand times stronger than the brain, to hijack the very thoughts of the brain and bring them into the pendulum motion of gratitude instead of the brain's programmed emotions of fear, worry, anger, bitterness, grief, depression, and so on. That is why Proverbs 4:23 instructs us to keep our heart with all diligence, for out of it flow the issues of life. If we keep gratitude, peace, joy, and love in our heart, then it is able to control the brain, and gratitude, peace, joy, and love will flow out of our mouths.

Did You Know...?

The heart is the strongest biological oscillator in the body with a magnetic field five thousand times stronger than the brain. It is literally able to draw the brain into sync with it.

According to the Institute of HeartMath, these core heart feelings of gratitude, joy, peace, and love increase synchronization and coherence in the heart rhythm patterns, and these in turn decrease stress. However, it is much more difficult for patients to experience joy and love, especially if they are anxious, depressed, angry, or grieving. But gratitude and thanksgiving are the entry emotions that are easier to experience and are powerful de-stressors. For more on this topic of HeartMath, see my book *Stress Less.*

"When Will I Feel Better?"

For some people reframing takes time, but often it doesn't. It depends on your willingness to let the old belief go. You may feel it's not safe to let it go, because if you do, the hurtful event might happen again. But I have news for you. If you don't let that distorted belief go, it's as if the hurtful event is happening to you over and over. It is similar to a thorn that is stuck in your flesh and has broken off, and now it is infected and festering.

The prospect of speaking to huge crowds when my pastor called me onstage kept me in a state of stress for a long time, so I had to reframe the situation. Instead of seeing it as an opportunity to embarrass myself,

I finally realized that it was an opportunity to give information on health that would help many people. In fact, it was a great opportunity to share my knowledge with thousands of other people. After a while I saw it as a golden opportunity, not a time to hit the panic button. Now I speak all over the country to crowds big and small. I even host a television program. None of it bothers me anymore. All other facts remain the same, but I have reframed my response.

I now frame my day each morning, and I encourage you to do the same. Live each day as if it were your last. From eternity's perspective, even "big" problems seem small. James wrote, "You do not know what will happen tomorrow. For what is your life? It is even a vapor that appears for a little time and then vanishes away" (James 4:14, NKJV).

By staying mindful of the present, thankful to God, and by reframing everything that happens to you according to the truth of God's Word, you will be able to cope with the major sources of stress in your life.

BUILDING BLOCKS TO A HEALTHY LIFE

POINTS TO PONDER: *Reframing is learning to shift your focus away from your present point of view in order to "see" another person or a situation from a new perspective. Like Frankl, imagine yourself coming out free on the other side of your circumstance. Envision all of the positive effects that will result from the situation. The heart's power to bring thoughts back into "sync" is a powerful tool to reframing the mind.*

ACTION STEP: *Instead of seeing disappointments, setbacks, and trials as a time to complain, worry, or criticize, begin to reframe and see these events as teachers. What did this situation teach you so that you can avoid that mistake next time around?*

DAY 46: The Power of Laughter and Joy

When people come into my office to be treated or placed on a nutritional program, I often ask them, "How often do you laugh?" You should see the looks they give me. A common response in cancer patients is, "I never laugh." I can tell they're thinking, *I have cancer, Dr. Colbert. What is there to laugh about?*

One of the most unusual prescriptions I give to many of my patients is to have at least ten belly laughs a day. True laughing offers one of the most powerful and natural healing methods without any side effects. Laughter lowers the stress hormones cortisol and epinephrine. It increases feel-good hormones. It keeps you squarely in the present moment. It helps you to reframe and feel thankful and helps you to see negative events in a more positive light. There's not a single bad thing laughter will do for your body and mind.

One study, however, stated that Americans feel happy just 54 percent of the time. They say they feel neutral about 25 percent of the time and sad 21 percent of the time.[1] If that's true, there are not a lot of happy people in the United States.

Has it ever occurred to you that you were created to be happy and filled with joy? The Bible declares:

> Rejoice in the Lord always. I will say it again: Rejoice!
>
> —Philippians 4:4, niv

The psalmist declared of God:

> In Your presence is fullness of joy; at Your right hand are pleasures forevermore.
>
> —Psalm 16:11, nkjv

Nehemiah told the workers who were rebuilding the walls of Jerusalem:

> The joy of the Lord is your strength.
>
> —Nehemiah 8:10

Jesus told the disciples:

> These things I have spoken to you, that My joy may remain in you, and that your joy may be full.
>
> —John 15:11, nkjv

Isn't it comforting to know that during His last night on Earth, Jesus' main concern was that His followers have joy?

Benefits of Happiness

I believe the Bible is so emphatic about joy because joy sustains life: "A cheerful heart is good medicine" (Proverbs 17:22, NIV). That is literally true. According to Rich Bayer, PhD, CEO of Upper Bay Counseling and Support Services, Inc., happy people have more social contact and better social relations than their unhappy counterparts. Studies of positive people show that they rate high on having good relationships with themselves and with others. Their love life is better as well. Happy people tend to be kinder to others and to express empathy more easily. They also have the ability to use their intelligence more effectively. Some studies show that people become better students when they are feeling happy.[2]

Of course, happy people are not "luckier" than other people. They experience tragedy and hardship, but studies show that happy people do a better job of reframing.[3] They remember the good events in their lives more readily, and when bad things happen, they believe things will eventually be all right. They have hope.

Happiness is one of the keys to a long, satisfying life. Studies also show that happy people have fewer health problems.[4] Research among older people indicates that folks with positive emotions outlive their sour counterparts. Happy people were shown to be half as likely to become disabled as sad people in the same age bracket. And happy people have a higher pain threshold than those who are sad.[5]

When you laugh, powerful chemicals called endorphins, which act much the same way as morphine, are released in the brain. Endorphins trigger a feeling of well-being throughout your entire body and relieve pain.

In the Department of Behavioral Medicine of the UCLA Medical School, a man named Norman Cousins conducted extensive research into

Chuckle for the Day

The new pastor was visiting in the homes of his parishioners. At one house it seemed obvious that someone was at home, but no answer came to his repeated knocks at the door. He took out a card and wrote Revelation 3:20, which says "Behold, I stand at the door and knock," and stuck it in the doorjamb.

The following Sunday when the offering was processed, he found that his card had been returned with this cryptic message, and he burst into laughter. The message added was from Genesis 3:10, which reads, "I heard your voice in the garden and I was afraid for I was naked."

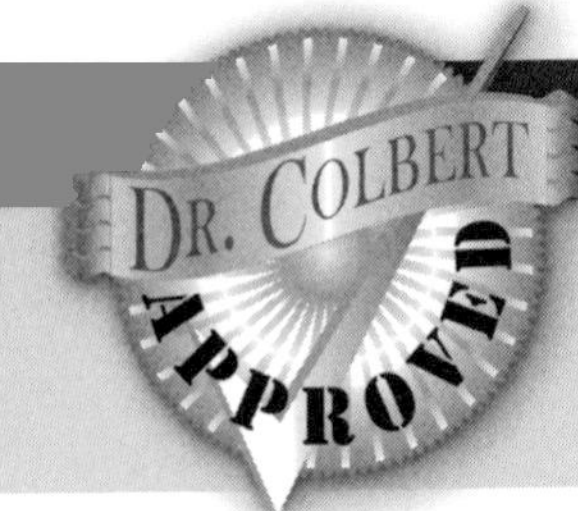

Dr. Colbert Approved

Get ten good belly laughs today. Good belly laughs are the equivalent of getting a good aerobic exercise workout.

the physical benefits of happiness. He established the Humor Research Task Force, which coordinated worldwide clinical research on humor. His research proved conclusively that laughter, happiness, and joy are perfect antidotes for stress.[6]

A good hearty laugh can help:

- Reduce stress
- Lower blood pressure
- Elevate mood
- Boost the immune system
- Improve brain functioning
- Protect the heart
- Connect you to others
- Foster instant relaxation
- Make you feel good[7]

According to the Association for Applied and Therapeutic Humor, "Without humor one's thought processes are likely to become stuck and narrowly focused, leading to increased distress."[8]

Did You Know...?

Some researchers contend that twenty seconds of belly laughter is equivalent to three minutes of working out on a rowing machine.[10]

Choosing a good attitude doesn't diminish the amount of suffering in your life or in the world, but it helps to lighten the load. Even when we suffer, we can choose to be joyful, because He is with us.[9]

Dr. Lee Berk and fellow researcher Dr. Stanley Tan of Loma Linda University in California studied the effects of laughter on the immune system and found a general decrease in stress hormones that constrict blood vessels and suppress immune activity in people exposed to humor. Levels of the stress hormone epinephrine were lower in the group both in anticipation of humor and after exposure to humor. Epinephrine levels remained down throughout the experiment.[11]

I recommend to all my patients ten belly laughs a day. I prescribe Carol Burnett DVDs, *Sanford and Son* DVDs, and other clean humor to my patients. Create a habit of happiness instead of a habit of worry. Your happiness is not at the mercy of other people or life circumstances and events. A merry heart is your greatest weapon against stress. For more information on this topic, please refer to my book *Deadly Emotions*.[12]

BUILDING BLOCKS TO A HEALTHY LIFE

POINTS TO PONDER: *Create a habit of happiness and laughter instead of a habit of worry. When you laugh, it lowers stress hormones and relieves stress. Laughter also boosts the immune system, protects the heart, and improves overall health. Ten belly laughs a day are equivalent to getting a good aerobic exercise workout, and they're the ultimate "stress buster."*

ACTION STEP: *Find a TV show DVD or movie with clean humor, watch it tonight, and laugh a lot!*

DAY 47: Forgive

A patient named Carrie came to me when she was in her mid-thirties. She had suffered from asthma for years, and sometimes her asthma attacks were so severe that they landed her in a hospital emergency room. Carrie had another problem as well: she was very easily offended. Sometimes when she was stressed out over an offense, she had an asthma attack. I asked her to tell me her earliest memory related to asthma, and she told me about being a toddler in a mist tent in the hospital. Another girl was in the same room under a mist tent. The other little girl received lots of toys and dolls as presents from her parents. But Carrie's parents only brought books for Carrie—no toys. Carrie was angry and offended at her parents for this incident. The offense was still so real in Carrie's mind—having rehearsed and retold her someone-done-me-wrong-song for so many years—that in just telling this story to me, it brought on an asthma attack!

I told Carrie that she was stuck in the past and that if she truly wanted to help her own asthmatic condition, she needed to quit repeating her grievance story and forgive this offense, which was primarily a perceived offense and nothing her parents ever intended to do to hurt her. Carrie agreed, and when she quit telling her grievance story, her asthma attacks decreased dramatically.

Rehashing

One of the secret causes of stress plaguing millions of people is unforgiveness. People rehash the wrong that was done to them, or that they misperceive was done to them, and their body immediately has a stress response. Your brain actually does not distinguish between short-term and long-term memories when it produces a biochemical stress response. It thinks the offense, which may have occurred decades ago, is happening right now. When you fail to forgive, you lock yourself into long-term stress similar to pulling a scab off a sore so that it never heals.

Most overstressed individuals are "rehashers." They constantly contemplate, relive, and meditate on painful experiences of their past. An upsetting event may have occurred fifteen years ago, but a rehasher can recall that experience as if it happened yesterday—and their body is literally stewing in its own stress juices every time they relive it.

I have discovered that, in dealing with severely ill patients, many of them began to spiral down into ill health at the precise time they began to harbor an offense. Their unforgiveness caused untold stress and cut them off from some of their most important relationships in life.

An offense is similar to a grudge. It is any circumstance or complaint that is perceived as unjust or hurtful. An offense usually produces what I call a "grievance story." A grievance story is when something happens in our life that we did not want to happen, and we deal with the problem by thinking about it too much and talking about it too much.

Real or Perceived?

Some offenses are real, even intentional. Most, however, are only perceived.

Years ago I had a very well-known actor come to my office to be seen as a patient. Although he was not scheduled for a visit, I worked him into the schedule as a courtesy. On this particular day, however, I had seen some very sick patients who required hospitalization, which took more of my time than normal. By the time I saw this man, I was a couple of hours late. A few weeks later I learned through a friend of his that he was highly offended and thought that I had deliberately caused him to wait, which was not the case at all. However, he perceived this offense to be real even though I had no way of knowing that I would treat such gravely ill patients.

The vast majority of offenses are imagined and not intentional; they are based on our own distorted thoughts. Please refer to my book *Deadly Emotions* for more insight into this.

When you feel you have been wronged or life has not been fair to you, resist the urge to allow this to turn into an offense. Be determined not to allow one or more negative events to define who you are. Instead, choose to forgive and "let it go." The tremendous damage of harboring an offense with the bitterness it brings keeps you stewing in stress chemicals.

This is also true when someone has hurt us intentionally. Accepting an offense is always optional. You don't have to own that grudge. It's like when the UPS man comes to your door. You can sign for the box, or you can refuse to take it. When you receive an offense, you may as well be signing for a box of rattlesnakes when it comes to your health. My friend Joyce Meyer says that bitterness and unforgiveness are like drinking poison and wishing the other person would die. I have said that bitterness and unforgiveness are like acid: they consume the very container in which they are stored. Unfortunately, that container may be you.

The apostle Paul wrote, "You must make allowance for each other's faults and forgive the person who offends you. Remember, the Lord forgave you, so you must forgive others" (Colossians 3:13, NLT).

To forgive does not mean that you didn't get hurt. Rather, it's choosing not to live in the feeling of unforgiveness. You can trust God to deal with the offense and the offender. Forgiving in its simplest form is letting go of old hurts and releasing people and situations into God's hands.

If you continue to hold on to unforgiveness toward someone else, you do not hurt that other person; rather, you damage your own health. Therefore, you should release your anger and bitterness for the sake of self-preservation. When you forgive, you release your right to judgment, punishment, and revenge related to the person who angered you.

For people struggling with stress caused by unforgiveness, I strongly recommend my books *Deadly Emotions* and *Stress Less.* What I want you to see is that forgiveness is part of the foundation of good health—and it will help to set you free from stress.

BUILDING BLOCKS TO A HEALTHY LIFE

POINTS TO PONDER: *When you fail to forgive an offense, you "rehash" that memory and keep yourself trapped in the stress of reliving that moment. Some offenses are real; some are perceived. It all comes down to your perception and whether or not you choose to forgive. Forgiveness is letting go of old hurts and people who wounded you, which will set you free from stress.*

ACTION STEP: *Use the sample declaration below to verbally forgive and release anyone who may have hurt you.*

A Declaration to Resolve Unforgiveness, Resentment, and Bitterness

It is helpful to first picture the person whom you wish to forgive with your eyes closed; then when you can see his/her face, say the name by which you called him/her when he/she first came into your life, and forgive him/her as described below.

Then in the same way, forgive all others, one by one, who have caused you anger, resentment, or pain, or who have caused pain or hurt in those you love. Do not forget to forgive yourself, God, biological parents, stepparents, adopted parents, grandparents, siblings, spouse, ex-spouse(s), children, and any others who have offended you, whether you remember specific events related to each one or not. You can release bitterness with either this affirmation or prayer below.

> *I choose to forgive* [[fill in the name]], *both consciously or subconsciously, for anything that he/she may have done or failed to do. I choose to forgive* [[fill in the name]] *for anything that he/she may have said or failed to say, which in my perception has caused pain in me or anyone else I care about. I also choose to forgive all of those whom I have unforgiveness and resentment toward for any reason. I choose to replace all bitterness with love, joy, and peace.*

Here's a sample prayer:

> *Father, I acknowledge that I have sinned against You by not forgiving those who have offended me. I also acknowledge my inability to forgive them apart from You. I understand Matthew 6:14–15, which says, "If ye forgive men their trespasses, your heavenly Father will also forgive you: But if ye forgive not men their trespasses, neither will your Father forgive your trespasses." Since Jesus forgave my sins and cancelled my debt by shedding His blood and dying on the cross for me, the least I can do is forgive [[fill in the name]] and cancel their debt against me. Therefore, with Your help and from my heart, I choose to forgive* [[fill in the name(s)]]. *I release them; they no longer owe me anything. I ask that You bless them and lead them into a closer relationship with You. In Jesus' name, amen.*

DAY 48: Margin

A few years ago I took my son, Kyle, to the airport, and we left the house two hours early, which was plenty of time to get him to the gate. As we started our drive my son said, "I'm starved. I've got to eat." So we stopped to get chicken at a Chick-fil-A restaurant, but the line was long and it took nearly half an hour to finally get our order. By that time it was 4:30 p.m. and five o' clock traffic had already started to line up on the interstate. Suddenly we were not as early as we thought. After sitting in almost standstill traffic, we realized he would miss his flight unless we took another route. Mary was driving, and she took a downtown exit and gunned our Hummer down side streets. Then we got behind a slow Coca-Cola truck. As my heart pounded, Mary passed it on a double yellow line. We seemed to hit every red light, and the chances of my son making his flight were shrinking by the minute.

Finally we made it to within a mile of the airport. Traffic was stuck again. But we were in a Hummer, so we had possibilities! There was an open turn lane so that we could get ahead of all the traffic, but a foot-tall curb was preventing us from going there, which would save us precious time. Mary drove over it and zoomed ahead of everyone. Angry drivers were yelling, shaking their fists, and honking at us, and I was glad I wasn't in the driver's seat. My son made his flight with not even a minute to spare. My heart was racing, I was perspiring profusely, and we all were arguing. We felt exhausted. But all of this exhausting stress could have been prevented if only we had allowed enough margin by simply leaving much earlier and allowing ourselves plenty of time.

A very practical and wise way to de-stress your life is to build margin into everything you do. Margin is that buffer between feeling overwhelmed and feeling at peace. Allowing yourself two hours to get to the airport when you only need one hour is margin. When you make a budget and spend only 80 percent of what you earn, that's margin.

I have learned about margin the hard way, in episodes like the one with my son's flight. Years ago, when Mary and I would travel, we would leave for the airport one hour before our flight, allowing a scant thirty minutes to get to the airport and thirty minutes to check in and get to the gate. It worked most of the time; however, it caused major stress because we were running late almost every time. A few years ago we learned that it is better to wait at the airport without stress than to arrive at the last minute worn out from stress.

Building Margin

In his book *The Overload Syndrome*, Dr. Richard Swenson contends that margin is the difference between vitality and exhaustion. It is where we gain breathing room and store up reserve energy.[1] If you are always in a hurry or always tired, it's usually because you haven't built enough margin into your schedule.

When you live without enough margin in your time, finances, and so on, you become instantly stressed. You may be overstressed simply because you are too busy. It may be overcommitment, too many activities, compounded by a growing "to-do" list added to an already hectic schedule.

Some people are on a "do-more-so-I-can-have-more" treadmill. The more some people have, the more they want, and so the harder they work. Recognize that eventually those things will own you instead of you owning them because they will consume your time and energy. It will rob you of peace and joy. People begin to irritate you, and you may become critical or complain too much, which causes even more stress. Developing margin breaks you out of this trap.

I have read through the Bible a number of times, and I have noticed that Jesus was never in a hurry. He knew how to build margin into His life. We need to slow down and get into God's rhythm.

Margin will not magically appear in your schedule or finances. You must plan it and put it there. Some people should cut back on their commitments by learning to say no or by being less ambitious. Others have plenty of time in their schedules, but they manage it poorly and are chronically late anyway. I have seen license plate frames that read, "Always late, but worth the wait." That is a selfish attitude. You stress other people out by being late, and you steal the margin they have built into their schedules. Learn to be punctual. Make a to-do list each evening before you go to bed, and build in time between your appointments. It will decrease your stress and the stress of people who might have to wait on you.

Other people desperately need to build margin into their finances. A third of Americans say money is a very significant source of stress for them.[2] Financial advice is beyond the scope of this book, but the most basic is often the best: spend less than you earn, pay off credit cards each month, build an emergency fund equal to four to six months of pay, and have health insurance. These things protect you when unexpected expenditures hit.

When you have margin in your life, you will sometimes find yourself at the doctor's office or other appointments five minutes early instead of late. Make the most of your time by bringing along work, something to read, or something to listen to.

When you purposely build margin into your life, your stress level will go down dramatically.

BUILDING BLOCKS TO A HEALTHY LIFE

DAY 48 DAY 48 DAY 48

POINTS TO PONDER: *Margin, according to Dr. Swenson, is the difference between vitality and exhaustion. I say it is the buffer between feeling overwhelmed and feeling at peace. When you fail to schedule adequate time between events or activities where you do have control, you set yourself up to experience stress. Get off the "do-more-so-I-can-have-more" treadmill! Margin is building time into your schedule, finances, and every area of your life so that you eliminate that unnecessary stress.*

ACTION STEP: *Whatever you need to accomplish today, allow for margin in your tasks. Make a "to-do" list; give yourself plenty of time to get from one destination to another. Prioritize your schedule and decide on what you can postpone for another day.*

DAY 49: Practice Stress-Reducing Habits

As we finish this final pillar of health, let me share several other very important habits that will help you cope with stress.

Some people wake up to loud music on the radio, watch soap operas, listen to gossipy morning talk shows while they get ready for the day, listen to music with depressing lyrics on the way to work, and reminisce about the dramatic television show they watched the previous night. Then they wonder why they're stressed out before they even get to work!

What enters your mind will be reflected in your health. The Bible says, "Keep thy heart with all diligence; for out of it are the issues of life" (Proverbs 4:23). If you are dumping other people's problems, fantasies, and lyrics into your head, what results do you expect?

The Bible says to "fix your thoughts on what is true and honorable and right. Think about things that are pure and lovely and admirable. Think about things that are excellent and worthy of praise" (Philippians 4:8, NLT).

Meditate on the Word of God

The most important foundation of a stress-less life is meditating on the Bible. It is the thread that runs through all the other advice—mindfulness, thankfulness, reframing, forgiving, laughter, margin, and more. I sometimes have my patients fast television, magazines, and radio for a certain period of time and memorize scriptures, especially 1 Corinthians 13, the "love chapter" you often hear recited at weddings. I tell them to read it aloud and insert their name into it: "I am patient. I am kind. I do not exalt myself." When your heart is filled with Scripture, there is not much room for stress.

You see, you can do everything this book advises, but if you do not follow moral biblical principles, your life will be full of stress. Live a life of high morals, be a person of your word, and be honest. Don't cheat yourself out of a wonderful, happy, peaceful life by sowing bad deeds. Do your best to treat others as you would have them treat you. You will then be living your best life.

Breathe

I have a friend who is a paramedic. One time I asked him what the difference was between people who died and people who lived after experiencing traumatic injuries. He thought a moment and then told me, "I have witnessed individuals with severe traumatic injuries live and others with significantly less severe injuries die because they simply quit breathing."

That's more profound than you might think. When I had a heat stroke and came close to dying, I kept hearing a voice say, "Just fall asleep. Quit breathing." I fought that impulse and made myself keep breathing, and I lived.

Proper breathing is one of the best ongoing relaxation and de-stressing techniques—and it is one of the least used. Most people don't know how to breathe properly. They go through life breathing shallowly, just as people do in times of stress. But proper breathing is a simple way to decrease your feeling of stress.

Watch any newborn baby in the nursery, and you will see its little belly rising and falling. This is abdominal or diaphragmatic breathing, and it is the way we are supposed to breathe. However, somewhere between childhood and adulthood we learn chest breathing, which is stress breathing. Usually only professional singers or musicians who play wind instruments continue to practice abdominal breathing. When we are severely stressed, usually we will initially hold our breath and then breathe rapid, shallow breaths.

Abdominal breathing has a calming effect on the brain and nervous system and helps to relieve pain and stress. It also helps muscles to relax.

To learn abdominal breathing, lie down on your back in a comfortable position. Place your left hand on your abdomen and your right hand on your chest. Since most Americans are chest breathers, their shoulders go up and down with each breath as opposed to the abdominal cavity moving in and out.

First, practice filling your lower lungs by allowing your abdomen to push out your left hand, which causes your abdominal cavity to expand. Your right hand on your chest should remain still. Make sure your breathing is slow and steady. About ten slow, deep abdominal breaths will leave you feeling relaxed and calm.

I recommend that you practice this nightly for five or ten minutes, and eventually you will be able to do it when stressed while sitting, standing, or even talking. Realize that you can't be relaxed and stressed out at

Dr. Colbert Approved

I play Christian music at my office to promote healing in my patients. Inspirational music can fill your inner person with peace and joy. While driving or working, softly play inspirational music. You will find that the peace of God will fill your heart.

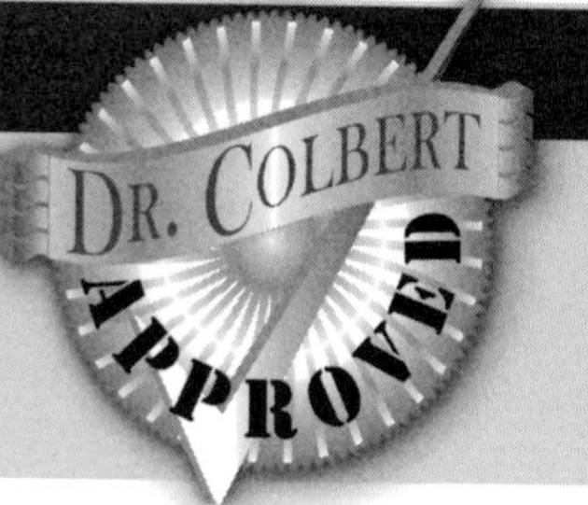

the same time, and abdominal breathing definitely relaxes the body. Don't wait until you are stressed to begin practicing abdominal breathing.

Remove Obvious Stressors

Each of us should regularly identify the stressors in our present environment and remove the ones we can. These might include clutter, our schedule, and our relationships.

First, order your world. Just as I finally ordered my office and home and tossed out stacks of stuff, you should embark on a campaign to order your life. Start with simple physical things around the house. Clean and organize the garage, your office, and the kids' rooms. Give yourself a pleasing environment in which to live. This will give you a sense of confidence and control, and it will reduce the day-to-day stress you feel. Studies prove that when people are given control over their home or work environments, they have far less stress.[1]

The Power of "No"

Then learn to say no. Proverbs 29:18 says, "Where there is no vision, the people perish." Once you get a vision for your life, you won't have room for someone else's goals for you, so you will have to become assertive. Assertive doesn't mean aggressive. It simply means being who you are and speaking your feelings, hopes, dreams, and desires confidently without fear of ridicule, reprimand, or punishment. Assertive people have a good self-image, high self-esteem, and well-defined personal boundaries—and they are less prone to stress than either passive or aggressive people.

If you tend to be passive, you will need to communicate your thoughts, feelings, wants, and needs more confidently. You may be accustomed to doing whatever people ask of you to avoid conflict. Then that person's problems have now become your problems simply because you were unable to say no. Those days must end. Even if you don't feel confident on the inside, speak more confidently. Tell people what you expect and what you like. Don't be mealy-mouthed or apologetic about it. Speak your mind happily and respectfully.

Learning to say no is one of the most powerful ways to decrease your stress level. In my book *Stress Less* I share ways of saying no. One of them is to add the phrase "right now" to your no. For example:

- "I don't think that is a good idea right now."
- "I'm not available to do that right now."
- "I'm not able to work that into my schedule right now."

Here are other useful phrases to use:

- "I have a different set of priorities."
- "I don't think that's a wise course of action for me."

When you understand your vision and goals, confidence will come easily. You will protect your time and energy because it is infinitely valuable to you.

Watch Your Friends, and Your Mouth

Finally, surround yourself with positive friends. Words, thoughts, and attitudes are contagious, so choose your friends carefully. Mary and I often say to each other, "You can tell rattlesnakes by their rattles. You can tell life-suckers by their whine." Life-suckers are people who are always singing the "somebody-done-me-wrong" song. The more time you spend with them, the more tired you will feel. It's like having a dead battery hooked up to you, draining you. With life-suckers, you always encourage them, and they always discourage you. You leave their presence thinking, *I always feel exhausted talking to that person.* But they tell you, "I always feel so good after talking to you." The Bible says to do all things without grumbling, fault-finding, or complaining.[2]

You are asking for unneeded stress if you surround yourself with life-suckers.

I'm not saying to completely avoid such people, but limit the time you spend with them. Don't let their negative attitude drain all of your energy, joy, and strength. Realize that a negative attitude, just like a positive one, is contagious. If you spend a lot of time with people who are negative, you will probably take on some of their characteristics.

And watch out! The most important life-sucker in your life may be you. Are you a whiner? Are you constantly thinking negatively in your own heart? Critiquing and criticizing yourself and others? The words you speak to yourself have a tremendous ability to cause or relieve stress.

I have found that it is extremely important for your health to love and accept yourself unconditionally.

Pleasant words add sweetness to the soul and bring health to the bones.[3] Choose attitudes and words of love, thankfulness, appreciation, and humility. As you practice this, you slam the door on stress and open the door for joy and peace.

BUILDING BLOCKS TO A HEALTHY LIFE

POINTS TO PONDER: *Think on good, positive things. Remember that old adage: "Accentuate the positive; eliminate the negative." Practice proper breathing techniques (abdominal breathing), which will help you de-stress. Learn the art of saying no. Do not volunteer or take on more activities than you are capable of handling. Limit the time spent with people who are pessimistic, whiners, or complainers. If you're not careful, they will drain the energy and life right out of you.*

ACTION STEP: *Take five minutes today to practice the abdominal breathing technique mentioned on page 256. If you find yourself in a stressful situation, take a moment to practice some deep breathing before you react.*

DAY 50: Your Day of Jubilee—The Chief Cornerstone

Isaiah 26:3 says, "Thou wilt keep him in perfect peace, whose mind is stayed on thee: because he trusteth in thee." Can you even imagine *perfect peace*? This is the same peace Jesus had in the midst of the storm at sea in Luke 8:23–25. The Amplified Version says, "A whirlwind revolving from below upwards swept down on the lake, and the boat was filling with water, and they were in great danger" (verse 23). This was most likely a tornado that was causing tremendous winds and waves, which were crashing on the boat and filling it with water. I can only imagine the violent rocking of the boat on the sea and the tremendous roar of the winds. But Jesus was in such a deep sleep that the disciples had to wake Him. *That* is perfect peace in the midst of the storm. You too can begin to experience peace in the midst of your storm.

The most important way to overcome stress is to keep our minds focused on the promises of God's Word and to trust His Word, which brings perfect peace. Unfortunately, most people are filling their minds with stress, fear, and worry from the news on TV; the programs they watch on TV; the magazines, books, and newspapers they read; the movies they watch; the friends they fellowship with; and by continually voicing their fears, worries, and stresses. The Word of God tells us in Joshua 1:8, "This Book of the Law shall not depart out of your mouth, but you shall *meditate* in it day and night..." (NKJV, emphasis added).

I teach my patients to meditate on God's Word especially for insomnia, but also to relieve stress and live in peace. Psalm 1:2 says a blessed man delights "in the law of the LORD, and in His law he *meditates* day and night" (NKJV, emphasis added). As we meditate on God's Word we replace our old distorted thought processes with God's thoughts, which is simply scriptural reframing or programming our mind with God's Word.

At the root of most of our stress is distorted thinking that was learned from our parents and figures of authority, such as a coach or teacher, as we were being raised. As we replace these old thought patterns, perceptions, and attitudes with God's thoughts, perceptions, and attitudes, a transformation takes place in our life. As we practice and meditate on His thoughts, the fruit of the Spirit is grown in our life. You see, fruit is grown and gifts are given. Too many Christians are praying for the fruit of the Spirit, when it actually comes only from passing the test of trials and tribulations with the attitude of gratitude. But with practice, patience, and the attitude of gratitude and meditation on His Word, the fruit of the Spirit grows *huge* in our life.

> But the fruit of the Spirit is love, joy, peace, longsuffering, gentleness, goodness, faith, meekness, temperance.
>
> —GALATIANS 5:22–23

Notice that stress, worry, anxiety, depression, grief, anger, and other toxic emotions are not even mentioned.

However, before receiving this peace that passes all understanding, you first need to receive Jesus Christ, the Prince of Peace, as your Lord and Savior. If you have never prayed this prayer, please pray with me now.

> *Lord Jesus, I want to know You as my Savior and Lord. I believe that You are the Son of God and You died for my sins. I also believe that You were raised from the dead and now sit at the right hand of the Father praying for me. I ask You to forgive my sins and change my heart so that I can be Your child and live with You eternally.*
>
> *Thank You for Your peace. Help me to walk with You so that I can begin to know You as my best friend and my Lord. Amen.*

If you prayed that prayer, we rejoice with you in your decision and your new relationship with Jesus. I strongly recommend that you get involved in a good Bible-believing church and start fellowshiping with other believers. Also, start reading the Bible every day. Get a New King James Version or another version that is easy to understand. Please contact us at pray4me@strang.com, and we will send you some materials that will help you become established in your new relationship with the Lord.

BUILDING BLOCKS TO A HEALTHY LIFE

POINTS TO PONDER: *Jesus is the Prince of Peace and offers you the peace that passes all understanding.*[1] *The best stress reliever is to pray and begin to learn to cast all your cares on Jesus.*[2] *Practice trusting in God's Word.*

ACTION STEP: *Today is your day of jubilee, so thank Him aloud for His goodness! By continuing to practice biblical principles of the Seven Pillars of Health, you will begin to walk in divine health.*

APPENDIX A
Recommended Products

Please mention Dr. Colbert as the referring physician for the companies listed below.

Divine Health Nutritional Products
1908 Boothe Circle
Longwood, FL 32750
Phone: (407) 331-7007
Web site: www.drcolbert.com
E-mail: info@drcolbert.com

Phytonutrient powders: *Divine Health Living Food (full phytonutrient rainbow protection and best tasting); Divine Health Living Fruit and Veggie (great-tasting green food); Divine Health Green Superfood*

Whole-food multivitamin: *Divine Health Living Multi*

B_{12}: *Divine Health B_{12} Complex (methylcobalamin, active form of folic acid, and B_6)*

Antioxidants: *Divine Health CoQ_{10}; Divine Health R-Form Alpha Lipoic Acid; Divine Health Comprehensive E (mixed tocopherols); Divine Health Buffered Vitamin C; Divine Health High Potency Turmeric; Divine Health Carnosine*

Omega-3 fats: *Divine Health Living Omega 3*

Enzymes and HCL: *Divine Health Digestive Enzyme; Divine Health Digestive Enzyme with HCL*

Natural sleep aids: *Divine Health Melatonin; Divine Health Sleep Formula (includes L-theanine); Divine Health 5HTP*

Bone health: *Divine Health Cal-Mag-D3 (calcium, magnesium, vitamin D_3)*

Liver detox: *Divine Health Milk Thistle*

High-potency DIM: *Divine Health Broccoli Balance*

Whole-food synbiotic nutrition (to repair the GI mucosa and provide beneficial microflora for the sensitive GI tract and whole food nutrition): *Rejuva Food (young sprouted green barley and synbiotic nutrients to heal the intestinal tract and provide whole food nutrition); De-Stress-B (organic, nutrient dense, alkaline-forming super foods)*

Integrative Therapeutics, Inc.
9 Monroe Parkway, Suite 250
Lake Oswego, OR 97035

To order these products contact:
Divine Health Nutritional Products
Phone: (407) 331-7007
Web site: www.drcolbert.com
E-mail: info@drcolbert.com

Antioxidant and liver detox: *Recancostat (glutathione)*

Antioxidant: *UBQH (reduced CoQ_{10})*

Living Fuel, Inc.
P.O. Box 1048
Tampa, FL 33601
Phone: (866) 580-FUEL (3835)
Web site: www.livingfuel.com
E-mail: info@livingfuel.com

Phytonutrient powders: *Living Fuel Super Greens; Living Fuel Super Berry*

Omega-3: *Omega 3 and E*

Metagenics
Web site: www.drcolbert.meta-ehealth.com

Liver detox: *UltraClear Plus PH*

Digestive aid: *Metagest (betaine hydrochloride and pepsin)*

Calcium supplements: *CalApatite with Magnesium; CalApatite with Boron*

Fiber: *MetaFiber (combination soluble and insoluble fiber from rice bran)*

Nutri-West
6223 Parkway Blvd.

Land O'Lakes, FL 34639
Phone: (813) 996-7322
Fax: (813) 996-2738
Web site: www.nutri-westfl.com
E-mail: info@nutri-westfl.com

Phytonutrient tab: *Total Veggie*

Digestive aids: *Total Enzyme; Hypo D (HCL)*

Vitalizer Plus

Order from Water and Air Essentials at:
Phone: (800) 399-4426
Fax: (214) 352-0585

Vital Nutrients

45 Kenneth Dooley Drive
Middleton, CT 06457
Phone: (888) 328-9992
Fax: (888) 328-9993
Web site: www.vitalnutrients.net

Liver detox: *DeTox Formula (an excellent liver detox formula); NAC (N-acetyl-cysteine)*

The Alkalizer Water Filter

24575A Hiawassee Rd, Suite 192
Orlando, FL 32835
Fax: 407-876-6893
E-mail: info@alkalizer.com

Jupiter Ionizers Water Filters

Web site: www.jupiterionizers.com

Bio-Identical Hormone Replacement Therapy

Access directory of physicians at the American Academy of Anti-Aging Medicine
Web site: www.worldhealth.net

Lifeline Therapeutics, Inc

6400 S. Fiddlers Green Circle, Suite 1750
Englewood, CO 80111
Phone: (877) 682-6346 (8-PROTANDIM)
Web site: www.protandim.com
E-mail: info@protandim.com

Antioxidants: *Protandim (turmeric and synergistic herbs)*

TheraSauna QCA Spas, Inc.

1021 State Street
Bettendor, IA 52722
Phone: (888) 729-7727
Web sites: www.therasauna.com; www.qcaspas.com
E-mail: sales@qcaspas.com

Wellness Shower Filter

Web site: www.wellnessfilter.com

Penta Water

6370 Nancy Ridge Drive, Suite 104
San Diego, CA 92121
Phone: (858) 452-8868
Fax: (858) 452-8890
Web sites: www.pentawater.com; www.hydrateforlife.com

Penta Water: *An excellent water that is made up of mostly smaller water clusters in order to better hydrate cells. Penta water is free of chlorine, fluoride, arsenic, bromate, chromium, MTBE, and hundreds of other chemicals that may be found in other waters.*

Neuroscience (for physicians only)

373 280th Street
Osceola, WI 54020
Phone: (888) 342-7272
Fax: (715) 294-3921
Web site: https://neurorelief.com/

APPENDIX B Vitamins, Minerals, and Their Recommended Intakes

In addition to the minerals I discussed in Pillar 6, your body also needs a few more essential and trace minerals. The first four minerals below—phosphorus, chloride, sulfur, and silicon—are major minerals we must have daily. The remaining minerals we need in smaller quantities.

1 *Phosphorus.* The American diet is high in phosphorus, and we do not need to supplement.

2. *Chloride.* Americans rarely are deficient in chloride due to their high intake of salt, which is sodium chloride.

3. *Sulfur* helps form our tissues and activates enzymes. It is also used for manufacturing many proteins, including those forming hair, skin, and muscles. It is a component of insulin and is needed to regulate blood sugar.

4. *Silicon* is essential for skeletal growth and development, and it plays a role in maintaining connective tissue.

5. *Iron* forms the oxygen-carrying portion of the red blood cell. Without adequate iron, you may become anemic and tired. Men and postmenopausal women, except those with iron-deficiency anemia, don't need extra iron. Also, iron can be a two-edged sword, because excessive amounts can cause oxidative damage to cells and organs.

6. *Zinc,* a very important mineral, is a component of more than three hundred enzymes. Zinc is needed to repair wounds, to improve immunity, to assist in fertility, to maintain vision, and to synthesize proteins. A deficiency of zinc is associated with skin problems, dermatitis, and healing problems.

7. *Copper.* A deficiency in copper is related to a decrease in energy production and decline in immune function and mental concentration. Like iron, copper needs to be care-

fully controlled, because too much copper can cause oxidative damage to your tissues.

8. *Manganese.* Deficiencies of manganese are associated with weakness, growth retardation, and bone malformations.
9. *Chromium* helps maintain normal blood sugar levels, regulates insulin, and may help control blood sugar in diabetics and patients with hypoglycemia.
10. *Vanadium.* Both chromium and vanadium are important in glucose and insulin metabolism. They have a positive effect on normalizing blood sugar for both hypoglycemia and diabetes.
11. *Selenium* supports your immune system and prevents cardiomyopathy—a heart-weakening disease.
12. *Molybdenum* helps the body use iron, promotes normal growth and development, and may prevent anemia, tooth decay, and impotency.

10\. *Boron* is essential for normal calcium and bone metabolism.

11\. *Cobalt.* You will have plenty of cobalt in your system as long as you take a multivitamin with B_{12}, which is cobalamin.

The following pages are charts from the National Academy of Sciences that give the dietary reference intakes (DRIs) for vitamins and minerals.[1]

Dietary Reference Intakes (DRIs): Recommended Intakes for Individuals, Vitamins *Food and Nutrition Board, Institute of Medicine, National Academies*													
Life Stage Group	**Vit A (µg/d)**	**Vit C (mg/d)**	**Vit D (µg/d)**	**Vit E (mg/d)**	**Vit K (µg/d)**	**Thiamine (Vit B_1) (mg/d)**	**Riboflavin (Vit B_2) (mg/d)**	**Niacin (Vit B_3) (mg/d)**	**Vit B_6 (mg/d)**	**Folate (µg/d)**	**Vit B_{12} (µg/d)**	**Pantothenic Acid (mg/d)**	**Biotin (µg/d)**
Infants													
0–6 mos	400*	40*	5*	4*	2.0*	0.2*	0.3*	2*	0.1*	65*	0.4*	1.7*	5*
7–12 mos	500*	50*	5*	5*	2.5*	0.3*	0.4*	4*	0.3*	80*	0.5*	1.8*	6*
Children													
1–3 yrs	**300**	**15**	5*	**6**	30*	**0.5**	**0.5**	**6**	**0.5**	**150**	**0.9**	2*	8*
4–8 yrs	**400**	**25**	5*	**7**	55*	**0.6**	**0.6**	**8**	**0.6**	**200**	**1.2**	3*	12*
Males													
9–13 yrs	**600**	**45**	5*	**11**	60*	**0.9**	**0.9**	**12**	**1.0**	**300**	**1.8**	4*	20*
14–18 yrs	**900**	**75**	5*	**15**	75*	**1.2**	**1.3**	**16**	**1.3**	**400**	**2.4**	5*	25*
19–30 yrs	**900**	**90**	5*	**15**	120*	**1.2**	**1.3**	**16**	**1.3**	**400**	**2.4**	5*	30*
31–50 yrs	**900**	**90**	5*	**15**	120*	**1.2**	**1.3**	**16**	**1.3**	**400**	**2.4**	5*	30*
51–70 yrs	**900**	**90**	10*	**15**	120*	**1.2**	**1.3**	**16**	**1.7**	**400**	**2.4**	5*	30*
› 70 yrs	**900**	**90**	15*	**15**	120*	**1.2**	**1.3**	**16**	**1.7**	**400**	**2.4**	5*	30*
Females													
9–13 yrs	**600**	**45**	5*	**11**	60*	**0.9**	**0.9**	**12**	**1.0**	**300**	**1.8**	4*	20*
14–18 yrs	**700**	**65**	5*	**15**	75*	**1.0**	**1.0**	**14**	**1.2**	**400**	**2.4**	5*	25*
19–30 yrs	**700**	**75**	5*	**15**	90*	**1.1**	**1.1**	**14**	**1.3**	**400**	**2.4**	5*	30*
31–50 yrs	**700**	**75**	5*	**15**	90*	**1.1**	**1.1**	**14**	**1.3**	**400**	**2.4**	5*	30*
51–70 yrs	**700**	**75**	10*	**15**	90*	**1.1**	**1.1**	**14**	**1.5**	**400**	**2.4**	5*	30*
› 70 yrs	**700**	**75**	15*	**15**	90*	**1.1**	**1.1**	**14**	**1.5**	**400**	**2.4**	5*	30*
Pregnancy													
14–18 yrs	**750**	**80**	5*	**15**	75*	**1.4**	**1.4**	**18**	**1.9**	**600**	**2.6**	6*	30*
19–30 yrs	**770**	**85**	5*	**15**	90*	**1.4**	**1.4**	**18**	**1.9**	**600**	**2.6**	6*	30*
31–50 yrs	**770**	**85**	5*	**15**	90*	**1.4**	**1.4**	**18**	**1.9**	**600**	**2.6**	6*	30*
Lactation													
14–18 yrs	**1,200**	**115**	5*	**19**	75*	**1.4**	**1.6**	**17**	**2.0**	**500**	**2.8**	7*	35*
19–30 yrs	**1,300**	**120**	5*	**19**	90*	**1.4**	**1.6**	**17**	**2.0**	**500**	**2.8**	7*	35*
31–50 yrs	**1,300**	**120**	5*	**19**	90*	**1.4**	**1.6**	**17**	**2.0**	**500**	**2.8**	7*	35*

NOTE: This table (taken from DRI reports, see www.nap.edu) presents Recommended Dietary Allowances (RDAs) in **bold type** and Adequate Intakes (AIs) in ordinary type followed by an asterisk (*). RDAs and AIs may both be used as goals for individual intake. RDAs are set to meet the needs of almost all (97–98 percent) individuals in a group. For healthy breastfed infants, the AI is the mean intake. The AI for other life stage and gender groups is believed to cover needs of all individuals in the group, but lack of data or uncertainty in the data prevent being able to specify with confidence the percentage of individuals covered by this intake.

Dietary Reference Intakes (DRIs): Recommended Intakes for Individuals, Elements
Food and Nutrition Board, Institute of Medicine, National Academies

Life Stage Group	Calcium (mg/d)	Chromium (μg/d)	Copper (μg/d)	Iodine (μg/d)	Iron (mg/d)	Magnesium (mg/d)	Manganese (mg/d)	Molybdenum (μg/d)	Phosphorus (mg/d)	Selenium (μg/d)	Zinc (mg/d)	Potassium (g/d)	Sodium (g/d)
Infants													
0–6 mos	210*	0.2*	200*	110*	0.27*	30*	0.003*	2*	100*	15*	2*	0.4*	0.12*
7–12 mos	270*	5.5*	220*	130*	**11**	75*	0.6*	3*	275*	20*	**3**	0.7*	0.37*
Children													
1–3 yrs	500*	11*	**340**	**90**	**7**	**80**	1.2*	**17**	**460**	**20**	**3**	3.0*	1.0*
4–8 yrs	800*	15*	**440**	**90**	**10**	**130**	1.5*	**22**	**500**	**30**	**5**	3.8*	1.2*
Males													
9–13 yrs	1,300*	25*	**700**	**120**	**8**	**240**	1.9*	**34**	**1,250**	**40**	**8**	4.5*	1.5*
14–18 yrs	1,300*	35*	**890**	**150**	**11**	**410**	2.2*	**43**	**1,250**	**55**	**11**	4.7*	1.5*
19–30 yrs	1,000*	35*	**900**	**150**	**8**	**400**	2.3*	**45**	**700**	**55**	**11**	4.7*	1.5*
31–50 yrs	1,000*	35*	**900**	**150**	**8**	**420**	2.3*	**45**	**700**	**55**	**11**	4.7*	1.5*
51–70 yrs	1,200*	30*	**900**	**150**	**8**	**420**	2.3*	**45**	**700**	**55**	**11**	4.7*	1.3*
> 70 yrs	1,200*	30*	**900**	**150**	**8**	**420**	2.3*	**45**	**700**	**55**	**11**	4.7*	1.2*
Females													
9–13 yrs	1,300*	21*	**700**	**120**	**8**	**240**	1.6*	**34**	**1,250**	**40**	**8**	4.5*	1.5*
14–18 yrs	1,300*	24*	**890**	**150**	**15**	**360**	1.6*	**43**	**1,250**	**55**	**9**	4.7*	1.5*
19–30 yrs	1,000*	25*	**900**	**150**	**18**	**310**	1.8*	**45**	**700**	**55**	**8**	4.7*	1.5*
31–50 yrs	1,000*	25*	**900**	**150**	**18**	**320**	1.8*	**45**	**700**	**55**	**8**	4.7*	1.5*
51–70 yrs	1,200*	20*	**900**	**150**	**8**	**320**	1.8*	**45**	**700**	**55**	**8**	4.7*	1.3*
> 70 yrs	1,200*	20*	**900**	**150**	**8**	**320**	1.8*	**45**	**700**	**55**	**8**	4.7*	1.2*
Pregnancy													
14–18 yrs	1,300*	29*	**1,000**	**220**	**27**	**400**	2.0*	**50**	**1,250**	**60**	**12**	4.7*	1.5*
19–30 yrs	1,000*	30*	**1,000**	**220**	**27**	**350**	2.0*	**50**	**700**	**60**	**11**	4.7*	1.5*
31–50 yrs	1,000*	30*	**1,000**	**220**	**27**	**360**	2.0*	**50**	**700**	**60**	**11**	4.7*	1.5*
Lactation													
14–18 yrs	1,300*	44*	**1,300**	**290**	**10**	**360**	2.6*	**50**	**1,250**	**70**	**13**	5.1*	1.5*
19–30 yrs	1,000*	45*	**1,300**	**290**	**9**	**310**	2.6*	**50**	**700**	**70**	**12**	5.1*	1.5*
31–50 yrs	1,000*	45*	**1,300**	**290**	**9**	**320**	2.6*	**50**	**700**	**70**	**12**	5.1*	1.5*

NOTE: This table presents Recommended Dietary Allowances (RDAs) in bold type and Adequate Intakes (AIs) in ordinary type followed by an asterisk (*). RDAs and AIs may both be used as goals for individual intake. RDAs are set to meet the needs of almost all (97–98 percent) individuals in a group. For healthy breastfed infants, the AI is the mean intake. The AI for other life stage and gender groups is believed to cover needs of all individuals in the group, but lack of data or uncertainty in the data prevent being able to specify with confidence the percentage of individuals covered by this intake.

APPENDIX C Bottled Water pH Comparisons

The first—and the most foundational—pillar to good health is water. Nothing can survive without water. Whenever possible, drink clean, natural bottled water rather than tap water. Below I have compiled a list of the best brands of bottled water. I've ranked them according to alkalinity and container (glass or plastic).[1] This is by no means exhaustive, but at least it will give you a head start on selecting the best water for you.

Very Alkaline 9+		
Evamor	9.0	Plastic
Trinity Springs Geothermal	9.0	Plastic
Comment: Look for the Geothermal bottled version (blue label). The mineral supplement brand (yellow label) has a high fluoride content. A one-liter bottle contains about 3.6 mg of fluoride.		
Alkaline 8.5–9		
Abita Springs	8.2	Plastic
8–8.5		
Noah*	8.4	Glass
hiOsilver*	8.4	Glass
BlueStar Sparkling*	8.4	Glass
Deer Park	8.05	Plastic
Arrowhead	7.8	Plastic
* Very high in magnesium also, all from Adobe Springs		
7.5–8		
Highland Spring	7.8	Glass
Ducale	7.8	Glass
Calistoga	7.64	Glass
Mountain Valley Spring Water	7.62	Glass
San Pellegrino	7.7	Glass
Speyside Glenlivet	7.7	Glass
Tipperary	7.7	Glass
San Benedetto	7.6	Glass
Cristaline	7.6	Glass

Zephyrhills	7.7	Plastic
Neutral 7–7.5		
Acqua Oligiminerale Lynx	7.5	Glass
Daggio	7.4	Glass
Panna	7.3	Glass
TAU	7.2	Glass
SOLE	7.2	Glass
Evian	7.2	Glass
Fiji	7.5	Plastic
Biota	7.3	Plastic
Mt. Olympus	7.3	Plastic
Contrex	7.3	Plastic
Glaceau Smart Water	7.0	Plastic
Penta	7.0	Plastic
6.5–7		
Saratoga	6.98	Glass
TyNant	6.8	Glass
Fiuggi	6.8	Glass
Voss	6.5	Glass
Ice Mountain	6.98	Plastic
Ozarka	6.6	Plastic
Great Bear	6.57	Plastic
Borsec	6.5	Plastic
6–6.5		
Badoit	6.0	Glass
Harghita	6.2	Plastic
Acidic 5.5–6		
Gerolsteiner	5.9	Glass
Remlosa	5.6	Glass

Some waters have been eliminated from the list due to high levels of bacteria, arsenic, or nitrates.

NOTES

Back Cover Statistics

Marjorie L. McCullough, RD, ScD, Frank M. Sacks, MD, and Eric B. Rimm, ScD, "Five Combined Health Habits Equal Lower Heart Disease Risk," *Circulation: Journal of the American Heart Association* (July 4, 2006): http://www.americanheart.org/presenter.jhtml?identifier=3040595 (accessed August 2, 2006); "News in Science: Lifestyle Can Almost Eliminate Heart Disease," November 9, 1999, access via Pandora, Australia's Web archive, http://pandora.nla.gov.au/pan/23316/20030723/www.abc.net.au/science/news/stories/s65068.htm (accessed August 21, 2006); and "Cancer Prevention by Nutritional Intervention," *Board Examination Review and Study Guide*, 2002 E1 ed.

Introduction

1. McCullough, Sacks, and Rimm, "Five Combined Health Habits Equal Lower Heart Disease Risk"; "News in Science: Lifestyle Can Almost Eliminate Heart Disease"; and "Cancer Prevention by Nutritional Intervention."

Pillar 1: Water

Day 1: Water and You

1. Don Colbert, MD, *The Bible Cure for Headaches* (Lake Mary, FL: Siloam, 2000), 40.
2. Tammy Darling, "Water Works," *Vibrant Life*, January 2001, http://www.findarticles.com/p/articles/mi_m0826/is_1_17/ai_69371786 (accessed February 3, 2006).
3. Environmental Protection Agency, "Where Does My Drinking Water Come From?" Drinking Water, http://www.epa.gov/region7/kids/drnk_b.htm (accessed February 3, 2006).
4. Barbara Levine, RD, PhD, "Hydration 101: The Case for Drinking Enough Water," Health and Nutrition News, http://www.myhealthpointe.com/health_Nutrition_news/index.cfm?Health=10 (accessed January 30, 2006).
5. Wellness Filter, "The Forgotten Secret of Health: Are You Missing the Most Important Ingredient for Optimum Health?" http://www.wellnessfilter.com/about/TheForgottenSecretofHealth.pdf (accessed February 3, 2006).
6. D. A. Mansfield, "What Percentage of the Human Body Is Water, and How Is This Determined?" *Boston Globe*, http://www.boston.com/globe/search/stories/health/how_and_why/011298.htm (accessed January 30, 2006).

Day 2: What Happens When You Don't Drink Water

1. Levine, "Hydration 101: The Case for Drinking Enough Water."
2. F. Batmanghelidj, MD, *Water for Health, for Healing, for Life* (New York: Time Warner Group, 2003), 32–35.
3. F. Batmanghelidj, MD, "Medical Report: A New Medical Discovery," Shirley's Wellness Café, http://www.shirleys-wellness-cafe.com/water.htm (accessed February 3, 2006).
4. Lori Ferme, "Water, Water Everywhere: How Much Should You Drink?" American Dietetic Association, http://www.eatright.org/cps/rde/xchg/ada/hs.xsl/media_3173_ENU_HTML.htm (accessed January 30, 2006).
5. Peyman Vaziri, Karen Dang, and G. Harvey Anderson, "Evidence for Histamine Involvement in the Effect of Histidine Loads on Food and Water Intake in Rats," *Journal of Nutrition* 127, no. 8 (August 8, 1997): 1519–1526. Also, F. Batmanghelidj, MD, *Your Body's Many Cries for Water* (Falls Church, VA: Global Health Solutions, Inc., 1997).
6. Batmanghelidj, *Your Body's Many Cries for Water*, 120.

Day 3: The Fountain of Youth

1. Mary Shomon, "Do You Need to Increase Your Metabolism?" About: Thyroid Disease, http://thyroid.about.com/od/loseweightsuccessfully/a/metabolism.htm (accessed February 2, 2006).
2. Dr. Mu Shik Jhon, *The Water Puzzle and the Hexagonal Key* (n.p.: Uplifting Press, 2004), 73.
3. W. D. Heiss et al., "Activation of PET as an Instrument to Determine Therapeutic Efficacy in Alzheimer's Disease," *Annals of the New York Academy of Sciences* 695: 327–331.
4. Batmanghelidj, *Your Body's Many Cries for Water*, 100.
5. AskDrSears.com, "All About Water: Why Your Body Needs Water," http://www.askdrsears.com/html/4/T045600.asp (accessed February 3, 2006).

Day 4: The Rap on Tap Water

1. ⊠Hidden Dangers in Water,⊠ Shirley⊠s Wellness Café, http://www.shirleys-wellness-cafe.com/water.htm (accessed February 3, 2006).

2. CAS Statistical Summary, 1907–2004, page 7, "Growth of the CAS Chemical Registry System," Chemical Abstracts Service, a division of the American Chemical Society.

3. Duff Conacher and Associates, *Troubled Waters on Tap: Organic Chemicals in Public Drinking Water Systems and the Failure of Regulation* (Washington, D.C.: Center for Study of Responsive Law, 1988), 114.

4. Posted response by Mike Adams on NewsTarget.com, "Natural Cellular Defense and Zeolite—Is It the Next Big Thing in Nutritional Therapies for Cancer and Chronic Disease?" posted December 1, 2005, http://www.newstarget.com/015232.html (accessed February 3, 2006).

5. Bobsilverstein.com, "Water = Life's Basic Building Block," Water Pollution, http://www.bobsilverstein.com/SaveHawaii-WaterPollution.htm (accessed February 3, 2006; site now discontinued).

6. Ibid.

7. Environmental Working Group, "Into the Mouths of Babes: Bottle-Fed Infants at Risk from Atrazine in Tap Water" (Washington, D.C.: Environmental Working Group, 1999), 3. Accessed at http://www.ewg.org/issues_content/risk_assessment/20030303/pdf/IntoMouthsofBabes.pdf on October 3, 2006.

8. U.S. Geological Survey, "Insecticides in Streams Were Highest in Urban Areas," *The Quality of Our Nation's Waters: Nutrients and Pesticides,* Circular 1225, http://pubs.usgs.gov/circ/circ1225/html/insecticides.html (accessed February 1, 2006).

9. Larry F. Land et al., "Summary of Major Issues and Findings in the Trinity River Basin," *Water Quality in the Trinity River Basin, Texas, 1992–95,* U.S. Geological Survey Circular 1171, http://pubs.usgs.gov/circ/circ1171/html/issfnd.htm (accessed February 1, 2006).

10. *Arizona Water Resource,* "Pharmaceuticals in Our Water Supplies," July–August 2000, http://ag.arizona.edu/AZWATER/awr/july00/feature1.htm (accessed February 3, 2006).

11. Rachel's Environment and Health News, "Drugs in the Water," Environmental Research Association, September 2, 1998, no. 614, http://www.rachel.org/bulletin/index.cfm?St=2 (accessed October 3, 2006). Provided by the Environmental Research Association, PO Box 5036, Annapolis, MD 21403; erf@rachel.org or info@rachel.org.

12. Betsy Mason, "River Fish Accumulate Human Drugs," Nature Science Update, November 5, 2003, Geological Society of America Meeting, Seattle, November 2003, http://www.mindfully.org/Water/2003/River-Fish-Human-Drugs5nov03.htm (accessed February 3, 2006).

13. Skin Deep, "Ingredient Report: Toluene," News About the Safety of Popular Health and Beauty Brands, a project of the Environmental Working Group, http://ewg.org/reports/skindeep2/report.php?type=INGREDIENT&id=4293 (accessed February 20, 2006).

14. *Arizona Water Resource,* "Pharmaceuticals in Our Water Supplies."

15. Phaedra S. Corso et al., "Cost of Illness in the 1993 Waterborne *Cryptosporidium* Outbreak, Milwaukee, Wisconsin," *Emerging Infectious Diseases* 9, no. 4 (April 2003): 426–431.

16. W. D. King and L. D. Marrett, "Case-Control Study of Bladder Cancer and Chlorination By-Products in Treated Water (Ontario, Canada)," *Cancer Causes and Control* 7, no. 6 (November 1996): 596–604. Abstract accessed at https://www.meb.uni-bonn.de/cgi-bin/mycite?ExtRef=MEDL/97086891 (accessed February 1, 2006).

17. Rachel's Environment and Health News, "Dangers of Chlorinated Water," Environmental Research Association, May 21, 1998, no. 599.

18. Wellness Filter, "The Forgotten Secret of Health: Are You Missing the Most Important Ingredient for Optimum Health?"

19. Environmental Working Group, "Environmental Groups Petition EPA to Retract Fluoride Pesticide Tolerances on Food," news release, September 21, 2005, http://ewg.org/issues/fluoride/20050921/index.php (accessed February 3, 2006).

20. Callum Coats, *Living Energies* (Bath, UK: Gateway Books, 1996), 194, as cited by Dan Stewart and Denise Routledge, "Water: Essential for Existence," *Explore,* vol. 8, no. 5, 1998, http://www.explorepub.com/articles/water.html (accessed February 3, 2006).

21. George Glasser, "Water: A Toxic Dump?" reprinted with permission from the Sarasota ECO Report, vol. 4., no. 12, December 1994, from *Health Freedom News,* July 1995, http://www.fluoridedebate.com/question32.html (accessed October 3, 2006).

22. New York State Coalition Opposed to Fluoridation, "Fluoride Linked to Dental Cavities," posted February 15, 2006, http://www.foodconsumer.org/777/8/Fluoride_linked_to_dental_cavities.shtml (accessed February 19, 2006). According to a report from the U.S. Centers for Disease Control, fluoride is delivered to two-thirds of Americans via public water supplies and virtually 100 percent via the food supply, yet 50 percent of six- to eight-year-olds, nationwide, have cavities.

23. Dan R. Rasmussen, "Professor's Research Reignites Fluoride-Cancer Correlation Debate With New Research," *The Harvard Crimson Online Edition*, September 28, 2005, http://www.thecrimson.com/printerfriendly.aspx?ref=50860 (accessed January 25, 2006).

24. Citizens for Safe Drinking Water, "Notable Quotes From Research Scientists and Medical Organizations," http://www.nofluoride.com/quotes.htm (accessed February 1, 2006).

25. John McDougall, MD, "Alzheimer's Disease: Dietary and Lifestyle Implications," McDougall Wellness Center, http://www.drmcdougall.com/science/alzheimers.html (accessed February 1, 2006).

26. United States Environmental Protection Agency, "Water on Tap: What You Need to Know," October 2003, http://www.epa.gov/safewater/wot/index.html (accessed February 17, 2006).

Day 5: Is Bottled Water Better?

1. Beverage Marketing Corporation, "Bottled Water Continues As Number 2 in 2004," International Bottled Water Association, http://www.bottledwater.org/public/Stats_2004.doc (accessed February 3, 2006).

2. Ibid.

3. NSF International, "The Facts About Bottled Water," NSF Water Safety Kit, http://www.nsf.org/consumer/newsroom/pdf/fact_water_bottledwater.pdf (accessed February 3, 2006).

4. Natural Resources Defense Council, "Bottled Water: Pure Drink or Pure Hype?" http://www.nrdc.org/water/drinking/bw/exesum.asp (accessed February 3, 2006).

5. Ibid.

6. Ibid.

7. NSF International, "The Facts About Bottled Water."

8. John Stossel, "Is Bottled Water Better Than Tap? Americans Are Spending Billions on a Drink That's Virtually Free," *ABC News: 20/20,* May 6, 2005, http://abcnews.go.com/2020/Health/story?id=728070&page=1 (accessed February 15, 2006).

9. Natural Resources Defense Council, "Bottled Water: Pure Drink or Pure Hype?"

10. Liza Gross, "The Hidden Life of Bottled Water," *Sierra Magazine*, May/June 1999, http://www.sierraclub.org/sierra/199905/water.asp (accessed February 15, 2006).

11. Michael Mascha, "Most Americans Unaware of the Many Choices in Bottled Waters," Fine Waters newsletter, July 2005, http://www.finewaters.com/Newsletter/July_2005/Most_Americans_Unaware_of_the_Many_Choices_in_Bottled_Waters.asp (accessed February 2, 2006).

12. *Now Online Edition,* "Plastic Problems," July 29, 2004, http://www.nowtoronto.com/issues/2004-07-29/goods_ecoholic.php (accessed October 3, 2006).

13. Elizabeth Weise, "Are Our Products Our Enemy?" *USA Today*, August 2, 2005, http://www.usatoday.com/news/health/2005-08-02-chemicals-hormones-cover_x.htm (accessed February 15, 2006).

14. Brenna Doheny, "Nalgene Plastic May Be Harmful: Studies Show That the Popular Water Bottle May Pose Serious Risks," *The Daily Barometer*, February 17, 2004, http://barometer.orst.edu/vnews/display.v/ART/2004/02/17/40324e5d40a14?in_archive=1 (accessed February 15, 2006).

15. Gross, "The Hidden Life of Bottled Water."

16. *Canadian Press,* "People Who Frequently Reuse Water Bottles May Be Risking Their Health," January 26, 2003, http://www.ghchealth.com/people-who-frequently-reuse-their-water-bottles-may-be-risking-their-health.html (accessed February 15, 2006).

17. Weise, "Are Our Products Our Enemy?"

18. Lauren M. Posnick, ScD, and Henry Kim, PhD, "Bottled Water Regulation and the FDA," *Food Safety Magazine*, August/September 2002, reprinted by the U.S. Food and Drug Administration, Center for Food Safety and Applied Nutrition, http://www.cfsan.fda.gov/~dms/botwatr.html (accessed January 25, 2006).

19. Thaddeus Herrick, "Microsoft Is Curbing Use of PVC, a Popular Plastic," *Wall Street Journal*, December 7, 2005, D7.

20. Allison Sloan, "Mothers and Others Magazine," International Plastics Task Force, http://www.ecologycenter.org/iptf/toxicity/mothersandothers.html (accessed October 3, 2006).

21. *Canadian Press*, "People Who Frequently Reuse Water Bottles May Be Risking Their Health."

Day 6: Filtered Water

1. Bill McTighe, "Water Filtration: Simple Carbon Filters Go a Long Way," Home Environmental, http://www.homeenv.com/art_wtr_filt.htm; Ion Life, Inc., "Apples with Apples: How to Choose a Water Filter System," Ion Life, http://www.ionizers.org/water-filters.html; and Denise Moffat, MD, "The Basics of Water," Health Basics, http://www.naturalhealthtechniques.com/Basics%20of%20Health/water_basics1.htm (all accessed February 3, 2006).

2. Moffat, "The Basics of Water."

3. Ion Life, Inc., "Apples with Apples: How to Choose a Water Filter System" and Moffat, "The Basics of Water."

4. Advanced Water Systems, "Frequently Asked Questions about Reverse Osmosis (RO) Systems," http://advancedh2o.com/products/brochures_html/domestic/faqs_ro.html (accessed February 3, 2006).

5. Ion Life, Inc., "Apples with Apples: How to Choose a Water Filter System."

6. Jhon, *The Water Puzzle and the Hexagonal Key*, 106–107.

7. Tools for Transformation, "Balancing Acid/Alkaline Foods," http://www.trans4mind.com/nutrition/pH.html (accessed February 3, 2006).

8. Ibid., 104.

Day 7: How Much, and When, to Drink

1. Mark Jeantheau, "Styrofoam Cups—Clouds in Your Coffee?" Grinning Planet, November 1, 2005, http://www.grinningplanet.com/2005/11-01/styrofoam-cups-article.htm (accessed August 10, 2006).

2. L. Maia and A. deMendonca, "Does Caffeine Intake Protect From Alzheimer's Disease?," *European Journal of Neurology* 9, no. 4 (July 2002): 377–382.

3. Eduardo Salazar-Martinez, MD, et al., "Coffee Consumption and Risk for Type 2 Diabetes Mellitus," *Annals of Internal Medicine* 140 (January 6, 2004), 1–8.

4. Susan Yara, "Coffee Perks," *Forbes Online*, October 11, 2005, http://www.forbes.com/health/2005/10/11/coffee-health-benefits-cx_sy_1012feat_ls.html (accessed February 3, 2006).

5. Victoria Gilman, "Coffee Buzz: Drink Is Top Antioxidant Source in U.S.," *National Geographic*, August 31, 2005, http://news.nationalgeographic.com/news/2005/08/0831_050831_coffee.html (accessed February 15, 2006). Also, *General Science*, "Coffee Is Number One Source of Antioxidants," August 29, 2005, http://www.physorg.com/news6067.html (accessed February 3, 2006).

6. Marc Leduc, "Is Coffee Good or Bad for Your Health?" Healing Daily Web site, http://www.healingdaily.com/detoxification-diet/coffee.htm (accessed February 3, 2006).

7. General Conference Nutrition Council, "A Position Statement on the Use of Caffeine," http://www.nadadventist.org/hm/gcnc/caffeine/caffeine.htm (accessed February 3, 2006).

8. J. Hintikka et. al., "Daily Tea Drinking Is Associated With a Low Level of Depressive Symptoms in the Finnish General Population," *European Journal of Epidemiology* 20, no. 4 (2005): 359–363.

9. Ion Health, "How Much Water Should You Drink?" http://www.ionhealth.ca/id70.html (accessed February 3, 2006). Also, Health4youonline.com, "Dehydration—the Benefits of Drinking Water," http://www.health4youonline.com/article_dehydration.htm (accessed February 3, 2006).

Pillar 2: Sleep and Rest

Day 8: Restoring Your Body With Sleep

1. National Sleep Foundation, "Sleep and Sports: Get the Winning Edge," Teens and Sleep, http://www.sleepfoundation.org/hottopics/index.php?secid=18&id=272 (accessed February 3, 2006).

2. Committee on Sleep Medicine and Research, *Sleep Disorders and Sleep Deprivation: An Unmet Public Health Problem*, The Institute of Medicine, April 4, 2006, press release, http://www.iom.edu/CMS/3740/23160/33668.aspx (accessed July 14, 2006).

3. Stephanie Saul, "Record Sales of Sleeping Pills Are Causing Worries," *New York Times*, February 7, 2006, http://www.nytimes.com/2006/02/07/business/07sleep.html?ex=115630560 0&en=b3db11459ac65eff&ei=5070 (accessed July 14, 2006).

4. National Sleep Foundation, "2000 Omnibus Sleep in America Poll,"1522 K Street NW, Suite 500, Washington, D.C., 20005.

5. Safety recommendation from James L. Kolstad, Chairman of the National Transportation Safety Board, to L. G. Rawl, Chairman of the Board, Exxon Corporation, September 18, 1990, http://www.ntsb.gov/recs/letters/1990/M90_26_31.pdf (accessed on July 25, 2006).

6. National Transportation Safety Board, *Korean Air Flight 801*, aircraft accident report, August 6, 1997, http://www.ntsb.gov/publictn/2000/AAR0001.pdf (accessed July 25, 2006).

7. Maria Thomas et al., "Neural Basis of Alertness and Cognitive Performance Impairments During Sleepiness: I. Effects of 24 h of Sleep Deprivation on Waking Human Regional Brain Activity," *Journal of Sleep Research* 9, no. 4 (December 2000): 335–352.

8. Summary of Findings, National Sleep Foundation 2005 Sleep in America Poll, http://www.sleepfoundation.org/_content/hottopics/2005_summary_of_findings.pdf (accessed February 3, 2006).

9. K. Spiegle, R. Leproult, and E. Van Cauter, "Impact of Sleep Debt on Metabolic and Endocrine Function," *Lancet* 354 (October 23, 1999): 1435–1439, referenced in "Backgrounder: Why Sleep Matters," http://www.sleepfoundation.org/NSAW/pk_background.cfm (accessed February 10, 2005).

10. A. A. Kuo, "Does Sleep Deprivation Impair Cognitive and Motor Performance as Much as Alcohol Intoxication?" *Western Journal of Medicine* 3, no. 174 (March 1, 2001): 180, referenced in "Backgrounder: Why Sleep Matters," http://www.sleepfoundation.org/NSAW/pk_background.cfm (accessed February 10, 2005).

11. Stephenie Overman, "Rise and Sigh—Sleep Deprivation," *HR Magazine*, May 1999, http://www.findarticles.com/p/articles/mi_m3495/is_5_44/ai_54711192 (accessed February 16, 2006).

12. Summary of Findings, National Sleep Foundation 2005 Sleep in America Poll.

13. *APA Online*, "Why Sleep Is Important and What Happens When You Don't Get Enough," http://www.apa.org/pubinfo/sleep.html#consequences (accessed February 2, 2006).

14. Shawn M. Talbott, PhD, *The Cortisol Connection* (Alameda, CA: Hunter House 2002), 52–54.

15. National Sleep Foundation, "Tools and Quizzes," http://www.sleepfoundation.org/quiz/quiz.php?id=6&qnum=2 (accessed October 3, 2006).

16. Don Colbert, MD, "7 Pillars of Health" PowerPoint presentation; also, Summary of Findings, National Sleep Foundation 2005 Sleep in America Poll.

17. Circadian Technologies, Inc., "Extended Hours Workers More Prone to Major Health Problems and Divorce," 2003 Health Study Release, http://www.circadian.com/media/2003_press_health.htm (accessed February 3, 2006).

Day 9: What Causes Insomnia

1. Summary of Findings, National Sleep Foundation 2005 Sleep in America Poll.

2. Center for Science in the Public Interest, "Caffeine Content of Food and Drugs," http://www.cspinet.org/new/cafchart.htm (accessed February 10, 2005); also, Center for Science in the Public Interest, "The Caffeine Corner: Products Ranked by Amount," Nutrition Action Health Letter, http://www.cspinet.org/nah/caffeine/caffeine_corner.htm (accessed February 10, 2005).

3. Summary of Findings, National Sleep Foundation 2005 Sleep in America Poll.

Day 10: How Much Sleep You Really Need

1. CNN.com, "Lack of Sleep America's Top Health Problem, Doctors Say," Health Story Page, March 17, 1997, http://www.cnn.com/HEALTH/9703/17/nfm/sleep.deprivation/ (accessed February 3, 2006).

2. CNN.com Transcripts, "Clinton Pardons: House Government Reform Committee Questions Former Clinton Aides," Special Event, aired March 1, 2001, http://transcripts.cnn.com/TRANSCRIPTS/0103/01/se.16.html (accessed February 3, 2006).

3. Kelly Myers, lecture notes for Psyc 2000 001, Louisiana State University, August 30, 2001, http://chancely29.tripod.com/lsunotes/id2.html (accessed February 24, 2006).

4. National Sleep Foundation, http://www.sleepfoundation.org (accessed February 6, 2006).

5. National Sleep Foundation, "Sleep and Aging: How Sleep Changes," http://www.sleepfoundation.org/hottopics/index.php?secid=12&id=183 (accessed February 6, 2006). Also, James Tighe, "Sleep Deprivation," *BBC Online,* first published June 2000, reviewed September 2006, http://www.bbc.co.uk/health/conditions/mental_health/coping_sleep.shtml (accessed February 6, 2006).

6. University of Chicago Hospitals, "Lack of Sleep Alters Hormones, Metabolism, Simulates Effects of Aging," press pelease, October 21, 1999, http://www.uchospitals.edu/news/1999/19991021-sleepdebt.html (accessed July 14, 2006).

7. "Sleep and Aging: How Sleep Changes"; also, Tighe, "Sleep Deprivation."

8. "Sleep and Aging: How Sleep Changes."

Day 11: Planning Your Perfect Night of Sleep

1. Jennifer Harper, "Portuguese Pull Most Late Nights, Sleep Poll Finds," *Washington Times,* March 10, 2005, http://www.washingtontimes.com/national/20050309-112252-5103r.htm (accessed February 6, 2006).

2. Don Colbert, MD, "7 Pillars of Health."

Day 12: Your Bedroom—Storage Unit or Sleep Haven?

1. Sheila Wray Gregoire, "When Sleeping Together Drives You Apart: Solutions to Marital Sleep Problems," *Marriage Partnership,* vol. 19, no. 2, Summer 2002, 32.

2. The Sleep Well, "Radio Frequency (RF) Procedure or Somnoplasty," Sleep Apnea Information and Resources, http://www.stanford.edu/~dement/apnea.html (accessed February 2, 2006).

Day 13: Sleep Aids

1. Frost & Sullivan Research Services, "U.S. Insomnia Therapies Market," April 16, 2004, http://www.frost.com/prod/servlet/report-brochure.pag?id=A747-01-00-00-00 (accessed February 6, 2006).

2. H. Dressing et al., "Insomnia: Are Valerian/Balm Combinations of Equal Value to Benzodiazepine [translated from German]?", *Therapiewoche* 42 (1992): 726–736.

3. G. Balderer and A. A. Borbely, "Effect of Valerian on Human Sleep," *Psycho-Parmacol* 87 (1985): 406–409.

4. U.S. Food and Drug Administration, "Milestones in U.S. Food and Drug Law History," FDA Backgrounder, May 3, 1999, updated August 2005, http://www.fda.gov/opacom/backgrounders/miles.html (accessed February 15, 2006).

5. Eliza-Jasmine Baotran Tran, "Drugs, Sex, and Politics," term paper manuscript, University of California—Berkeley, May 5, 1999, http://sulcus.berkeley.edu/mcb/165_001/papers/manuscripts/_180.html (accessed February 15, 2006).

6. Phyllis A. Balch, CNC, *Prescription for Nutritional Healing,* rev. and expanded edition (New York: Avery Books, 2000), 473–474.

7. Joseph E. Pizzorno Jr. and Michael T. Murray, eds., *Textbook of Natural Medicine* (New York: Churchill Livingston, 1999), 920–923.

8. Holisticonline.com, "Alternative and Integral Therapies for Insomnia," http://www.holistic-online.com/remedies/Sleep/sleep_ins_nutrition.htm (accessed February 6, 2006).

9. L. R. Juneja et al., "L-theanine—a Unique Amino Acid of Green Tea and Its Relaxation Effect in Humans," *Trends in Food Science and Technology* 10 (1999): 199–204.

10. Ibid.

11. Julie Thibeau, "Suntheanine," NutriScience Innovation, http://www.nutriscienceusa.com/productinfo_123.htm (accessed February 16, 2006).

12. Balch, *Prescription for Nutritional Healing,* 75, 474.

Day 14: Learn to Rest

1. Summary of Findings, National Sleep Foundation 2005 Sleep in America Poll.

2. Tighe, "Sleep Deprivation."

3. National Sleep Foundation, "The Short Story on Napping," http://www.sleepfoundation.org/hottopics/index.php?secid=18&id=278 (accessed February 6, 2006).

4. Ibid.

5. Don Colbert, MD, *The Bible Cure for Sleep Disorders* (Lake Mary, FL: Siloam, 2001).

Pillar 3: Living Food

Day 15: Living Food vs. Dead Food

1. *Rural Migration News*, "How We Eat," vol. 3, no. 4, October 1996, http://migration.ucdavis.edu/rmn/more.php?id=158_0_5_0 (accessed February 21, 2006).

2. *California Healthline*, "Life Expectancy Increases to 77.6 Years in U.S., Study Finds," December 9, 2005. *California Healthline* is published for the California HealthCare Foundation by the Advisory Board Company.

Day 16: Your Body Is a Temple

1. C. C. Cowie et al., "Prevalence of Diabetes and Impaired Fasting Glucose in Adults in the U.S. Population: National Health and Nutrition Examination Survey (NHANES) 1999–2000," *Diabetes Care* 29, no. 6 (June 2006): 1263–1268.

2. Roy Walford, *Beyond the 120 Year Diet* (New York: Four Walls Eight Windows, 2000), 45–49, referenced in K. C. Craichy, *Super Health* (Minneapolis, MN: Bronze Bow Publishing, 2005), 57.

3. Kenneth F. Ferraro, "Firm Believers? Religion, Body Weight, and Well-Being," *Review of Religious Research* 39, no. 3 (March 1998): 224ff, referenced in Beth Forbes, "Firm Believers More Likely to Be Flabby, Purdue Study Finds," *Purdue News*, March 1998, http://news.uns.purdue.edu/html4ever/9803.Ferraro.fat.html (accessed February 21, 2006).

4. Adapted from the National Heart, Lung, and Blood Institute's body mass index table in the *Clinical Guidelines on the Identification, Evaluation, and Treatment of Overweight and Obesity in Adults.* Used by permission.

Day 17: What the Bible Says About Food

1. Jeanie Lerche Davis, "America's Food Trends: People Eating Healthy, Eating at Home," WebMD Medical News, http://www.webmd.com/content/article/72/81891.htm (accessed February 21, 2006).

2. T. J. Key et al., "Mortality in Vegetarians and Non-Vegetarians: A Collaborative Analysis of 8300 deaths Among 76,000 Men and Women in Five Prospective Studies," *Public Health Nutrition* 1, no. 1 (March 1998): 33–41.

3. G. E. Fraser and D. J. Shavlik, "Ten Years of Life: Is It a Matter of Choice?" *Archives of Internal Medicine* 161, no. 13 (2001): 1645–1652.

Day 18: What to Avoid—the Dark Side of the Food World

1. TruthinLabeling.org, "Collected Reports of Endocrine Disorders, Retinal Degeneration, and Adverse Reactions Caused by MSG," http://www.truthinlabeling.org/adversereactions.html (accessed May 8, 2006).

2. MedlinePlus Encyclopedia, s.v. "Chinese Restaurant Syndrome," http://www.nlm.nih.gov/medlineplus/ency/article/001126.htm (accessed August 2, 2006).

3. Becky Hand, "The Hunt for Hidden Sugar: How Much of the Sweet Stuff Is Hiding Your Foods?" BabyFit.com, http://www.babyfit.com/articles.asp?id=685 (accessed August 14, 2006).

4. S. J. Schoenthaler and I. D. Bier, "The Effect of Vitamin-Mineral Supplementation on Juvenile Delinquency Among American Schoolchildren: A Randomized, Double-blind Placebo-controlled Trial," *The Journal of Alternative and Complementary Medicine* 6, no. 1 (February 2000): 7–17.

5. Don Colbert, MD, *The Bible Cure for Candida and Yeast Infections* (Lake Mary, FL: Siloam, 2001).

6. Educate-Yourself.org, "Sugar," Nutrition, the Key to Energy, http://educate-yourself.org/nutrition/#sugar (accessed February 21, 2006).

7. NewsTarget.com, "The Politics of Sugar: Why Your Government Lies to You About This Disease-Promoting Ingredient," July 21, 2005, www.newstarget.com/z009797.html (accessed January 28, 2006).

8. Daniel DeNoon, "Drink More Diet Soda, Gain More Weight?" WebMD Medical News, June 13, 2005, http://www.webmd.com/content/Article/107/108476.htm?printing=true (accessed September 28, 2006).

9. Russell Blaylock, *Excitotoxins: The Taste That Kills* (Santa Fe, NM: Health Press, 1997), 180.

10. Stephen Fox, "New Mexico Senate Bill to Ban Artificial Sweetener Aspartame as Neurotoxic Carcinogen," *Newswire Today* - /newswire/ - Santa Fe, New Mexico, January 17, 2006.

11. Joseph Mercola, MD, "The Potential Dangers of Sucralose: Reader Testimonials," http://www.mercola.com (accessed July 25, 2006).

12. Food and Diet, "Splenda," http://www.foodanddiet.com/NewFiles/splenda.html (accessed January 29, 2006).

13. Federal Register of the U.S. Food and Drug Administration, Center for Food Safety and Applied Nutrition, "Food Additives Permitted for Direct Addition to Food for Human Consumption; Sucralose," vol. 63, no. 64, April 3, 1998, pages 16417–16433, http://www.cfsan.fda.gov/%7Elrd/fr980403.html (accessed February 27, 2006).

A six-month clinical study (E157) was performed investigating the effect of sucralose (667 mg/d through oral administration) on glucose homeostasis in patients with NIDDM (type 2 diabetes). The study was divided into a screening phase, a testing phase, and a follow-up phase. Forty-one patients participated in the testing phase of the study. The forty-one patients were divided into two groups: twenty patients whose diabetes was managed by insulin, and twenty-one managed by oral hypoglycemic agents (OHAs). Each of these two groups were further subdivided into a sucralose group and a placebo group. Percent concentration of glycosylated hemoglobin (HbA1c) was the primary measure of long-term glycemic control in this study. In addition, the following parameters of glucose homeostasis were measured: (1) Fasting levels of plasma glucose, serum C-peptide, and serum insulin; and (2) postprandial measures of plasma glucose, serum C-peptide, and serum insulin. These parameters were measured after zero, one, three, and six months of treatment with either sucralose or a placebo (cellulose). The results from this study showed a small but statistically significant increase in the glycosylation of hemoglobin (HbA1c) from baseline levels in the sucralose-treated group compared to that seen in the placebo group (dataset 1: mean difference of 0.007 percent, p =0.005; dataset 2: mean difference of 0.006 percent, p = 0.012) (Ref.42). This HbA1c effect was observed in the sucralose-treated group at 1 month of treatment and did not significantly increase to higher levels throughout the remainder of the study (mean difference range of 0.006 to 0.008 percent, p<ls-thn-eq> 0.0043). Overall, during the test phase of the study, no statistically significant changes from baseline were observed in any of the secondary measurements of glucose homeostasis (ie., plasma glucose and serum C-peptide and insulin concentrations). Because of the small patient group sizes in this study, the ultimate clinical significance of the observed HbA1c effect could not be determined (Ref. 42). *However, generally speaking, increases in glycosylation in hemoglobin imply lessening of control of diabetes.*

14. Ibid.

15. Eric Schlosser, *Fast Food Nation* (New York: Houghton Mifflin, 2001).

16. McDonalds USA, "McDonald's USA Nutrition Facts for Popular Menu Items/French Fries," http://www.mcdonalds.com/app_controller.nutrition.index1.html#1 (accessed February 11, 2006).

17. Paul Appleby, "Do Vegetarians Live Longer?" lecture notes for a talk given to student members of the Oxford Green Party, Friends Meeting House, Oxford, UK, March 1, 2002, http://www.ivu.org/oxveg/Talks/veglongevity.html (accessed February 8, 2006); also, T. J. Key, G. K. Davey, and P. N. Abbleby, "Health Benefits of a Vegetarian Diet," *The Proceedings of the Nutrition Society* 58, no. 2 (May 1999): 271–275.

18. Cancer Prevention Coalition, "Hot Dogs and Nitrites," http://www.preventcancer.com/consumers/food/hotdogs.htm (accessed August 3, 2006).

19. Kristen Philipkoski, "Meat Stripper Gets Third Degree," *Wired Magazine*, January 19, 2004, as reported at OrganicConsumers.org, http://www.organicconsumers.org/madcow/stripper11904.cfm (accessed May 7, 2006).

20. "Nutritional Information from Bob Evans Menu," provided by the company Web site, http://www.bobevans.com, accessed February 16, 2006. The information provided was last updated February 16, 2006.

21. Ban Trans Fats, "New Labeling," http://www.bantransfats.com/newlabeling.html (accessed February 21, 2006).

22. Stephanie Lingafelter, "Supersized Fat in America," Mother Earth Living, http://www.motherearthliving.com/issues/motherearthliving/whole_foods/Trans-Fat-Risks_227-1.html (accessed September 28, 2006).

23. CalorieKing by Allan Borushek, "Calories and Carbs in Fats: Animal Fats or Lards, Meat drippings," http://www.calorieking.com/foods/food/carbs-calories-in-fats-animal-fats-or-lards-meat-drippings_Y2lkPTMzNDIxJmJpZD0xJmZpZD02ODA1NSZlaWQ9Mzc1MDIyNTQmcG9zPTgmcGFyPSZrZXk9YmFjb24.html (accessed March 2, 2006).

24. Prostate Cancer Foundation, "Dietary Fats and Red Meat: Rethinking the American Way," http://www.prostatecancerfoundation.org/site/c.itIWK2OSG/b.788359/k.6989/Dietary_Fats_and_Red_Meat.htm (accessed August 2, 2006).

25. American Heart Association, "Limiting Fats and Cholesterol," http://www.americanheart.org/presenter.jhtml?identifier=323 (accessed August 23, 2006).

Day 19: What to Eat—the Living Foods List

1. American Chemical Society, "Research at Great Lakes Meeting Shows More Vitamin C in Organic Oranges Than Conventional Oranges," press release, June 2, 2002, http://www.sciencedaily.com/releases/2002/06/020603071017.htm (accessed February 21, 2006).

2. U.S. Department of Health and Human Services and the U.S. Department of Agriculture, "Dietary Guidelines for Americans 2005," http://healthierus.gov/dietaryguidelines (accessed March 22, 2006).

3. Harvard School of Public Health, "Fruits and Vegetables," http://www.hsph.harvard.edu/nutritionsource/fruits.html (accessed February 21, 2006).

4. Health 101 Institute, "Enzymes' Role in Health," taken from the Life Extension Foundation, accessed via Health101.org, http://www.health101.org/art_enzymes.htm (accessed February 21, 2006).

5. Don Colbert, MD, *Toxic Relief* (Lake Mary, FL: Siloam, 2003).

6. Better Health Channel, "Food Processing and Nutrition Fact Sheet," http://www.betterhealth.vic.gov.au/bhcv2/bhcarticles.nsf/pages/Food_processing_and_nutrition?OpenDocument (accessed February 22, 2006).

7. E. Giovannucci et al., "A Prospective Study of Tomato Products, Lycopene, and Prostate Cancer Risk," *Journal of the National Cancer Institute* 94, no. 5 (March 6, 2002): 391–398.

8. Educate-Yourself.org, "Fiber," Nutrition, the Key to Energy, http://www.educate-yourself.org/nutrition/#fiber (accessed February 22, 2006).

9. U.S. Department of Health and Human Services and the U.S. Department of Agriculture, "Dietary Guidelines for Americans 2005."

10. Best Diet Tips, "Glycemic Index List of Foods," http://www.bestdiettips.com/html/glycemic_index.html (accessed February 22, 2006).

11. T. A. Mori and L. J. Beilin, "Omega-3 Fatty Acids and Inflammation," *Current Atherosclerosis Reports* 6, no. 6 (November 2004): 461–467; W. Elaine Hardman, "(n-3) Fatty Acids and Cancer Therapy," *The Journal of Nutrition* 134, suppl. 12 (December 2004): 3427S–3430S; A. A. Berbert et al., "Supplementation of Fish Oil and Olive Oil in Patients With Rheumatoid Arthritis," *Nutrition* 21, no. 2 (February 2005): 131–136; P. Guesnet et al., "Analysis of the 2nd Symposium: Anomalies of Fatty Acids, Ageing and Degenerating Pathologies," *Reproduction Nutrition Development* 44, no. 3 (May–June 2004): 263–271; J. A. Conquer et al., "Fatty Acid Analysis of Blood Plasma of Patients With Alzheimer's D, Other Types of Dementia, and Cognitive Impairment," *Lipids* 35, no. 12 (December 2000): 1305–1312; L. A. Horrocks and Y. K. Yeo, "Health Benefits of Docosahexaenoic Acid (DHA)," *Pharmacological Research* 40, no. 3 (September 1999): 211–225; E. M. Hjerkinn et al., "Influence of Long-Term Intervention With Dietary Counseling, Long-Chain n-3 Fatty Acid Supplements, or Both on Circulating Markers of Endothelial Activation in Men With Long-Standing Hyperlipidemia," *Alternative Medicine Review* 81, no. 3 (March 2005): 583–589; and Joyce A. Nettleton and Robert Katz, "n-3 Long-Chain Polyunsaturated Fatty Acids in Type 2 Diabetes: A Review," *Journal of the American Dietetic Association* 105, no. 3 (March 2005): 428–440.

12. Prostate Cancer Foundation, "Dietary Fats and Red Meat: Rethinking the American Way."

13. M. G. Enig, *Trans Fatty Acids in the Food Supply: A Comprehensive Report Covering 60 Years of Research*, 2nd edition (Silver Spring, MD: Enig Associates, Inc., 1995).

14. Don Colbert, MD, *What Would Jesus Eat?* (Nashville, TN: Thomas Nelson, 2001).

Day 20: What to Eat With Caution—Meat and Dairy

1. University Of Michigan Integrative Medicine, "Healthy Fats," http://www.med.umich.edu/umim/clinical/pyramid/fats.htm (accessed February 22, 2006).

2. PublicCitizen.org, "Is Irradiated Food Safe?" http://www.citizen.org/print_article.cfm?ID=1423 (accessed February 22, 2006).

3. J. D. Decuypere, MD, "Radiation, Irradiation and Our Food Supply," The Decuypere Report, http://www.healthalternatives2000.com/food_supply_report.html (accessed February 22, 2006).

4. Ibid.

5. PublicCitizen.org, "Is Irradiated Food Safe?"

6. Decuypere, "Radiation, Irradiation and Our Food Supply."

7. Joseph Mercola, "The Problems With Irradiated Food: What the Research Says," http://www.mercola.com/article/irradiated/irradiated_research.htm (accessed February 22, 2006).

8. MayoClinic.com, "Irradiation: One Tool for Improving Food Safety," as printed by International Council on Food Radiation, "News & Views," April 20, 2004, http://www.icfi

.org/newsandviews.php?PHPSESSID=20b0a84d64e2e532edadbd570aacc1b5. Also, PCC Natural Markets, "Irradiated Foods," http://www.pccnaturalmarkets.com/issues/irradiated.html (accessed February 22, 2006).

9. "Irradiated Foods."

10. Ibid.

11. "Irradiation: One Tool for Improving Food Safety."

12. C. A. Daley et al., "A Literature Review of the Value-Added Nutrients Found in Grass-fed Beef Products," California State University—Chico, draft manuscript, June 2005, http://www.csuchico.edu/agr/grassfedbeef/health-benefits/index.html (accessed September 2, 2005).

13. Emily Oken, MD, et al., "Decline in Fish Consumption Among Pregnant Women After a National Mercury Advisory," *Obstetrics and Gynecology* 102 (2003): 346–351, http://www.greenjournal.org/cgi/content/full/102/⅔46 (accessed February 22, 2006).

14. Lynn R. Goldman, MD, MPH, et al., "American Academy of Pediatrics: Technical Report: Mercury in the Environment: Implications for Pediatricians," *Pediatrics* 108, no. 1 (July 2001): 197–205.

15. Educate-Yourself.org, "Dairy Products," Nutrition, the Key to Energy, http://www.educate-yourself.org/nutrition/#dairyproducts (accessed February 22, 2006).

16. George Mateljan Foundation, "Pasteurization," http://www.whfoods.com/genpage.php?tname=george&dbid=149#answer (accessed August 17, 2006).

17. I-Min Lee and Ralph S. Paffenbarger Jr., "Life Is Sweet: Candy Consumption and Longevity," *British Medical Journal* 317 (December 19, 1998): 1683–1684.

18. University of Alabama–Birmingham Health System, "Chocolate Works Against Hypertension," http://www.health.uab.edu/show.asp?durki=84606 (accessed February 22, 2006).

19. PreventDisease.com, "Study Tracks Lead Level in Chocolate," November 1, 2005, http://preventdisease.com/news/articles/110105_lead_chocolate.shtml (accessed February 22, 2006).

Day 21: "Dinner's Ready!": How to Prepare and Serve Food

1. Janet Raloff, "Microwaves Bedevil a B Vitamin—Research Indicates Overcooking and Microwaving Meat and Dairy Foods Inactivate Vitamin B_{12}—Brief Article," *Science News*, February 14, 1998, http://www.findarticles.com/p/articles/mi_m1200/is_n7_v153/ai_20346932 (accessed February 22, 2006).

2. Good Eats Fan Page, "Cooking Oil Smoke Points," http://www.goodeatsfanpage.com/CollectedInfo/OilSmokePoints.htm (accessed March 2, 2006).

3. Ralph W. Moss, PhD, "How Food Preparation Affects Nutrients," *Weekly Cancer Decisions* 114, January 2004, http://annieappleseedproject.org/howfoodprepa.html (accessed February 22, 2006).

4. B. H. Blanc and H. U. Hertel, "Comparative Study of Food Prepared Conventionally and in the Microwave Oven," published by Raum & Zeit, 1992, in *Journal of the Science of Food and Agriculture* 3, no. 2 (2003): 43.

5. Malaria Foundation International, "FAQs: Is DDT Still Effective and Needed to Control Malaria?" http://www.malaria.org/DDTcosts.html (accessed February 3, 2006).

6. University of Dayton Research Institute, "Olive Oil, Lower Temperatures Less Toxic in Frying," *UDRI News*, September 2003, http://www.udri.udayton.edu/News/news0903.htm (accessed February 22, 2006).

7. Better Health Channel, "Food Processing and Nutrition Fact Sheet."

8. Environmental Protection Agency, "EPA Settles PFOA Case Against DuPont for Largest Environmental Administrative Penalty in Agency History," December 14, 2005, http://yosemite.epa.gov/opa/admpress.nsf/68b5f2d54f3eefd28525701500517fbf/fdcb2f665cac66bb852570d7005d6665!OpenDocument (accessed January 26, 2006).

9. Associated Press, "DuPont Settles EPA's Teflon Charges for $10M Fine," FOXNews.com, December 14, 2005, http://www.foxnews.com/printer_friendly_story/0,3566,178756,00.html (accessed January 26, 2006).

10. National Center on Addiction and Substance Abuse at Columbia University, "Casa and TV Land/Nick at Nite Report Shows Frequent Family Dinners Cut Teens' Substance Abuse Risk in Half," press release, September 13, 2005, http://66.135.34.236/absolutenm/templates/PressReleases.aspx?articleid=405&zoneid=64 (accessed August 17, 2006).

Pillar 4: Exercise

Day 22: Let's Stir the Waters

1. Colbert, *What Would Jesus Eat?* 168.
2. Ibid., 168–169.

Day 23: The Benefits of Exercise, Part I

1. PreventDisease.com, "More Evidence that Exercise Prevents Cancer," July 2004 http://preventdisease.com/home/tips42.shtml (accessed August 18, 2006).
2. International Agency for Research on Cancer, *IABC Handbooks of Cancer Prevention, Volume 6: Weight Control and Physical Activity* (Lyon. France: IABC Press, 2001).
3. National Cancer Institute, "Cancer Trends Progress Report—2005 Update," http://progressreport.cancer.gov (accessed January 29, 2006).
4. Anne McTiernan, MD, PhD, et al., "Recreational Physical Activity and the Risk of Breast Cancer in Postmenopausal Women," *Journal of the American Medical Association* 290, no. 10 (September 10, 2003): 1331–1336.
5. Brian McGovern, MD, "MADIT II Trial—Prophylactic Implantation of a Defibrillator in Patients With Myocardial Infarction and Reduced Ejection Fraction," American Heart Association, http://www.americanheart.org/presenter.jhtml?identifier=3007300 (accessed February 16, 2006).
6. James A. Levine, N. L. Eberhardt, and M. D. Jensen, "Role of Nonexercise Activity Thermogenesis in Resistance to Fat Gain in Humans," *Science* 283 (January 8, 1999): 212–214.
7. Judy Ismach, "No Two Genders About It, a Heart Is Just a Heart," *Physician's Weekly,* vol. 14, no. 10, February 10, 1997, http://www.physweekly.com/archive/97/02_10_97/itn1.html (accessed February 16, 2006).
8. *Harvard University Gazette,* "It's Never Too Late: Joslin Study Shows Diabetes Sufferers See Major Benefits From Minor Exercise, Weight Loss," December 11, 2003, http://www.news.harvard.edu/gazette/2003/12.1½5-diabetes.html (accessed February 8, 2006).
9. Christiaan Leeuwenburgh et al., "Oxidized Amino Acids in the Urine of Aging Rats: Potential Markers for Assessing Oxidative Stress in Vivo," *American Journal of Physiology: Regulatory, Integrative and Comparative Physiology* 276 (January 1999): R128–R135.

Day 24: The Benefits of Exercise, Part II

1. Levine, "Hydration 101: The Case for Drinking Enough Water."
2. Leeuwenburgh et al., "Oxidized Amino Acids in the Urine of Aging Rats: Potential Markers for Assessing Oxidative Stress in Vivo."
3. Tom Lloyd, PhD, study published in *The Journal of Pediatrics,* as referenced in Jeanie Lerche Davis, "Got Exercise? Workouts Better for Bone Health," WebMD, June 11, 2004, http://www.webmd.com/content/Article/88/100005.htm (accessed July 21, 2006).
4. Aetna InteliHealth, "Exercise," Diseases and Conditions: Digestive, http://www.intelihealth.com/IH/ihtIH/WSIHW000/8270/8759/189154.html?d=dmtContent (accessed February 8, 2006).
5. Robert Preidt, "Exercise Eases Digestion Problems in the Obese," HealthDay News, October 4, 2005, http://www.medicinenet.com/script/main/art.asp?articlekey=54770 (accessed February 8, 2006).
6. S. S. Tworoger et al., "Effects of a Yearlong Moderate-Intensity Exercise and a Stretching Intervention on Sleep Quality in Postmenopausal Women," *Sleep* 26, no. 7 (November 2003): 830–836.
7. Ibid.
8. Associated Press, "Working Out May Help Prevent Colds, Flu: Moderate Exercise Can Boost Body's Defenses, but Too Much Can Be Harmful," MSNBC.com, January 17, 2006, http://www.msnbc.msn.com/id/10894093/ (accessed July 31, 2006).
9. James Blumenthal et al., "Effects of Exercise Training in Older Patients With Major Depression," *Archives of Internal Medicine* 159, no. 19 (1999): 2349–2356.
10. Christine Brownlee, "Buff and Brainy: Exercising the Body Can Benefit the Mind," *Science News Online,* vol. 169, no. 8, February 25, 2006, http://www.sciencenews.org/articles/20060225/bob10.asp (accessed July 24, 2006).
11. Free Health Encyclopedia, "Physical Fitness—Benefits of Physical Activity and Exercise on the Body," http://www.faqs.org/health/Healthy-Living-V1/Physical-Fitness.html (accessed October 3, 2006).

12. Mayo Clinic Staff, "Chronic Pain: Exercise Can Bring Relief," MayoClinic.com, August 31, 2005, http://www.mayoclinic.com/health/chronic-pain/AR00017 (accessed August 16, 2006).

13. Mayo Clinic Staff, "Aerobic Exercise: What 30 Minutes a Day Can Do for Your Body," MayoClinic.com, March 4, 2005, http://www.mayoclinic.com/health/aerobic-exercise/EP00002 (accessed August 29, 2006).

Day 25: Aerobic Exercise

1. Jackie Berning, PhD, RD, "Strategies for Weight Loss," University of Michigan Health System, http://www.med.umich.edu/1libr/sma/sma_weight_sma.htm (accessed February 8, 2006).

2. Susan Steeves, "Don't Sweat It: Ten Minutes Several Times May Get You in Shape," WebMD.com, February 8, 2001, http://www.webmd.com/content/article/18/1676_52466.htm (accessed February 17, 2006).

3. Ralph S. Paffenberger et. al., "The Association of Changes in Physical-Activity Level and Other Lifestyle Characteristics with Mortality Among Men," *The New England Journal of Medicine* 328, no. 8 (February 1993): 538–545.

4. U.S. Department of Health and Human Services and the U.S. Department of Agriculture, "Dietary Guidelines for Americans 2005: Chapter 4, Physical Activity," http://www.health.gov/dietaryguidelines/dga2005/document/html/chapter4.htm (accessed December 4, 2005).

5. American College of Sports Medicine, "Calculate Your Exercise Heart Rate Range," http://www.acsm.org/pdf/Calculate.pdf (accessed February 16, 2006).

6. Elizabeth Quinn, "Delayed Onset Muscle Soreness: Dealing With Muscle Pain After Exercise," About: Sports Medicine, http://sportsmedicine.about.com/cs/injuries/a/aa010600.htm (accessed February 17, 2006).

Day 26: Anaerobic Exercise

1. National Osteoporosis Foundation, "Fast Facts: Prevalence," http://www.nof.org/osteoporosis/diseasefacts.htm (accessed February 17, 2006).

2. Ibid.

3. Wikipedia, s.v. "Weight Training," http://en.wikipedia.org/wiki/Weight_training (accessed February 17, 2006).

4. You may also contact them at PO Box 412, Berea, KY 40403. Their phone number is (859) 986-2181; fax, (859) 986-7580.

Day 27: Fun, Alternative Exercises

1. SahajaYoga.org, "Medical Research on Effects of Sahaja Yoga on Hypertension," Stress Management, http://www.sahajayoga.org.in/StressMgmt.asp (accessed February 14, 2005).

2. Marian S. Garfinke et al., "Yoga-Based Intervention for Carpal Tunnel Syndrome," *Journal of the American Medical Association* 280 (November 11, 1998): 1601–1603.

3. Judith Horstman, "Tai Chi," *Arthritis Today*, http://www.arthritis.org/resources/arthritistoday/2000_archives/2000_07_08_taichi.asp (accessed February 14, 2005). Jacqueline Stenson, "Tai Chi Improves Lung Function in Older People," Medical Tribune News Service (1995). Also, D. D. Brown et al., "Cardiovascular and Ventilatory Responses During Formalized Tai Chi Chuan Exercise," *Research Quarterly for Exercise and Sport* 60, vol. 3 (1989): 246–250.

4. P. Jin, "Changes in Heart Rate, Noradrenaline, Cortisol and Mood During Tai Chi," *Journal of Psychosomatic Research* 33, vol. 2 (1989): 197–206.

5. The Pilates Center, "A History of Joseph Hubertus Pilates," http://www.thepilatescenter.com/jhpilates.htm (accessed February 17, 2006).

6. Wikipedia, s.v. "Pilates," http://en.wikipedia.org/wiki/Pilates (accessed February 7, 2006).

Day 28: Exercise for Life!

1. MU News Bureau, "Daily Dog Walks Work Off Weight for Owners, MU Researchers Find," University of Missouri—Columbia, Sinclair School of Nursing, September 28, 2005, http://www.missouri.edu/~nursing/pressroom/releases/092805.php (accessed February 8, 2006).

2. RX Refunds, "Calories Burned by Exercise," Exercise and Calories Chart, http://www.rxrefunds.com/health/calories-burned.htm (accessed February 17, 2006).

3. CalorieKing by Allan Borushek, "Nutritional Information," http://www.calorieking.com/foods/ (accessed March 2, 2006).

Pillar 5: Detoxification

Day 29: Believe It or Not—You're Probably Toxic

1. Dr. Paul Yanick, *Quantum Repatterning Technique—II*, copyright © 2006 by Quantafoods, LLC.

2. Environmental Working Group, "Body Burden—the Pollution in Newborns," July 14, 2005, www.ewg.org/reports/bodyburden2 (accessed February 20, 2006).

3. Lynn Goldman, MD, "A Special Report on Toxic Chemicals and Children's Health in North America," Commission for Environmental Cooperation of North America, March 2004.

4. Duff Conacher and Associates, "Troubled Waters on Tap: Organic Chemicals in Public Drinking Water Systems and the Failure of Regulation."

Day 30: Where Toxins Come From

1. American Lung Association, "State of the Air 2005," http://lungaction.org/reports/stateoftheair2005.html (accessed February 20, 2006).

2. Alicia DiRado, "Smog May Speed Atherosclerosis," USC Public Relations Newsroom, November 12, 2004, http://www.usc.edu/uscnews/stories/10761.html (accessed February 20, 2006).

3. G. T. Sterling et al., "Health Effects of Phenoxy Herbicides," *Scandinavian Journal of Work Environmental Health* 12 (1986): 161–173, referenced in Don Colbert, MD, "Curbing the Toxic Onslaught," *NutriNews*, August 2005, http://www.hmscrown.com/Health_Research/DetoxificationIII.pdf#search=%22nutrinews%20colbert%22 (accessed October 4, 2006).

4. American Cancer Society, "Cigarette Smoking," revised February 13, 2006, http://www.cancer.org/docroot/PED/content/PED_10_2X_Cigarette_Smoking.asp?sitearea=PED&viewmode=print& (accessed August 4, 2006).

5. Harvard Reports on Cancer Prevention, "Volume I: Human Causes of Cancer," *Cancer Causes and Control* 7 (Supplement) (November 1996): http://www.hsph.harvard.edu/cancer/resources_materials/reports/HCCPreport_1fulltext.htm (accessed August 1, 2006).

6. American Cancer Society, "The Facts About Secondhand Smoke" http://www.cancer.org/docroot/COM/content/div_TX/COM_11_2x_The_Facts_about_Secondhand_Smoke.asp?sitearea=COM (accessed August 4, 2006).

7. Michael F. Roizen, *YOU: The Owner's Manual* (New York: HarperCollins, 2005), 172.

8. Associated Press, "Toxic Chemical Found in Cows' Milk," *USA Today*, June 22, 2004, www.usatoday.com/news/nation/2004-06-22-milk_x.htm, referenced in Colbert, "Curbing the Toxic Onslaught."

9. Associated Press, "Rocket Fuel Chemical Found in Organic Milk," ABC News, http://www.abcnews.go.com/Health/print?id=293356 (accessed February 20, 2006), referenced in Colbert, "Curbing the Toxic Onslaught."

10. Robert Preidt, "Pesticide Exposure Causes Damage to Nervous System, Brain" HealthDay News, August 4, 2006, http://www.refluxissues.com/ms/news/534119/main.html (accessed October 4, 2006).

11. Alberto Ascherio et al., "Pesticide Exposure and Risk of Parkinson's Disease," *Annals of Neurology* (July 2006): referenced in "Pesticide Exposure Associated With Incidence of Parkinson's Disease," press release from EurekAlert.com, June 26, 2006, http://www.eurekalert.org/pub_releases/2006-06/jws-pea061906.php (accessed August 19, 2006).

12. A. Blair et al., "Clues to Cancer Etiology From Studies of Farmers," *Scandinavian Journal of Work, Environment, and Health* 18, no. 4 (1992): 209–215, referenced in National Cancer Institute, "Risk Factors," http://rex.nci.nih.gov/NCI_Pub_Interface/raterisk/risks99.html (accessed August 20, 2006).

13. Gene Marine and Judith Van Allen, *Food Pollution—the Violation of Our Inner Ecology* (Canada: Holt, Rinehart, and Winston, 1972), referenced in Judy Campbell, BSc, et al., "Nutritional Characteristics of Organic, Freshly Stone-ground, Sourdough and Conventional Breads," Ecological Agricultural Projects, http://www.eap.mcgill.ca/Publications/EAP35.htm (accessed February 20, 2006), referenced in Colbert, "Curbing the Toxic Onslaught."

14. *Idaho Observer*, "Bleaching Agent in Flour Linked to Diabetes," July 2005, http://proliberty.com/observer/20050718.htm (accessed February 20, 2006), referenced in Colbert, "Curbing the Toxic Onslaught."

15. Educate-Yourself.org, "Nutrition, the Key to Energy."

16. Mark Peplow, "US Rice May Carry an Arsenic Burden," *News@nature.com*, August 2, 2005, www.nature.com/news/2005/05081/pf/05081-5_pf.htm, referenced in Colbert, "Curbing the Toxic Onslaught."

17. Pollution in People, "PCBs and DDT: Banned but Still with Us" July 2006, http://www.pollutioninpeople.org/toxics/pcbs_ddt (accessed August 17, 2006).

18. Ibid.

19. T. S. Johnson, "Diagnosis and Treatment of Five Parasites: Enterobus vermicularis, Giardia lamblia, Trichuris trichuira, Ascaris lumbricoides, Entamoeba histolytica," *Drug Intelligence and Clinical Pharmacy* 15, no. 2 (1981): 103–110.

20. Michael D. Gershon, MD, *The Second Brain* (New York: HarperPernnial, 1999), 152–153.

21. Michael Epitropoulos and Cal Streeter, "Detoxification in Relationship to Alkaline- and Acid-Forming Foods," *Dynamic Chiropractic*, October 21, 2002.

Day 31: Unexpected Sources of Toxins

1. Informed Choice, "Vaccine Ingredients," http://www.informedchoice.info/cocktail.html (accessed February 20, 2006), referenced in Colbert, "Curbing the Toxic Onslaught."

2. U.S. Food and Drug Administration, Center for Biologics Evaluation and Research, "Thimerosal in Vaccines," http://www.fda.gov/cber/vaccine/thimerosal.htm (accessed February 20, 2006), referenced in Colbert, "Curbing the Toxic Onslaught."

3. Ibid.

4. Don Colbert, MD, *What You Don't Know May Be Killing You* (Lake Mary, FL: Siloam, 2004); also, Don Colbert, MD, *Get Healthy Through Detox and Fasting* (Lake Mary, FL: Siloam, 2006).

5. Greg Ciola, "Mercury: The Unsuspected Killer!" *Crusader Special Report*, April/May 2004, 3, referenced in Colbert, "Curbing the Toxic Onslaught."

6. Donald W. Miller Jr., MD, "Mercury on the Mind," LewRockwell.com, http://www.lewrockwell.com/miller/miller14.html (accessed February 20, 2006), referenced in Colbert, "Curbing the Toxic Onslaught."

7. Walter J. Crinnion, ND, "Environmental Medicine, Part Three: Long-Term Effects of Chronic Low-Dose Mercury Exposure," http://www.thorne.com/altmedrev/fulltext/enviro5-3.html (accessed February 20, 2006).

8. Agency for Toxic Substances and Disease Registry, "A Toxicology Curriculum for Communities Trainer's Manual," lecture notes for module four, http://www.atsdr.cdc.gov/training/toxmanual/modules/4/lecturenotes.html (accessed February 20, 2006).

9. Fact Sheet, "Safe Substitutes at Home: Non-toxic Household Products," http://es.epa.gov/techinfo/facts/safe-fs.html (accessed February 20, 2006), excerpted from Gary A. Davis and Em Turner, "Safe Substitutes at Home: Non-toxic Household Products," working paper, University of Tennessee—Knoxville Waste Management Institute.

10. Ibid.

11. Ibid.

12 Environmental Working Group, "Ethyl Benzene," http://www.ewg.org/bodyburden/cheminfo.php?chemid=90001 (accessed May 20, 2006); Christian Nordqvist, "High Benzene Levels Found in Some Soft Drinks," *Medical News Today*, May 20, 2006, http://www.medicalnewstoday.com/healthnews.php?newsid=43763 (accessed August 2, 2006).

13. Nordqvist, "High Benzene Levels Found in Some Soft Drinks."

14. Agency for Toxic Substances and Disease Registry (ATSDR), "ToxFAQs for Tetrachloroethylene (PERC)," September 1997, http://www.atsdr.cdc.gov/tfacts18.html (accessed August 7, 2006).

15. N. Hanioka et al., "Interaction of 2,4,4'-trichloro-2'-hydroxydiphenyl Ether With Microsomal Cytochrome P450-dependent Monooxygenases in Rat Liver," *Chemosphere* 33, no. 2 (July 1996): 265–276; H. N. Bhargava and P. A. Leonard, "Triclosan: Applications and Safety," *American Journal of Infection Control* 24, no. 3 (June 1996): 209–218.

16. Garth H. Rauscher, David Shore, and Dale P. Sandler, "Hair Dye Use and Risk of Adult Acute Leukemia," *American Journal of Epidemiology* 160, no. 1, (2004): 19–25.

Day 32: What Toxins Do to the Body

1. D. L. Davis et al., "Medical Hypothesis: Xenoestrogens as Preventable Causes of Breast Cancer," *Environmental Health Perspectives* 101, no. 5 (October 1993): 372–377.

2. Fact Sheet, "Safe Substitutes at Home: Non-toxic Household Products."

3. Theo Colborn, *Our Stolen Future* (New York: Penguin Group, 1997), 150–152.

4. BreastCancer.org, "Ovarian and Breast Cancer," http://www.breastcancer.org/prv_hist_risk_ovarian.html (accessed March 8, 2006). Also, American Cancer Society, "Overview: Prostate Cancer: How Many Men Get Prostate Cancer?" http://www.cancer.org/docroot/CRI/content/CRI_2_2_1X_How_many_men_get_prostate_cancer_36.asp?sitearea (accessed March 8, 2006).

5. Sterling et al., "Health Effects of Phenoxy Herbicides."

6. Don Colbert, MD, *Fasting Made Easy* (Lake Mary, FL: Siloam, 2004).

Day 33: It's Time to Get Rid of Toxic Trash

1. P. Angulo et al., "Independent Predictors of Liver Fibrosis in Patients With Nonalcoholic Steatohepatitis," *Hepatology* 30 (1999): 1356–1362.

2. ConsumerReports.org, "When Buying Organic Pays (and Doesn't)," February 2006, http://www.consumerreports.org/cro/food/organic-products-206/when-buying-organic-pays-and-doesnt/index.htm (accessed August 31, 2006).

3. HyScience.com, "Farmed Salmon May Increase Cancer Risk," December 1, 2005, http://www.hyscience.com/archives/2005/12/farmed_salmon_m.php (accessed March 4, 2006).

4. R. Hites et al., "Farm-Raised Salmon Contain More Toxins Than Wild Salmon," *Science*, January 9, 2004, http://www.breastcancer.org/research_farm_raised_salmon.html (accessed February 20, 2006).

5. Environmental Working Group, "Summary—PCBs in Farmed Salmon," http://www.ewg.org/reports/farmedPCBs/printversion.php (accessed March 7, 2006).

6. Essence-of-Life.com, compiled from "Shifting Your pH Toward Alkaline" food chart, http://www.essense-of-life.com/info/foodchart.htm (accessed March 4, 2006).

Day 34: Detoxing Through the Skin

1. Alison Cullen, "Save Your Skin," *Healthy Way Online*, http://www.healthywaymagazine.com/issue32/06_skin_conditions.html (accessed February 20, 2006).

2. Department of Health and Human Services, Substance Abuse and Mental Health Services Administration Drug Testing Advisory Board, scientific meeting notes for "Drug Testing of Alternative Specimens and Technologies," http://www.health.org/workplace/dtabday2.aspx (accessed February 21, 2006).

3. JigsawHealth.com, "Sweat," http://www.jigsawhealth.com/sweat.aspx (accessed February 21, 2006).

4. Craig C. Freudenrich, "How Sweat Works," HowStuffWorks.com, http://health.howstuffworks.com/sweat2.htm (accessed February 21, 2006).

Day 35: Other Important Detoxifiers

1. Pacific Rim Vaccine Initiative, "Scouring the Air," http://www.ohsu.edu/prvi/tour4.html (accessed March 4, 2006).

2. *Consumer Reports*, "Ratings: Room Air Cleaners," October 2005, http://www.consumerreports.org/cro/appliances/air-cleaners-1005/ratings/ratings-room-models.htm (accessed March 4, 2006).

3. U.S. Environmental Protection Agency, National Academy of Science, "Indoor—Asthma: Take the Asthma Quiz!," http://www.epa.gov/iaq/asthma/quiz/q7.htm (accessed October 7, 2003).

4. Fact Sheet, "Safe Substitutes at Home: Non-toxic Household Products."

Pillar 6: Nutritional Supplements

Day 36: Your Nutritional Deficit

1. Robert H. Fletcher, MD, MSc, and Kathleen M. Fairfield, MD, DrPH, "Vitamins for Chronic Disease Prevention in Adults," *Journal of the American Medical Association* 287 (2002): 3127–3129.

2. Ibid.

3. The Results Project, "Why You Can't Eat Well," http://www.resultsproject.net/Why_you_cant_eat_well.html (accessed February 1, 2006), referenced in Colbert, "Curbing the Toxic Onslaught."

4. The Silver Gecko Company, Ltd., "About Colloidal Minerals," http://www.silver-gecko.com/extrainfo.asp?LinkNo=21 (accessed February 1, 2006).

5. *Life Extension*, "Vegetables Without Vitamins," Cover Story, March 2001, http://www.lef.org/magazine/mag2001/mar2001_report_vegetables.html (accessed February 22, 2006).

6. University of Maine News, "Acid Rain Study Confirms Soil Nutrient Depletion," March 23, 2004, http://www.umaine.edu/News/Archives/2004/April04/041204/AcidRain.htm (accessed February 22, 2006).
7. The George Mateljan Foundation, "The World's Healthiest Foods List, A–Z," http://www.whfoods.org/foodstoc.php (accessed October 4, 2006).
8. LifeExtension.org, "Digestive Disorders," updated June 5, 2003, http://www.lef.org/protocols/prtcl-044.shtml (accessed February 22, 2006).

Day 37: The Most Common Nutrient Deficiencies

1. Alanna Moshfegh, Joseph Goodman, and Linda Cleveland, "What We Eat in America, NHANES 2001–2002: Usual Nutrient Intakes From Food Compared to Dietary Reference Intakes," U.S. Department of Agriculture, Agricultural Research Service, http://www.ars.usda.gov/Services/docs.htm?docid=14018#2001-02 (accessed October 4, 2006).
2. Ohio State University, "Extension Fact Sheet: Vitamin E," http://ohioline.osu.edu/hyg-fact/5000/5554.html (accessed October 4, 2006).
3. National Institutes of Health Office of Dietary Supplements, "Dietary Supplement Fact Sheet: Vitamin E," NIH Clinical Center, http://ods.od.nih.gov/factsheets/vitamine.asp (accessed February 23, 2006).
4. Eva Lonn, MD, MSc, et al., "Effects of Long-Term Vitamin E Supplementation on Cardiovascular Events and Cancer," *Journal of the American Medical Association* 293, no. 11 (March 16, 2005): 1338–1347.
5. National Cancer Institute, "Alpha-Tocopherol, Beta-Carotene Cancer Prevention (ATBC) Trial," press release, July 22, 2003, http://www.cancer.gov/newscenter/pressreleases/ATBCfollowup (accessed February 23, 2006).
6. K. J. Helzlsouer et. al., "Association Between Alpha-Tocopherol, Gamma-Tocopherol, Selenium, and Subsequent Prostate Cancer," *Journal of the National Cancer Institute* 92, no. 24 (December 2000): 1966–1967.
7. Moshfegh, Goodman, and Cleveland, "What We Eat in America, NHANES 2001–2002."
8. National Institutes of Health Office of Dietary Supplements, "Dietary Supplement Fact Sheet: Magnesium," NIH Clinical Center, http://ods.od.nih.gov/factsheets/magnesium.asp (accessed February 23, 2006).
9. National Institutes of Health Office of Dietary Supplements, "Dietary Supplement Fact Sheet: Calcium," NIH Clinical Center, http://ods.od.nih.gov/factsheets/calcium.asp (accessed February 23, 2006).
11. Ibid.
12. CalciumInfo.com, "Important News on Osteoporosis and Bone Health," http://www.calciuminfo.com/, referencing *Bone Health and Osteoporosis: A Report of the Surgeon General,* available at http://www.surgeongeneral.gov/topics/bonehealth/ (accessed September 1, 2006).
13. Moshfegh, Goodman, and Cleveland, "What We Eat in America, NHANES 2001–2002."
14. Balch, *Prescription for Nutritional Healing,* 14–15.
15. National Institutes of Health Office of Dietary Supplements, "Dietary Supplement Fact Sheet: Vitamin A and Carotenoids," NIH Clinical Center, http://ods.od.nih.gov/factsheets/vitamina.asp (accessed February 23, 2006).
16. Ibid.
17. K. J. Rothman, L. L. Moore, and M. R. Singer, "Tertogenecity of High Vitamin A Intake," *New England Journal of Medicine* 333 (1995): 1369–1373.
18. Pizzorno and Murray, eds., *Textbook of Natural Medicine,* 1013.
19. From an e-mail from Cathy Leet, BSN, Director of Market Development, Integrative Therapeutics Inc., to author's office, Tuesday, January 31, 2006.
20. National Institutes of Health Office of Dietary Supplements, "Dietary Supplement Fact Sheet: Vitamin A and Carotenoids."
21. Pizzorno and Murray, eds., *Textbook of Natural Medicine,* 1007–1013.
22. Moshfegh, Goodman, and Cleveland, "What We Eat in America, NHANES 2001–2002."
23. Ohio State University, "Extension Fact Sheet: Vitamin C (Ascorbic Acid)," http://ohioline.osu.edu/hyg-fact/5000/5552.html (accessed October 4, 2006).
24. WrongDiagnosis.com, "Symptoms of Vitamin C deficiency," http://www.wrongdiagnosis.com/v/vitamin_c_deficiency/symptoms.htm (accessed February 23, 2006).
25. Pizzorno and Murray, eds., *Textbook of Natural Medicine,* 549, 836, 915–916.
26. Moshfegh, Goodman, and Cleveland, "What We Eat in America, NHANES 2001–2002."

27. Balch, *Prescription for Nutritional Healing*, 22–23. Also, Linus Pauling Institute Micronutrient Information Center, "Vitamin K," Oregon State University, http://lpi.oregonstate.edu/infocenter/vitamins/vitaminK/index.html (accessed February 23, 2006).

28. NorthwesterNutrition, "Nutrition Fact Sheet: Vitamin K," Northwestern University, http://www.feinberg.northwestern.edu/nutrition/factsheets/vitamin-k.html (accessed February 23, 2006).

29. Ibid.

30. Balch, *Prescription for Nutritional Healing*, 23.

31. Y. Seyama and H. Wachi, "Atherosclerosis and Matrix Dystrophy," *Journal of Artherosclerosis and Thrombosis* 11, no. 5 (2004): 236–245.

32. A. M. Stapleton and R. L. Rydall, "Crystal Matrix Protein—Getting Blood Out of a Stone," *Mineral and Electrolyte Metabolism* 20, no. 6 (1994): 399–409.

33. NorthwesterNutrition, "Nutrition Fact Sheet: Dietary Fiber," Northwestern University, http://www.feinberg.northwestern.edu/nutrition/factsheets/fiber.html (accessed February 23, 2006).

34. Moshfegh, Goodman, and Cleveland, "What We Eat in America, NHANES 2001–2002."

35. NorthwesterNutrition, "Nutrition Fact Sheet: Dietary Fiber."

36. Ibid.

37. Ibid.

38. Moshfegh, Goodman, and Cleveland, "What We Eat in America, NHANES 2001–2002."

39. J. E. Leklem, "Vitamin B_6," in M. E. Shils, et al., ed., *Modern Nutrition in Health and Disease*, 9th ed. (Baltimore: Williams and Wilkins, 1999), 413–421.

40. National Institutes of Health Office of Dietary Supplements, "Dietary Supplement Fact Sheet: Vitamin B_6," NIH Clinical Center, http://ods.od.nih.gov/factsheets/vitaminb6.asp (accessed January 24, 2006); and George Mateljan Foundation, "Vitamin B_6," World's Healthiest Foods, A–Z, http://www.whfoods.com/genpage.php?tname=nutrient&dbid=108#foodsources (accessed January 24, 2006).

41. Ibid.

42. Janet Raloff, "Understanding Vitamin D Deficiency," *Science News Online*, April 30, 2005, http://www.sciencenews.org/articles/20050430/food.asp (accessed February 23, 2006).

43. Balch, *Prescription for Nutritional Healing*, 21.

44. National Institutes of Health Office of Dietary Supplements, "Dietary Supplement Fact Sheet: Vitamin D," NIH Clinical Center, http://ods.od.nih.gov/factsheets/vitamind.asp (accessed February 23, 2006).

45. According to an analysis published in 2004 and based on the Third National Health and Nutrition Examination Survey (NHANES III).

46. Raloff, "Understanding Vitamin D Deficiency."

47. National Institutes of Health Office of Dietary Supplements, "Dietary Supplement Fact Sheet: Vitamin D."

48. Ibid.

49. National Osteoporosis Foundation, "Prevention: Calcium and Vitamin D," http://www.nof.org/prevention/calcium.htm (accessed September 29, 2006).

50. National Institutes of Health Office of Dietary Supplements, "Dietary Supplement Fact Sheet: Vitamin D."

51. Moshfegh, Goodman, and Cleveland, "What We Eat in America, NHANES 2001–2002."

52. University of Maryland Medical Center, "Potassium," fact sheet, http://www.umm.edu/altmed/ConsSupplements/Potassiumcs.html (accessed February 23, 2006).

53. Hopkins Technology, LLC, "Food Sources of Potassium," http://www.hoptechno.com/bookfoodsourceK.htm (accessed February 23, 2006).

54. Joseph G. Hollowell et al., "Iodine Nutrition in the United States. Trends and Public Health Implications: Iodine Excretion Data from National Health and Nutrition Examination Surveys I and III (1971–1974 and 1988–1994)," *Journal of Clinical Endocrinology & Metabolism* 83, no. 10 (October 1998): 3401–3408, http://jcem.endojournals.org/cgi/content/full/83/10/3401 (accessed September 1, 2006).

55. New Hampshire Natural Health Clinic, "Iodine Insufficiency," http://www.nhnatural.com/Iodine.htm (accessed September 1, 2006).

Day 38: Your Need for Antioxidants

1. P. Mecocci et al., "Plasma Antioxidants and Longevity: a Study on Healthy Centenarians," *Free Radical Biology and Medicine* 28, no. 8 (September 2000): 1243–1248.

2. V. P. Chernyshov et al., "Effects of Rec. Comp. on Immune System on Chernobyl Children with RRD," *International Journal of Immunorehabilitation* 5 (May 1997): 72.

3. Sally K. Nelson et al., "The Induction of Human Superoxide Dismutase and Catalase in Vivo: A Fundamentally New Approach to Antioxidant Therapy," *Free Radical Biology and Medicine* 40 (2006): 341–347.

4. Lester Packer, PhD, *The Antioxidant Miracle* (New York: John Wiley and Sons, Inc., 1999).

5. Linus Pauling Institute Micronutrient Information Center, "Alpha-Lipoic Acid," Oregon State University, http://lpi.oregonstate.edu/infocenter/othernuts/la/index.html (accessed February 23, 2006).

6. C. W. Shults et al., "Effects of Coenzyme Q_{10} in Early Parkinson Disease," *Archives of Neurology* 59 (2002): 1541–1550. The Huntington Study Group, "A Randomized, Placebo-Controlled Trial of Coenzyme Q10 and Remacemide in Huntington's Disease," *Neurology* 57 (2001): 397–404. P. Langsjoen et al., "The Aging Heart: Reversal of Diastolic Dysfunction Through the Use of Oral CoQ_{10} in the Elderly," in *Anti-Aging Medical Therapeutics,* R. M. Klatz and R. Goldman, eds. (n.p.: Health Quest Publications, 1997), 113–120. C. W. Shults, "Absorption, Tolerability, and Effects on Mitochondrial Activity of Oral Coenzyme Q_{10} in Parkinsonian Patients," *Neurology* 50 (1998): 793–795. K. Folkers, "Lovastatin Decreases Coenzyme Q Levels in Humans," *Proceedings of the National Academy of the Sciences of the United States of America* 87, no. 22 (1990): 8931–8934. C. W. Shults et al., "Pilot Trial of High Dosages of Coenzyme Q_{10} in Patients With Parkinson's Disease," *Experimental Neurology* 188, no. 2 (August 2004): 491–494.

Day 39: The Power of Phytonutrients

1. George Mateljan Foundation, *"What Is the Special Nutritional Power Found in Fruits and Vegetables?"* http://www.whfoods.com/genpage.php?tname=faq&dbid=4 (accessed August 20, 2006).

2. Balch, *Prescription for Nutritional Healing,* 9.

3. Greenpeace Aotearoa/New Zealand, "Threats and Solutions," http://www.greenpeace.net.nz/campaigns/forests/amazon_threats_solutions.asp (accessed September 5, 2006).

4. Department of Health and Human Services, Centers for Disease Control and Prevention, "5 A Day: Data and Statistics Display," http://apps.nccd.cdc.gov/5ADaySurveillance (accessed August 17, 2006)

5. E. Giovannucci et al., "Intake of Carotenoids and Retinol in Relation to Risk of Prostate Cancer," *Journal of the National Cancer Institute* 87 (December 6, 1995): 1767–1776.

6. Tracy Shuman, MD, ed., "Prostate Cancer: Prostate Cancer Risk Factors," WebMD.com, http://www.webmd.com/content/article/45/1688_50826.htm (accessed February 8, 2006).

7. Wikipedia, s.v "Tomato: Fruit or Vegetable?" http://en.wikipedia.org/wiki/Tomato#Fruit_or_vegetable.3F (accessed February 4, 2006).

8. Bolton Evening News, "Carrots Cut Cancer Risk," February 9, 2005, abstract accessed at http://archive.thisislancashire.co.uk/2005/02/09/445271.html (accessed February 23, 2006).

9. "The Effect of Vitamin E and Beta-Carotene on the Incidence of Lung Cancer and Other Cancers in Male Smokers," *New England Journal of Medicine* 330, no. 15 (April 14, 1994): 1029–1035.

10. J. Michael Gaziano, MD, et al., "A Prospective Study of Consumption of Carotenoids in Fruits and Vegetables and Decreased Cardiovascular Mortality in the Elderly," *Annals of Epidemiology* 5, no. 4 (July 1995): 255–260.

11. J. M. Seddon et al., "Dietary Carotenoids, Vitamins A, C, and E, and Advanced Age-Related Macular Degeneration," *Journal of the American Medical Association* 272 (1994): 1413–1420.

12. B. B. Aggarwal and H. Ichikawa, "Molecular Targets and Anticancer Potential of Indole-3-Carbinol and Its Derivatives," *Cell Cycle* 4, no. 9 (September 2004): 1201–1215.

13. H. Lucille, "Assessing the Underlying Cause," in *Creating and Maintaining Balance: A Woman's Guide to Safe, Natural, Hormone Health* (Boulder CO: IMPAKT Health, 2004), 15–25.

14. Alzheimersupport.com, "Research: Can Curcumin Help Prevent Alzheimer's Disease," http://www.alzheimersupport.com/library/showarticle.cfm/id/2173 (accessed February 23, 2006).

15. LifeExtension.org, "Cholesterol Reduction: Benefits of Curcumin," http://www.lef.org/protocols/prtcl-032b.htm (accessed February 23, 2006).

16. American Cancer Society, "Soy's Effect May Lower Breast Cancer Risk," ACS News Center, March 29, 2002, http://www.cancer.org/docroot/NWS/content/NWS_1_1x_Soys_Effect_May_Lower_Breast_Cancer_Risk.asp?sitearea=NWS&viewmode=print& (accessed February 23, 2006).

17 Judy McBride, "High-ORAC Foods May Slow Aging," United States Department of Agriculture, Agricultural Research Service, February 8, 1999, http://www.ars.usda.gov/is/pr/1999/990208.htm (accessed August 28, 2006).

18. Ronald L. Prior et al., "Can Foods Forestall Aging?" *Agricultural Research Magazine*, February 1999, http://www.ars.usda.gov/is/AR/archive/feb99/aging0299.htm?pf=1 (accessed August 28, 2006).

19. X. Wu et al., "Lipophilic and Hydrophilic Antioxidant Capacities of Common Foods in the United States," Journal of Agricultural and Food Chemistry 52, no. 12 (June 9, 2004): 4026–4037.

20. Tiesha D. Johnson, BSN, RN, "All About Supplements: Blueberries," *Life Extension*, September 2006, 88.

21. Ibid.

Day 40: Vitamin Confusion

1. Daniel H. Chong, ND, "Real or Synthetic: The Truth Behind Whole-Food Supplements," http://www.mercola.com/2005/jan/19/whole_food_supplements.htm (accessed February 23, 2006).

2. American Stroke Association and American Heart Association, "Heart Disease and Stroke Statistics—2005 Update," http://www.americanheart.org/downloadable/heart/1105390918119HDSStats2005Update.pdf (accessed February 23, 2006).

3. American Cancer Society, *Cancer Facts & Figures 2005* (Atlanta: American Cancer Society, 2005), 3; http://www.cancer.org/downloads/STT/CAFF2005f4PWSecured.pdf (accessed February 3, 2006).

4. Balch, *Prescription for Nutritional Healing*, 13.

5. Dr. Ben Kim, "Synthetic vs. Natural Vitamins," Life Essentials Health Clinic, http://chetday.com/naturalvitamin.htm (accessed February 23, 2006).

6. Dr. Ben Kim, "Hidden Hazards of Vitamin and Mineral Tablets," Life Essentials Health Clinic, http://chetday.com/vitaminhazards.htm (accessed February 23, 2006).

7. Ibid.

8. Dominique Patton, "Oxidised Fish Oils on Market May Harm Consumer, Warns Researcher," NutraIngredients.com/Europe, October 20, 2005, http://www.nutraingredients.com/news/ng.asp?id=63341-fish-oil-antioxidant (accessed February 23, 2006).

9. Ibid.

10. Ibid.

Day 41: Mega-Dosing

1. Kim, "Hidden Hazards of Vitamin and Mineral Tablets."

2. WrongDiagnosis.com, "Symptoms of Pyridoxine Deficiency," http://www.wrongdiagnosis.com/p/pyridoxine_deficiency/symptoms.htm (accessed February 23, 2006).

3. National Institutes of Health Office of Dietary Supplements, "Dietary Supplement Fact Sheet: Vitamin A and Carotenoids."

4. Balch, *Prescription for Nutritional Healing*, 32.

5. Lonn, MD, MSc, et al., "Effects of Long-Term Vitamin E Supplementation on Cardiovascular Events and Cancer."

6. Shands Health Care, "Vitamin C," in the Illustrated Health Encyclopedia, http://www.shands.org/health/information/article/002404.htm (accessed February 23, 2006).

7. National Institutes of Health Office of Dietary Supplements, "Dietary Supplement Fact Sheet: Vitamin D."

8. Fletcher and Fairfield, "Vitamins for Chronic Disease Prevention in Adults."

9. National Cancer Institute, "Alpha-Tocopherol, Beta-Carotene Cancer Prevention (ATBC) Trial."

10. Ibid.

Day 42: How to Pick the Right Supplements

1. Paavo Airola, MD, PhD, *How to Get Well* (Scottsdale, AZ: Health Plus Publishers, 1974), in Jane Sheppard, "The Baffling World of Nutritional Supplements," Healthy Child Online,

http://www.healthychild.com//database/the_baffling_world_of_nutritional_supplements.htm (accessed February 23, 2006).

2. MayoClinic.com, "Vitamin B_{12}," http://www.mayoclinic.com/print/vitamin-B12/Ns_patient-vitaminb12/METHOD=print (accessed February 8, 2006).

Pillar 7: Coping With Stress

Day 43: Stress and Your Health

1. Tara Parker-Pope, "Health Journal: Secrets of Successful Aging," *Wall Street Journal*, June 20, 2005, R3.

2. D. A. Snowdon et al., "Linguistic Ability in Early Life and Cognitive Function and Alzheimer's Disease in Late Life. Findings From the Nun Study," *Journal of the American Medical Association* 275 (February 21, 1996): 528–532.

3. S. Kennedy, J. K. Kiecolt-Glaser, and R. Glaser, "Immunological Consequences of Acute and Chronic Stressors: Mediating Role of Interpersonal Stressors," *British Journal of Medical Psychology* 61 (1988): 77–85.

4. H. J. Eysenck et al., "Personality Type, Smoking Habit, and Their Interaction as Predictors of Cancer and Coronary Disease," *Personality and Individual Difference* 9, no.2 (1988): 479–495.

5. Ibid.

6. Ibid.

7. P. M. Plotsky, et al., "PsychoNeural Endocrinology of Depression: Hypothalamic-Pituitary-Adrenal Axis," *Psychoneurology* 21, no. 2 (1998): 293–306.

8. D. Wayne, "Reactions to Stress," Identifying Stress, Health-Net & Stress Management, February 1998, in Vincent M. Newfield, "Defeating Deadly Emotions," Enjoying Everyday Life, April 2004, http://www.thehealingdoctor.com/articles.htm (accessed March 22, 2005).

9. Don Colbert, MD, *Stress Less* (Lake Mary, FL: Siloam, 2005).

Day 44: Practicing Mindfulness

1. Mind/Body Medical Institute, "Mindfulness," http://www.mbmi.org/pages/wi_mslaa.asp (accessed April 13, 2005).

2. University of Maryland Medical Center, "Who Is at Risk for Chronic Stress or Stress-Related Diseases and How Can the Risks Be Reduced: General Factors That Increase Susceptibility," http://www.umm.edu/patiented/articles/who_at_risk_chronic_stress_or_stress-related_diseases_000031_6.htm (accessed February 19, 2006).

Day 45: Reframing

1. Albert Ellis, *A New Guide to Rational Living* (New York: Institute for Rational-Emotive Therapy, 1975).

2. Viktor E. Frankl, *Man's Search for Meaning* (New York: Touchstone, 1984).

3. Doc Childre and Deborah Rozman, PhD, *Transforming Anxiety: The HeartMath Solution for Overcoming Fear and Worry and Creating Serenity* (Oakland, CA: New Harbinger Publicatons, Inc., 2006), 45.

Day 46: The Power of Laughter and Joy

1. Rich Bayer, PhD, "Benefits of Happiness," Upper Bay Counseling and Support Services, Inc., http://www.upperbay.org/benefits_of_happiness.htm (accessed April 11, 2005).

2. Ibid.

3. Ibid.

4. Ibid.

5. Ibid.

6. Norman Cousins, *Head First: The Biology of Hope and the Healing Power of the Human Spirit* (New York: Penguin, 1990), reference in P. Wooten, "An Antidote for Stress," *Holistic Nursing Practice* 10, no. 2 (1996): 49–56.

7. Helpguide.com, "Humor and Laughter: Health Benefits and Online Sources," http://www.helpguide.org/aging/humor/humor_laughter_health.htm (accessed April 11, 2005).

8. Ibid.

9. "In the world you will have tribulation; but be of good cheer, I have overcome the world" (John 16:33, NKJV).

10. W. F. Fry et al., *Make 'Em Laugh* (Palo Alto, CA; Science and Behavior Books, 1972).

11. HolisticOnline.com, "Therapeutic Benefits of Laughter," http://www.holistic-online.com/Humor_Therapy/humor_therapy_benefits.htm (accessed February 19, 2006).

12. Don Colbert, MD, *Deadly Emotions* (Nashville: Thomas Nelson, 2003).

Day 48: Margin

1. Richard A. Swenson, *The Overload Syndrome* (Colorado Springs, CO: NavPress, 1998).

2. *Medical News Today,* "Money Is Number One Cause of Stress Say Americans," April 1, 2004, http://www.medicalnewstoday.com/medicalnews.php?newsid=6934 (accessed February 19, 2006).

Day 49: Practice Stress-Reducing Habits

1. Parker-Pope, "Health Journal: Secrets of Successful Aging."

2. "Do all things without murmurings and disputings" (Philippians 2:14).

3. "Pleasant words are like a honeycomb, sweetness to the soul and health to the bones" (Proverbs 16:24, NKJV).

Day 50: Your Day of Jubilee—the Chief Cornerstone

1. "And the peace of God, which passeth all understanding, shall keep your hearts and minds through Christ Jesus" (Philippians 4:7).

2. "Casting all your care upon him; for he careth for you" (1 Peter 5:7).

Appendix B: Vitamins, Minerals, and Their Recommended Intakes

1. Reprinted with permission from *Dietary Reference Intakes for Vitamin A, Vitamin K, Arsenic, Boron, Chromium, Copper, Iodine, Manganese, Molybdenum, Nickel, Silicon, Vanadium, and Zinc,* copyright © 2000 by the National Academy of Sciences, courtesy of the National Academies Press, Washington DC.

Appendix C: Bottled Water pH Comparisons

1. This chart is compiled from various Web sites giving information on water brands, including the sites listed in text and www.finewaters.com.

INDEX